New Frontiers in Critical Care

New Frontiers in Critical Care

Edited by Anderson Murphy

hayle
medical

New York

Hayle Medical,
750 Third Avenue, 9th Floor,
New York, NY 10017, USA

Visit us on the World Wide Web at:
www.haylemedical.com

ISBN: 978-1-63241-593-6

Cataloging-in-Publication Data

New frontiers in critical care / edited by Anderson Murphy.
    p. cm.
Includes bibliographical references and index.
ISBN 978-1-63241-593-6
1. Critical care medicine. 2. Emergency medicine. 3. Intensive care units.
I. Murphy, Anderson.
RC86.7 .N49 2019
616.025--dc23

Table of Contents

Preface

It is often said that books are a boon to mankind. They document every progress and pass on the knowledge from one generation to the other. They play a crucial role in our lives. Thus I was both excited and nervous while editing this book. I was pleased by the thought of being able to make a mark but I was also nervous to do it right because the future of students depends upon it. Hence, I took a few months to research further into the discipline, revise my knowledge and also explore some more aspects. Post this process, I begun with the editing of this book.

Critical care medicine is a branch of medicine that is concerned with the diagnosis and management of critical health issues, which may require advanced life support and dedicated monitoring. The ultimate goal of life support is to sustain life, while the underlying diseases or injury is being evaluated or treated. Some of the diverse therapies and techniques involved in the care of patients in intensive care are mechanical ventilation, defibrillation, cardiopulmonary resuscitation, dialysis, total parenteral nutrition, etc. The care of premature or ill newborn infants is undertaken in a neonatal intensive care unit. Administration of high-risk medications and antibiotics, management of infants requiring ventilator support, surgical care and resuscitation, etc. are crucial to neonatal critical care. There are psychiatric intensive care units in psychiatric wards. These are designed to care for patients who pose a degree of risk to themselves or others. Patients are cared for in such units until their mental state is stable. Critical care is an upcoming field of medicine that has undergone rapid development over the past few decades. This book aims to shed light on some of the unexplored aspects of critical care and the recent researches in this field. It will help new researchers by foregrounding their knowledge in this field.

I thank my publisher with all my heart for considering me worthy of this unparalleled opportunity and for showing unwavering faith in my skills. I would also like to thank the editorial team who worked closely with me at every step and contributed immensely towards the successful completion of this book. Last but not the least, I wish to thank my friends and colleagues for their support.

Editor

Urine Biochemistry in the Early Postoperative Period after Cardiac Surgery: Role in Acute Kidney Injury Monitoring

Alexandre Toledo Maciel and Daniel Vitório

Intensimed Research Group, Adult Intensive Care Unit, Hospital São Camilo, Pompéia Avenue, 1178 Pompéia, 05022-001 São Paulo, SP, Brazil

Correspondence should be addressed to Alexandre Toledo Maciel; alexandre.toledo@intensimed.com

Academic Editors: C. Lazzeri and G. Pichler

We have recently suggested that sequential urine electrolyte measurement in critically ill patients may be useful in monitoring kidney function. Cardiac surgery is one of the leading causes of acute kidney injury (AKI) in the intensive care unit (ICU). In this paper, we describe the sequential behavior of urine electrolytes in three patients in the early (first 60 hours) postoperative period after cardiac surgery according to AKI status: no AKI, transient AKI, and persistent AKI. We have found that the patient with no AKI had stable and high concentrations of sodium (NaU) and chloride (ClU) in sequential spot samples of urine. AKI development was characterized in the other two patients by decreases in NaU and ClU, which have started early after ICU admission. Transient AKI was marked by also transient and less severe decreases in NaU and ClU. Persistent AKI was marked by the less favorable clinical course with abrupt and prolonged declines in NaU and ClU values. These electrolytes in urine had a behavior like a "mirror image" in comparison with that of serum creatinine. We suggest that sequential urine electrolytes are useful in monitoring acute kidney injury development in the early postoperative period after cardiac surgery.

1. Introduction

Acute kidney injury (AKI) is frequent among patients undergoing cardiac surgery [1, 2]. It seems to be an independent risk factor for increased intensive care and hospital mortality [3]. Serum creatinine level and urine output are still the cornerstones for AKI diagnosis in all settings, including postoperative AKI. Urine biochemistry, although a major tool in AKI diagnosis and management in the past, is nowadays considered not useful [4] especially due to evidence showing its dissociation from renal hemodynamics [5]. However, sequential evaluation of urine electrolytes (basically, sodium, potassium, and chloride) in the course of early postoperative period has never, to our knowledge, been performed. We have recently observed that alterations in the concentration of these electrolytes measured in spot urine samples may be related to kidney function and AKI development, sometimes preceding elevations in serum creatinine [6, 7]. In this paper, we report the sequential behavior of urine electrolytes in a 60 h period in three patients after undergoing cardiac surgery.

2. Case Presentation

We will briefly present the 3 cases separately. In all cases, there was no previous history of kidney disease, and the surgical procedure consisted in on-pump coronary artery bypass graft (CABG), and all patients had their serum creatinine as well as urine sodium (NaU), chloride (ClU), and potassium (KU) measured at 0 (T_0), 6 (T_6), 12 (T_{12}), 24 (T_{24}), 36 (T_{36}), 48 (T_{48}), and 60 (T_{60}) hours after ICU admission. These measurements are part of a research protocol in our ICU of which these patients were the first three included. All patients were admitted in the ICU immediately after the surgery. An indwelling urinary catheter was in place during the entire observation period. AKIN creatinine-based criteria were used to define AKI [8]. Baseline creatinine was considered the creatinine value at ICU admission. Oliguria was defined as a urine output less than 0.5 mL/kg/h in a 6 h period. AKI reversal was defined as a creatinine value lower than baseline creatinine +0.3 (mg/dL). Day 1 (D1) is the day of ICU admission.

2.1. Patient 1 (P1). P1 was a 67-year-old female with a past medical history of hypertension, dyslipidemia, and hypothyroidism in which CABG was electively indicated due to stable angina. Three coronary bypasses were performed in 67 minutes of cardiopulmonary bypass (CPB) and 51 minutes of aortic clamping (AC). No vasopressors were needed neither intraoperatively nor postoperatively. She was extubated 5 hours after ICU admission. Creatinine remained stable around 1 mg/dL in all measurements (unfortunately, creatinine value at T_{24} was missed) (Figure 1). Oliguria occurred between T_{12} and T_{24}, for which furosemide was administered. It was also administered between T_{48} and T_{60}. NaU increased progressively from T_0 to T_{12}, decreasing a little between T_{12} and T_{24}, remaining stable after that, and increasing again at T_{60}. ClU behavior was similar to that of NaU (Figure 1). KU increased progressively until T_{24}, decreasing progressively after that. The rest of ICU stay was unremarkable, and P1 was discharged at D4.

2.2. Patient 2 (P2). P2 was a 74-year-old female with a past medical history of hypertension, diabetes mellitus, dyslipidemia, and hypothyroidism in which CABG was indicated electively a few days after an acute coronary syndrome. The patient was stable before the procedure. Three coronary bypasses were performed in 105 minutes of CPB and 78 minutes of AC. No vasopressors were needed intraoperatively. She was extubated 9 hours after ICU admission. Norepinephrine infusion was initiated due to hypotension between T_{12} and T_{24}, remaining in low doses until T_{60}. No diuretics were needed between T_0 and T_{60}, although oliguria also occurred between T_{24} and T_{36}. Creatinine increased progressively until it reached AKIN stage 1 at T_{24} (Figure 1). Peak creatinine was reached at T_{36}, and AKI reversal occurred at T_{60}. NaU and ClU had small decreases between T_0 and T_{24} and reached their lowest values at T_{36}. KU increased progressively until T_{24}, decreasing progressively until T_{60}. Norepinephrine infusion was stopped at D4, and P2 was discharged at D5.

2.3. Patient 3 (P3). P3 was a 71-year-old female with a past medical history of hypertension, diabetes mellitus, chronic pulmonary obstructive disease, and ischemic stroke in which CABG was also indicated electively a few days after an acute coronary syndrome. The patient was stable before the procedure. Four coronary bypasses were performed in 85 minutes of CPB and 64 minutes of AC. Norepinephrine was needed both intraoperatively and postoperatively (including doses above 0.5 mcg/kg/min), during the entire observation period (T_0–T_{60}). She was extubated 5 hours after ICU admission. Furosemide and bicarbonate were infused between T_6 and T_{12} due to metabolic acidosis and oliguria. Furosemide was also repeated frequently between T_{12} and T_{60} due to oliguria and pulmonary edema. Creatinine increased fast, and AKIN stage 1 was present at T_6 (Figure 1). Peak creatinine was reached at T_{24}, decreasing slowly in the subsequent measurements but without reaching AKI reversal criterion until T_{60}. Both NaU and ClU decreased fast and to very low

levels (<10 mEq/L) at T_{48}–T_{60} (Figure 1). KU increased progressively reaching its peak at T_{36}. Norepinephrine infusion was stopped at D5, and P3 was discharged at D6.

3. Discussion

The 3 reported cases described above show 3 distinct evolutions during and after CABG surgery. P1 had a more benign course with no need of vasopressors at anytime and no significant elevations in creatinine. Urine biochemistry was marked by high values of NaU and ClU at all times, increasing until T_{12} followed by a small fall between T_{12} and T_{24}, coinciding with oliguria and high KU. Unfortunately, we cannot exclude an increase in creatinine at T_{24}, but, even if it has happened, it decreased back to normal values in 12 hours. P2 had a worse clinical course than P1, characterized by longer periods of CPB and AC and the need of vasopressors in low doses in the postoperative period. Creatinine has gradually and transitorily increased, which was simultaneous with gradual but also transitory decreases in NaU and ClU, both reaching lower values than those reached by P1 (Figure 1). P3 had the worst clinical course characterized by prolonged use of vasopressors in high doses including the intraoperative period. An earlier and more persistent AKI developed, which was accompanied by early and abrupt decreases in NaU and ClU values until very low levels, which remained low during the entire AKI course. This may reflect the severity of the disease and might be a sign of microcirculatory impairment in the kidneys in association with activation of sympathetic and renin-angiotensin-aldosterone systems. Curiously, KU had a very similar behavior in all patients; it progressively increased reaching a peak between T_{24} and T_{36}, decreasing thereafter. All these data suggest that sequential urine electrolyte measurement in the early postoperative period has standardized behaviors according to renal function: relatively preserved (oliguria without increases in creatinine) as occurred in P1 with high values of NaU and ClU, possibly due to higher glomerular filtration rate and lower microcirculatory stress. Furosemide could have contributed to increases in urine electrolytes, but P3 has used furosemide in similar doses but more frequently, and this has not increased NaU and ClU values. In fact, patients who had a more severe compromise of renal function and systemic circulation also had more significant decreases in NaU and ClU. AKI recovery was followed by increases in NaU and ClU probably due to glomerular filtration recovery and microcirculatory improvement. Very low values of NaU and ClU should not be interpreted as markers of "prerenal" impairment. This old concept seems flawed [9, 10], and low values of these electrolytes are probably markers of glomerular function impairment (regardless of total renal blood flow) together with an avid sodium retentive state in the tubules. It is noteworthy that, although many previous studies have demonstrated early increase in markers of tubular injury in postoperative AKI, including cardiac surgery [2], P3 was a case of persistent AKI that seemed to be predominantly hemodynamic, which presupposes preservation of global tubular function but does not exclude some degree of tubular

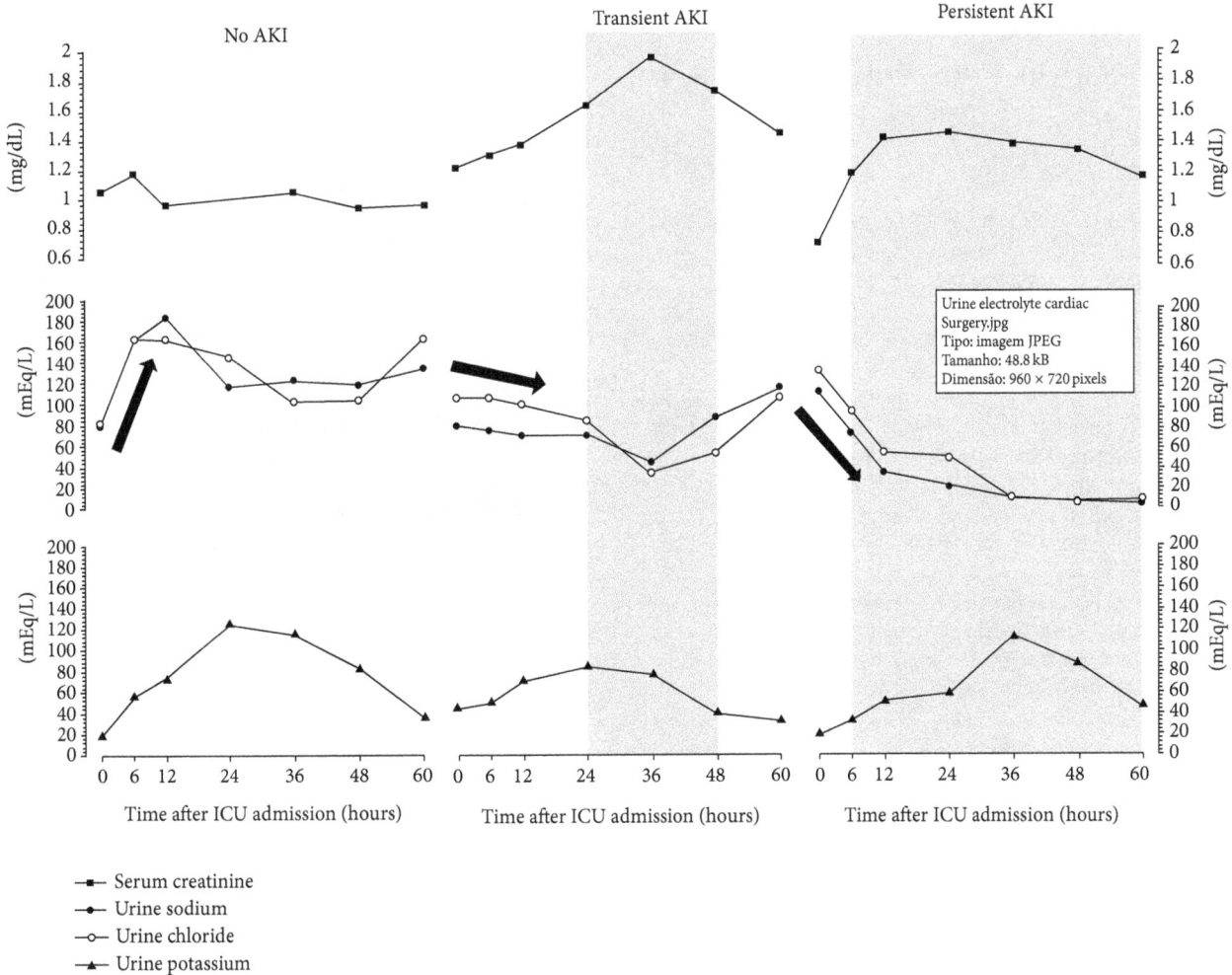

FIGURE 1: Sequential serum creatinine and urine electrolyte concentrations in the first 60 hours after intensive care unit admission of 3 patients in the postoperative period of cardiac surgery. Patient 1 did not develop creatinine-based AKI (left); patient 2 developed a transient AKI (middle), and patient 3 developed a persistent AKI (right). AKI: acute kidney injury.

injury [11]. In fact, back leak of solutes in the tubules cannot be discarded as a contributor to low NaU and ClU values in P3.

4. Conclusions

Urine electrolyte concentrations in the early postoperative period after cardiac surgery are closely related to renal function and systemic hemodynamic compromise. NaU and ClU had similar behaviors, which were generally in the opposite direction of that of creatinine (as "mirror images"— see Figure 1). Decreases in NaU and ClU levels should be viewed as alert signs. An abrupt fall in NaU and ClU values is probably related to a more severe ongoing renal impairment. Transient AKI had equally transitory alterations in these electrolytes. On the other hand, persistent AKI had persistent low values of NaU and ClU. The cases reported here should be viewed as examples of the potential relevance of urine electrolyte measurement in AKI monitoring after

cardiac surgery. Of particular interest is the evaluation of these electrolytes in the first 6–12 hours after surgery (black arrows in Figure 1)—NaU and ClU increase in P1 suggested preserved renal function, and decrease in P2 and especially P3 suggested some degree of renal impairment. All of these findings must be tested in a large scale as well as in other scenarios such as noncardiac postoperative period and sepsis.

Abbreviations

AKI: Acute kidney injury
CABG: Coronary artery bypass graft
CPB: Cardiopulmonary bypass
AC: Aortic clamping
P1, P2, P3:   Patients 1, 2, and 3, respectively
NaU: Spot urine sodium
ClU: Spot urine chloride
KU: Spot urine potassium.

Acknowledgment

The authors thank Dr. Marcelo Park for his help in the elaboration of Figure 1.

References

[1] E. A. J. Hoste, J. A. Kellum, N. M. Katz, M. H. Rosner, M. Haase, and C. Ronco, "Epidemiology of acute kidney injury," *Contributions to Nephrology*, vol. 165, pp. 1–8, 2010.

[2] G. Coppolino, P. Presta, L. Saturno, and G. Fuiano, "Acute kidney injury in patients undergoing cardiac surgery," *Journal of Nephrology*, vol. 26, no. 1, pp. 32–40, 2013.

[3] C. Ronco, J. A. Kellum, and R. Bellomo, "Cardiac surgery-associated acute kidney injury," *International Journal of Artificial Organs*, vol. 31, no. 2, pp. 156–157, 2008.

[4] J. Prowle, S. M. Bagshaw, and R. Bellomo, "Renal blood flow, fractional excretion of sodium and acute kidney injury: time for a new paradigm?" *Current Opinion in Critical Care*, vol. 18, no. 6, pp. 585–592, 2012.

[5] C. Langenberg, L. Wan, S. M. Bagshaw, M. Egi, C. N. May, and R. Bellomo, "Urinary biochemistry in experimental septic acute renal failure," *Nephrology Dialysis Transplantation*, vol. 21, no. 12, pp. 3389–3397, 2006.

[6] A. T. Maciel and M. Park, "Early diagnosis of acute kidney injury in a critically ill patient using a combination of blood and urinary physicochemical parameters.," *Clinics(Sao Paulo)*, vol. 67, no. 5, pp. 525–526, 2012.

[7] A. T. Maciel, M. Park, and E. Macedo, "Urinary electrolyte monitoring in critically ill patients: a preliminary observational study," *Revista Brasileira de Terapia Intensiva*, vol. 24, no. 3, pp. 236–245, 2012.

[8] R. L. Mehta, J. A. Kellum, S. V. Shah et al., "Acute Kidney Injury Network: report of an initiative to improve outcomes in acute kidney injury," *Critical Care*, vol. 11, no. 2, article R31, 2007.

[9] R. Bellomo, S. Bagshaw, C. Langenberg, and C. Ronco, "Pre-renal azotemia: a flawed paradigm in critically ill septic patients?" *Contributions to Nephrology*, vol. 156, pp. 1–9, 2007.

[10] J. A. Kellum, "Prerenal azotemia: still a useful concept?" *Critical Care Medicine*, vol. 35, no. 6, pp. 1630–1631, 2007.

[11] M. Nejat, J. W. Pickering, P. Devarajan et al., "Some biomarkers of acute kidney injury are increased in pre-renal acute injury," *Kidney International*, vol. 81, no. 12, pp. 1254–1262, 2012.

Acute Hepatic Failure as a Leading Manifestation in Exertional Heat Stroke

Qi Jin, Erzhen Chen, Jie Jiang, and Yiming Lu

Department of Emergency, Shanghai Rui Jin Hospital, Shanghai Jiao Tong University School of Medicine, Shanghai 20025, China

Correspondence should be addressed to Yiming Lu, luyiming@rjh.com.cn

Academic Editors: Y. D. Durandy, K. Klouche, and K. Lenz

Background. Acute hepatic failure (AHF) is uncommon as a leading symptom in patients with exertional heat stroke (EHS). Which stage to perform the liver transplantation for severe hepatic failure in EHS is still obscure at clinical setting. The conservative management has been reported to be successful in treating heat-stroke-associated AHF even in the presence of accepted criteria for emergency liver transplantation. *Case Presentation.* Here, we reported a 35-year-old male who presented with very high transaminases, hyperbilirubinemia, significant prolongation of the prothrombin time, and coma. No other causes for AHF could be identified but physical exhaustion and hyperthermia. Although the current patient fulfilled London criteria for emergency liver transplantation, he spontaneously recovered under conservative treatment including intravenous fluids, cooling, diuretics as mannitol, and hepatocyte growth-promoting factors. *Conclusions.* Meticulous supportive management could be justified in some selected cases of AHF due to EHS.

1. Introduction

Exertional heat stroke (EHS) is a life-threatening condition caused by excess heat generated from muscular exercise that exceeds the body's ability to dissipate it at the same rate [1]. Potential complications of EHS include acute renal failure, acute hepatic failure (AHF), rhabdomyolysis, disseminated intravascular coagulation (DIC), and multiorgan dysfunction [2, 3].

While mild and moderate hepatic injury is a relatively common feature of EHS [4], few patients undergo fatal extensive hepatocellular damage [5, 6]. To date, no definite indications for liver transplantation to AHF in heat stroke have been established. Three patients with EHS experiencing liver transplantation died within one year [6–8], and one case was reported to survive for more than one year [9]. The conservative management has been described to be successful in treating heat-stroke-associated AHF even in the presence of accepted criteria for emergency liver transplantation [10, 11]. Recently, we experienced a patient who had AHF as a leading symptom during the course of EHS and who survived with the complete recovery of liver function under conservative treatment. Here we reported this unusual case with a review of literature.

2. Case Report

A previously healthy 35-year-old male was found unconscious after a 24 h consecutively physical work under heavy heat load and was delivered to the resuscitation room and our Intensive Care Unit of the Department of Emergency, Rui Jin hospital, Shanghai Jiao Tong University School of Medicine, 2 days later in July 2008. On admission, the patient had spontaneous respiration at the rate of 36 breaths per min, and his pulse was about 130 beats per min with regular rhythm. He was found to be comatose at grade 5 on the Glasgow Coma Scale (GCS; E1V1M3). The patient's surface temperature was more than 40°C. Complete blood count showed white blood cell 14,300/μL, hemoglobin 13.9 g/dL, hematocrit 40%, platelet 19,000/μL. The results of blood biochemistry exhibited very high transaminases, 2336 U/L alanine aminotransferase (ALT) (normal < 64 U/L), 1841 U/L aspartate aminotransferase

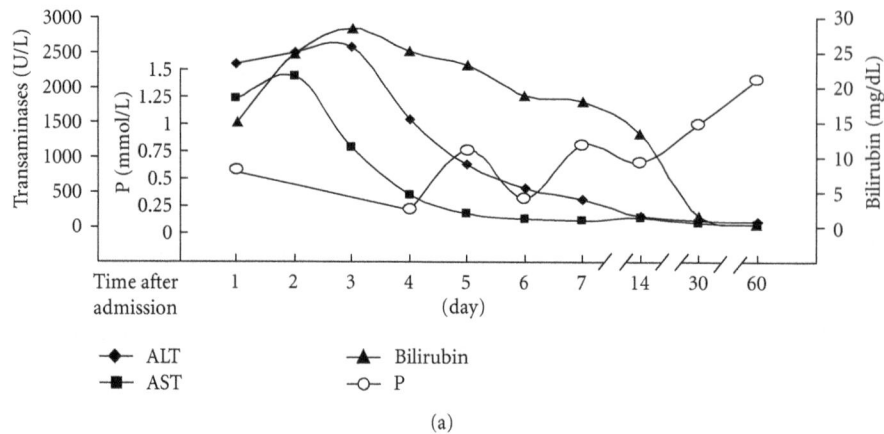

(a)

Cr(mg/dL)	0.9	0.8	0.8	0.7	0.8	0.7	0.6	0.7	0.4	0.3
LDH(U/L)	1465	1761	1064	696	—	510	—	571	—	—
Myoglobin(ng/mL)	555	788	494	684	—	503	—	1297	—	—
CK(U/L)	2729	1389	693	715	—	368	—	687	—	—
PT(s)	70.2	60.0	32.9	18.7	—	12.8	—	—	12.2	—
pH	7.39	—	7.45	7.51	—	7.5	7.45	—	—	—
PaCO$_2$	4.15	—	5.77	4.41	—	4.84	5.22	—	—	—

(b)

FIGURE 1: Basic laboratory parameters of the patient presenting with AHF during the course of EHS. In (a), ALT and AST began to be decreased from day 3 after admission in our ICU and recovered to be normal within 2 weeks. Total bilirubin declined more slowly than transaminases. In the early stage of EHS, hypophosphatemia was evident. (b) Showed the dynamic change of Cr, LDH, CK, PT and arterial blood gas analysis with pH and PaCO$_2$ within 2 months in our hospital. ALT, alanine aminotransferase; AST, aspartate aminotransferase; P, phosphonium; Cr, creatinine; LDH, lactate dehydrogenase; CK, creatinine kinase; PT, prothrombin time.

(AST) (normal < 42 U/L), and significantly elevated total bilirubin 14.9 mg/dL (normal < 1.4 mg/dL) (Figure 1). Further laboratory parameters showed an evident prolongation of the prothrombin time (PT) (70.2 s, control 13 ± 3 s), D-dimer (1.22 mg/L, normal < 0.5 mg/L), an elevated lactate dehydrogenase (LDH) (1465 U/L, normal < 192 U/L), creatinine kinase (CK) (2729 U/L, normal < 269 U/L), and myoglobin (555 ng/mL, normal < 70 ng/mL) (Figure 1). His electrocardiogram showed ST elevation in lead I, II, III, aVL, aVF, and V1-5.

To exclude other causes for AHF, virus serological tests were performed. There were no positive findings for acute or chronic hepatitis A, B, C, E or human immunodeficiency virus (HIV). Also, acute infection with Epstein-Barr virus (EBV) and cytomegaly virus (CMV) was ruled out. The autoimmune antibodies (ANA, ANCA, ENA, RF) were negative. In addition, an abdominal ultrasound and CT scan did not exhibit the evidence of dilated bile ducts. After normalization of prothrombin time and platelet count, a liver biopsy was performed for exact staging of the severity of hepatic damage. Liver histology showed that the areas of liver cell necrosis contain a mild inflammatory infiltrate consisting of lymphocytes, plasma cells, and neutrophilic leukocyte. Liver cell vacuolization and fatty degeneration were present to differing extents. The immunohistochemical results indicated negative for HBsAg and HBcAg as well as negative HCV.

The patient was further monitored in our ICU and accepted the treatment of cooling that included cold saline infusion from gastric tube, ice cap, ice pack to axillae, neck and groin, and cold alcohol applied to the patient's skin. Meanwhile, we also administrated other supportive therapy with intravenous fluids, mannitol, and hepatocyte growth-promoting factors, and so on. The abnormal laboratory parameters returned slowly to normal within a few days while the renal function was always normal after admission (Figure 1). Because of the continual elevation of the ST segment in ECG and elevated myocardial enzymes, the echocardiography was performed and it indicated regional wall motion abnormality with a 43% ejection fraction.

The patient regained consciousness on day 7 from the onset of coma. He was delayed to be transferred to a regular ward because of toxic epidermis necrosis induced by vancomycin for treating respiratory tract infection caused by methicillin-resistant staphylococcus aureus. After the skin erosion disappeared and new epidermis covered the body, he was admitted to an internal medicine ward. Finally, at the time of discharge from our hospital, the patient's laboratory parameters had returned to normal values.

3. Discussion

In the present case study, we described a young patient with severe EHS that was mainly complicated with AHF as well as DIC, the failure of heart and central nervous system. The success in treating this EHS case suggested that the physicians and intensivists could consider appropriate supportive therapy to AHF as a predominant manifestation under the intensive investigation during the course of EHS.

The clinical manifestations of heat stroke are variable. Hyperthermia and central nervous system dysfunction must be present for a diagnosis of heat stroke. Hepatic injury in most cases of EHS is usually asymptomatic and can be reversed [4]. Approximately 5% of EHS experienced fulminant hepatic failure, which might be fatal [12]. Orthotopic liver transplantation (OLT) has been suggested as a potential therapy despite that even the extensive may recover spontaneously. However, to the best of our knowledge, the outcome of OLT in the four reported cases seemed to be disappointed. The first three patients underwent OLT on 8 days, 72 h, and 48 h respectively, after heat stroke and died of systemic infection, chronic transplantation rejection, and cardiopulmonary arrest respectively, within one year after liver transplantation [6–8]. Only one patient survived for more than one year after living donor liver transplantation [9]. Although the current patient fulfilled accepted London criteria [13] for emergency liver transplantation on day 2 after admission (PT longer than 50 s, bilirubin higher than 17.5 mg/dL, and non-A, non-B hepatitis (Figure 1)), we did not decide to perform liver transplantation immediately. The reasons that we decided upon watchful waiting for one more day are as follows: (1) while acute renal failure and acute respiratory distress are frequently seen in EHS, this patient did not have to receive the invasive mechanical ventilation and his plasma creatinine was always in the normal range; (2) the poor and limited outcome of liver transplantation in heat stroke in the previous case studies; (3) a previous study demonstrated, in the conservatively managed group of EHS-induced liver failure, 61.5% patients recovered spontaneously [11], (4) despite that the patient's PT was longer than 50 s, impaired coagulation tests were overestimated because of concomitant heat-induced endothelial injury and the consequent DIC.

EHS is a medical emergency that results in multiorgan dysfunction, which carries a high mortality. Very recently, a retrospective study [14] demonstrated that high levels of CK (>1000 U/L), metabolic acidosis, and elevated liver enzymes were predictive for multiorgan dysfunction among the various parameters during heat stroke. The overall case fatality rate was more than 70% and the mortality was even higher (85%) in patients with dysfunction of two or more organs. Accurate estimation of prognosis in AHF is a paramount goal. Evaluations of the prognostic criteria have had varied results; while some appear promising, more researches are needed to determine their reliability [15]. The predictor of AHF during EHS remains less clear. Recently, Gracin JM et al. reported that hypophosphatemia (<0.5 mmol/L) was the only independent predictive factor of AHF in confirmed EHS patients by multivariate analysis (RR 3.8, 95% CI 1.1–6.2). Consistent with Gracin's study, this patient appeared to be a marked hypophosphatemia that altered from 0.22 mmol/L to 0.81 mmol/L (normal 0.8–1.6 mmol/l) during the first two weeks after admission

(Figure 1), although physiological phosphorus requirement was administrated each day. Hypophosphatemia has been observed consistently in patients with conditions characterized by fever or hyperthermia. The mechanism of hypophosphatemia in acute heat stroke is still elusive. The possible mechanisms are as follows. (1) Heat-stroke-related hypophosphatemia was associated with abnormal phosphaturia independent of the parathyroid hormone level. (2) Acute respiratory alkalosis induced by hyperthermia increased intracellular pH and caused phosphorus to shift from the extracellular to the intracellular compartment. (3) The elevation of body temperature increased intracellular utilization of phosphate in the glycolytic pathway, causing phosphorus to shift from the extracellular fluid into cells. In this patient, respiratory alkalosis presenting in the early stage of EHS could be one of the causes that resulted in hypophosphatemia. But it was unlikely to be the sole explanation for the observed hypophosphatemia because it sometimes occurred without respiratory alkalosis (Figure 1). However, to the best of our knowledge, there is no evidence that hypophosphatemia by itself could result in important liver dysfunction. Therefore, phosphatemia should be measured systematically on admission and 1-2 weeks later, and phosphorus should be supplied and evaluated as a predictor for AHF secondary to EHS.

In conclusion, appropriate supportive therapy in some cases could be justified in the early stage of AHF due to EHS and substantially reduce the mortality. It is now necessary to establish a scoring system for stratification of severity and prediction of mortality. Further clinical experience is needed to weigh the risk and benefit of conservative therapy or organ transplantation to treat AHF associated with heat stroke

References

[1] World Health Organization, *Manual of International Statistical Classification of Diseases, Injuries, and Causes of Death*, vol. 9, World Health Organization, Geneva, Switzerland, 1977.

[2] A. Bouchama and J. P. Knochel, "Medical progress: heat stroke," *The New England Journal of Medicine*, vol. 346, no. 25, pp. 1978–1988, 2002.

[3] J. L. Glazer, "Management of heatstroke and heat exhaustion," *American Family Physician*, vol. 71, no. 11, pp. 2133–2140, 2005.

[4] T. Hassanein, A. Razack, J. S. Gavaler, and D. H. Van Thiel, "Heatstroke: its clinical and pathological presentation, with particular attention to the liver," *American Journal of Gastroenterology*, vol. 87, no. 10, pp. 1382–1389, 1992.

[5] C. Ichai, J. F. Ciais, H. Hyvernat, Y. Labib, P. Fabiani, and D. Grimaud, "Fatal acute liver failure: a rare complication of exertional heat stroke," *Annales Francaises d'Anesthesie et de Reanimation*, vol. 16, no. 1, pp. 64–67, 1997.

[6] J. Berger, J. Hart, M. Millis, and A. L. Baker, "Fulminant hepatic failure from heat stroke requiring liver transplantation," *Journal of Clinical Gastroenterology*, vol. 30, no. 4, pp. 429–431, 2000.

[7] T. Hassanein, J. A. Perper, L. Tepperman, T. E. Starzl, and D. H. Van Thiel, "Liver failure occurring as a component of exertional heatstroke," *Gastroenterology*, vol. 100, no. 5, part 1, pp. 1442–1447, 1991.

[8] J. M. Saissy, "Liver transplantation in a case of fulminant liver failure after exertion," *Intensive Care Medicine*, vol. 22, no. 8, p. 831, 1996.

[9] K. I. Takahashi, K. Chin, K. Ogawa et al., "Living donor liver transplantation with noninvasive ventilation for exertional heat stroke and severe rhabdomyolysis," *Liver Transplantation*, vol. 11, no. 5, pp. 570–572, 2005.

[10] M. Wagner, P. Kaufmann, P. Fickert, M. Trauner, C. Lackner, and R. E. Stauber, "Successful conservative management of acute hepatic failure following exertional heatstroke," *European Journal of Gastroenterology and Hepatology*, vol. 15, no. 10, pp. 1135–1139, 2003.

[11] E. Hadad, Z. Ben-Ari, Y. Heled, D. S. Moran, Y. Shani, and Y. Epstein, "Liver transplantation in exertional heat stroke: a medical dilemma," *Intensive Care Medicine*, vol. 30, no. 7, pp. 1474–1478, 2004.

[12] J. P. Knochel and G. Reed, "Disorders of heat regulation," in *Maxwell and Kleemans Clinical Disorders of Fluid and Electrolyte Metabolism*, R. G. Narins, Ed., pp. 1549–1590, McGraw-Hill, New York, 1994.

[13] A. Pauwels, N. Mostefa-Kara, C. Florent, and V. G. Levy, "Emergency liver transplantation for acute liver failure. Evaluation of London and Clichy criteria," *Journal of Hepatology*, vol. 17, no. 1, pp. 124–127, 1993.

[14] G. M. Varghese, G. John, K. Thomas, O. C. Abraham, and D. Mathai, "Predictors of multi-organ dysfunction in heatstroke," *Emergency Medicine Journal*, vol. 22, no. 3, pp. 185–187, 2005.

[15] J. Polson and W. M. Lee, "AASLD position paper: the management of acute liver failure," *Hepatology*, vol. 41, no. 5, pp. 1179–1197, 2005.

3

Ciprofloxacin-Induced Thrombotic Thrombocytopenic Purpura: A Case of Successful Treatment and Review of the Literature

Hafiz Rizwan Talib Hashmi,[1] **Gilda Diaz-Fuentes,**[1]
Preeti Jadhav,[2] **and Misbahuddin Khaja**[1]

[1]*Division of Pulmonary and Critical Care Medicine, Bronx Lebanon Hospital Center, Bronx, NY 10457, USA*
[2]*Department of Internal Medicine, Bronx Lebanon Hospital Center, Albert Einstein College of Medicine, Bronx, NY 10457, USA*

Correspondence should be addressed to Hafiz Rizwan Talib Hashmi; rizwan404@hotmail.com

Academic Editor: Caterina Mammina

A 49-year-old African American woman was admitted to our hospital with abdominal pain, nausea, vomiting, lethargy, and confusion. She was receiving ciprofloxacin for a urinary-tract infection prior to admission. Laboratory examination revealed anemia, thrombocytopenia, elevated lactate dehydrogenase, and serum creatinine. Peripheral smear showed numerous schistocytes, and the patient was diagnosed with thrombotic thrombocytopenic purpura (TTP). Ciprofloxacin was identified as the offending agent. The patient received treatment with steroids and plasmapheresis, which led to rapid clinical recovery. This is the first case to our knowledge of successfully treated ciprofloxacin-induced TTP; previously reported cases had fulminant outcomes. Quinolones are an important part of the antibiotic armamentarium, and this case can raise awareness of the association between quinolones and TTP. A high index of suspicion for detection and early and aggressive management are vitally important for a successful outcome.

1. Introduction

Ciprofloxacin is a DNA gyrase inhibitor that provides excellent coverage of gram-negative bacteria with marginal effectiveness against gram-positive bacteria. It is generally used to treat infections of bones and joints, endocarditis, gastroenteritis, malignant otitis externa, respiratory-tract infections, cellulitis, urinary-tract infections, prostatitis, anthrax, and chancroid. Common side effects include neurological symptoms (dizziness, insomnia, and nervousness), gastrointestinal symptoms (diarrhea, dyspepsia, and nausea), and transaminitis [1].

Quinolones should be prescribed with caution to patients with HIV infection because of the potential for associated hypersensitivity reaction [2]. Uncommon adverse effects of ciprofloxacin include renal failure, agranulocytosis, anemia, bone-marrow suppression, and thrombocytopenia. Although full manifestation of fluoroquinolone-induced thrombotic thrombocytopenic purpura (TTP) requiring plasmapheresis is extremely rare, there are documented cases of life-threatening complications of TTP due to moxifloxacin [3].

There is sparse literature on TTP caused by other fluoroquinolones including ciprofloxacin. Here, we report an unusual case of TTP associated with the use of ciprofloxacin that was successfully treated with steroids and plasmapheresis.

2. Case Presentation

A 49-year-old African American woman presented to the emergency room with complaints of nausea, vomiting, abdominal pain, and altered sensorium. The abdominal pain was poorly localized, dull, and associated with nonbloody, nonbilious vomiting. The patient reported subjective fever and chills. Her medical history was remarkable for hypertension controlled with diet and lifestyle modifications. She was seen in another hospital 5 days earlier for urinary-tract infection and was prescribed ciprofloxacin and discharged. The patient denied taking any other prescribed or nonprescribed medications. She was a light smoker and denied any history of illicit or recreational drug use. On physical examination, she was in mild distress and confused but had normal vitals, and

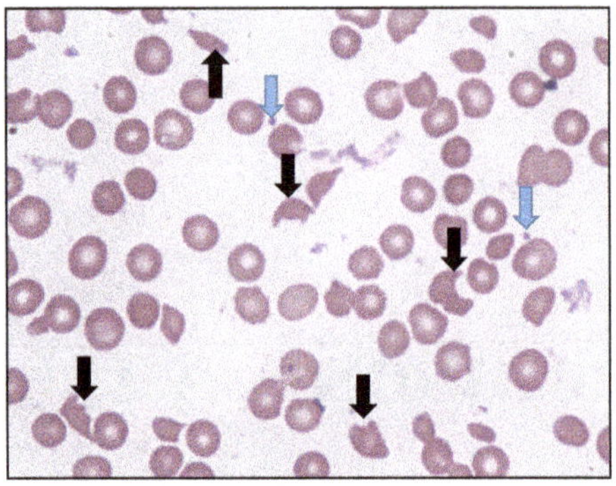

FIGURE 1: Peripheral smear shows moderate to severe schistocytes (black arrows) and very few platelets (blue arrows).

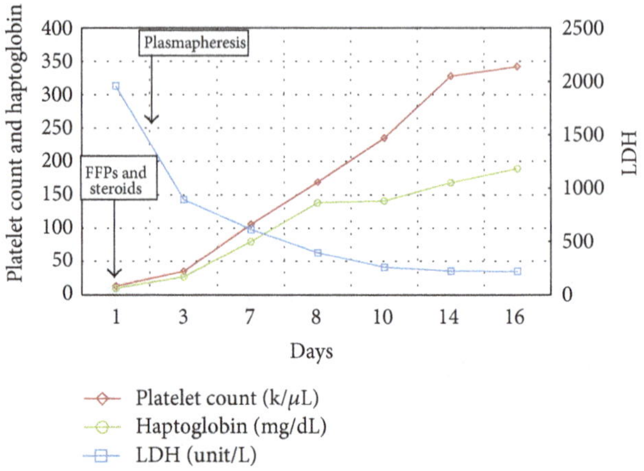

FIGURE 2: Platelet count, haptoglobin, and LDH over the course of treatment.

neurological examination did not reveal sensory or motor deficit. Cardiorespiratory examination was unremarkable. Abdominal examination revealed minimal diffuse tenderness without guarding, rigidity, or other signs of peritonitis. Bowel sounds were present, and no visceromegaly was appreciated. Skin examination did not reveal any petechiae or rash.

Laboratory examination revealed anemia (hemoglobin: 8.1 g/dL, Ref.: 12–16 g/dL) and thrombocytopenia (platelets: 13 k/μL, Ref.: 150–450 k/μL) with 1959 U/L lactate dehydrogenase (Ref.: 100–190 U/L). Serum haptoglobin was 10 mg/dL (Ref.: 30–200 mg/dL), and the patient had reticulocyte count of 14%. Peripheral smear revealed moderate to severe schistocytosis and few platelets (Figure 1). Serum creatinine was 1.3 mg/dL with a baseline of 0.8 mg/dL (Ref.: 0.5–1.5 mg/dL). Serum lipase level was normal. Chest roentgenogram and computed tomography of the brain and abdomen were unremarkable. A clinical diagnosis of TTP was made, and the patient was admitted to the medical intensive care unit.

Coomb's test, HIV antibody test, hepatitis panel, and septic work-up including blood, urine, and stool were negative. The patient's ADAMTS 13 activity was <3 (Ref.: 68–163). During hospitalization, the patient received fresh frozen plasma while awaiting plasmapheresis. Eight sessions of plasmapheresis with one volume exchange in each session were done. In addition, patient received intravenous methylprednisolone 62.5 mg two doses and 40 mg of intravenous methylprednisolone twice a day for two weeks (until a sustained rise in platelet was seen), followed by a gradual taper with oral prednisone. During the course of treatment, the hematological abnormalities, that is, platelets, LDH, and haptoglobin, returned to normal (Figure 2). The patient was discharged and remained asymptomatic with stable hematological profile during follow-up in the ambulatory clinic.

3. Discussion

TTP, first described by Moschcowitz in 1924 [4], is a form of thrombotic microangiopathy characterized by systemic microvascular platelet aggregation and erythrocyte destruction. It has an estimated annual incidence in the United States of 4 to 11 cases per million people and is more common

in women and individuals of African descent [5]. TTP is associated with a pentad of clinical signs and symptoms including thrombocytopenia, microangiopathic hemolytic anemia, neurological abnormalities, renal failure, and fever. Since a randomized control trial demonstrated the efficacy of plasma exchange therapy in the treatment of TTP [6], microangiopathic hemolytic anemia and thrombocytopenia without any alternate etiology have been considered sufficient for diagnosis [7]. The use of those criteria for diagnosis has resulted in a 7-fold increase in the number of patients treated for TTP [8].

TTP has diverse etiologies including infections, medications, and idiopathic and familial causes. Drug-associated TTP represents about 12% of all cases [9]. Before the advent of plasma therapy, most of the patients presenting with acute TTP died: the case-fatality rate reported in clinical series was near 100% until the 1960s [10, 11].

A test for severe deficiency (activity < 5) of von Willebrand factor- (vWF-) cleaving protease called ADAMTS 13 is 100% sensitive and specific for the diagnosis of TTP. ADMATS 13 cleaves vWF multimers, and its absence results in large vWF multimers that react with platelets, resulting in the widespread formation of platelet thrombi, which are responsible for the clinical presentation of TTP [12]. Although it is not always detected, the presence of ADAMTS 13 inhibitor suggests the acquired forms of TTP. Congenital TTP usually presents in early childhood in individuals with a positive family history of similar disorders.

For adults, plasma exchange is the only treatment supported by well-founded data. The effectiveness of plasma exchange is attributed to the removal of ADAMS 13 autoantibodies and the restoration of ADAMTS 13 activity [4, 13]. Plasma exchange is effective, however, even in patients who do not have severe ADAMTS 13 deficiency [14].

Current guidelines recommend daily plasma exchange with replacement of 1.0 to 1.5 times the predicted plasma volume of the patient [15, 16]. Further recommendations include the use of glucocorticoids in all patients with TTP and continued plasma exchange therapy for at least 2 days after the platelet count returns to normal [16, 17].

Many commonly prescribed drugs and pharmacological substances have been associated with the development of TTP. It is difficult to evaluate case reports describing associations between various drugs and the disease entity, however, because there are no standardized criteria to document the drugs as the probable cause of TTP. The incidence of TTP remains poorly defined and is dependent on voluntary reporting. Moreover, the case reports of drug-induced TTP have not been reviewed systemically to determine a formal cause-effect relation, as has been done for drug-induced thrombocytopenia [18].

Fluoroquinolones are an emerging but underrecognized cause of drug-induced thrombocytopenia. Cheah et al. described fluoroquinolone-induced thrombocytopenia [19]. Here, we focus on fluoroquinolones as a cause of TTP. Fluoroquinolones have a wide range of immune-hematopathologic effects, and the exact mechanisms for most of those effects remain unclear. It has been hypothesized that similarities in the chemical structures of quinolones and quinine might be contributory [19], because quinines are a well-recognized cause of thrombocytopenia [20].

Fluoroquinolones have been associated with TTP and the hemolytic-uremic syndrome. One of the largest published series described "temafloxacin syndrome" in which 95 patients developed hemolytic anemia, thrombocytopenia, and renal failure following treatment with temafloxacin, which was subsequently withdrawn from the market [21]. A comprehensive review of the existing literature on immune thrombocytopenia and TTP secondary to drugs did not indicate fluoroquinolones as a causative agent [7, 22, 23]. The few previous reports of ciprofloxacin-induced TTP described a fulminant course with very high mortality. Mouraux et al. described a case of a 43-year-old female who developed fulminant TTP early in a course of ciprofloxacin therapy. That patient was initially suspected to have meningoencephalitis because of marked thrombocytopenia, however, and spinal tap was delayed. Later on, cerebrospinal fluid analysis was unremarkable, and the patient was diagnosed with TTP; however, the patient died due to systemic complications [24]. Tuccori et al. described a case of TTP in a 30-year-old female receiving ciprofloxacin treatment for a urinary-tract infection, who died within 17 hours of diagnosis [25].

4. Conclusion

Ciprofloxacin is a common and widely used antibiotic with excellent tissue penetration and gastrointestinal absorption. Our patient highlighted a rare but, if unrecognized, potentially fatal complication that clinicians should be aware of. There are no established risk factors to prospectively determine which patients are at increased risk of developing TTP due to ciprofloxacin. Therefore, early recognition and aggressive management are of paramount importance for survival.

References

[1] D. H. Deck and L. G. Winston, "Sulfonamides, trimethoprim, & quinolones," in *Basic & Clinical Pharmacology*, B. G. Katzung and A. J. Trevor, Eds., McGraw-Hill Education, New York, NY, USA, 13th edition, 2015.

[2] J. Bertino Jr. and D. Fish, "The safety profile of the fluoroquinolones," *Clinical Therapeutics*, vol. 22, no. 7, pp. 798–817, 2000.

[3] S. P. Surana, Z. Sardinas, and A. S. Multz, "Moxifloxacin (Avelox) induced thrombotic thrombocytopenic purpura," *Case Reports in Medicine*, vol. 2012, Article ID 459140, 3 pages, 2012.

[4] J. L. Moake, "Thrombotic microangiopathies," *The New England Journal of Medicine*, vol. 347, no. 8, pp. 589–600, 2002.

[5] D. R. Terrell, L. A. Williams, S. K. Vesely, B. Lämmle, J. A. K. Hovinga, and J. N. George, "The incidence of thrombotic thrombocytopenic purpura-hemolytic uremic syndrome: all patients, idiopathic patients, and patients with severe ADAMTS-13 deficiency," *Journal of Thrombosis and Haemostasis*, vol. 3, no. 7, pp. 1432–1436, 2005.

[6] G. A. Rock, K. H. Shumak, N. A. Buskard et al., "Comparison of plasma exchange with plasma infusion in the treatment of thrombotic thrombocytopenic purpura," *The New England Journal of Medicine*, vol. 325, no. 6, pp. 393–397, 1991.

[7] J. N. George, "Clinical practice. Thrombotic thrombocytopenic purpura," *The New England Journal of Medicine*, vol. 354, no. 18, pp. 1927–1935, 2006.

[8] W. F. Clark, A. X. Garg, P. G. Blake, G. A. Rock, A. P. Heidenheim, and D. L. Sackett, "Effect of awareness of a randomized controlled trial on use of experimental therapy," *The Journal of the American Medical Association*, vol. 290, no. 10, pp. 1351–1355, 2003.

[9] S. Bapani, N. Epperla, Y. Kasirye, R. Mercier, and R. Garcia-Montilla, "ADAMTS13 deficiency and thrombotic thrombocytopenic purpura associated with trimethoprim-sulfamethoxazole," *Clinical Medicine and Research*, vol. 11, no. 2, pp. 86–90, 2013.

[10] E. L. Amorosi and J. E. Ultmann, "Thrombotic thrombocytopenic purpura: report of 16 cases and review of the literature," *Medicine*, vol. 45, no. 2, pp. 139–159, 1966.

[11] T. J. Torok, R. C. Holman, and T. L. Chorba, "Increasing mortality from thrombotic thrombocytopenic purpura in the United States—analysis of national mortality data, 1968-1991," *American Journal of Hematology*, vol. 50, no. 2, pp. 84–90, 1995.

[12] H.-M. Tsai, "Physiologic cleavage of von Willebrand factor by a plasma protease is dependent on its conformation and requires calcium ion," *Blood*, vol. 87, no. 10, pp. 4235–4244, 1996.

[13] J. E. Sadler, J. L. Moake, T. Miyata, and J. N. George, "Recent advances in thrombotic thrombocytopenic purpura," *Hematology/The Education Program of the American Society of Hematology. American Society of Hematology. Education Program*, pp. 407–423, 2004.

[14] S. K. Vesely, J. N. George, B. Lämmle et al., "ADAMTS13 activity in thrombotic thrombocytopenic purpura-hemolytic uremic syndrome: relation to presenting features and clinical outcomes in a prospective cohort of 142 patients," *Blood*, vol. 102, no. 1, pp. 60–68, 2003.

[15] J. W. Smith, R. Weinstein, and K. L. Hillyer, "Therapeutic apheresis: a summary of current indication categories endorsed by the AABB and the American Society for Apheresis," *Transfusion*, vol. 43, no. 6, pp. 820–822, 2003.

[16] M. Scully, B. J. Hunt, S. Benjamin et al., "Guidelines on the diagnosis and management of thrombotic thrombocytopenic purpura and other thrombotic microangiopathies," *British Journal of Haematology*, vol. 158, no. 3, pp. 323–335, 2012.

[17] S. L. Allford, B. J. Hunt, P. Rose, and S. J. Machin, "Guidelines on the diagnosis and management of the thrombotic microangiopathic haemolytic anaemias," *British Journal of Haematology*, vol. 120, no. 4, pp. 556–573, 2003.

[18] J. N. George, G. E. Raskob, S. R. Shah et al., "Drug-induced thrombocytopenia: a systematic review of published case reports," *Annals of Internal Medicine*, vol. 129, no. 11, pp. 886–890, 1998.

[19] C. Y. Cheah, B. De Keulenaer, and M. F. Leahy, "Fluoroquinolone-induced immune thrombocytopenia: a report and review," *Internal Medicine Journal*, vol. 39, no. 9, pp. 619–623, 2009.

[20] N. F. Crum and P. Gable, "Quinine-induced hemolytic-uremic syndrome," *Southern Medical Journal*, vol. 93, no. 7, pp. 726–728, 2000.

[21] M. D. Blum, D. J. Graham, and C. A. McCloskey, "Temafloxacin syndrome: review of 95 cases," *Clinical Infectious Diseases*, vol. 18, no. 6, pp. 946–950, 1994.

[22] R. Cathomas, A. Goldhirsch, and R. von Moos, "Drug-induced immune thrombocytopenia," *The New England Journal of Medicine*, vol. 357, no. 18, pp. 1870–1871, 2007.

[23] P. J. Medina, J. M. Sipols, and J. N. George, "Drug-associated thrombotic thrombocytopenic purpura-hemolytic uremic syndrome," *Current Opinion in Hematology*, vol. 8, no. 5, pp. 286–293, 2001.

[24] A. Mouraux, M. Gille, F. Piéret, and I. Declercq, "Fulminant thrombotic thrombocytopenic purpura in the course of ciprofloxacin therapy," *Revue Neurologique*, vol. 158, no. 11, pp. 1115–1117, 2002.

[25] M. Tuccori, B. Guidi, G. Carulli, C. Blandizzi, M. D. Tacca, and M. Di Paolo, "Severe thrombocytopenia and haemolytic anaemia associated with ciprofloxacin: a case report with fatal outcome," *Platelets*, vol. 19, no. 5, pp. 384–387, 2008.

4

Fatal Pulmonary Tumor Embolic Microangiopathy in Young Lady without Known Primary Malignancy

Adel Hammodi,[1] M. Ali Al-Azem,[2] Ahmed Hanafy,[1] and Talal Nakkar[1]

[1] King Fahad Specialist Hospital, P.O. Box 15215, Dammam 31444, Saudi Arabia
[2] Critical Care Department, King Fahad Specialist Hospital, P.O. Box 15215, Dammam 31444, Saudi Arabia

Correspondence should be addressed to Adel Hammodi; adelali34@gmail.com

Academic Editor: Zsolt Molnár

Pulmonary embolism (PE) is a common cause of morbidity and mortality in hospitalized patients. Malignancy, prolonged recumbence, and chemotherapy are renowned risk factors for development of clinically significant PE. Cancer exerts a multitude of pathophysiological processes, for example, hypercoagulability and abnormal vessels with sluggish circulation that can lead to PE. One of the peculiar characteristics of tumor cells is their ability to reach the circulation and behave as blood clot—not a metastasis-occluding the pulmonary circulation. We present a case of fatal pulmonary embolism diagnosed histologically to be due to tumor cell embolism.

1. Introduction

Hypoxemia and tachypnea are the most serious signs of critical illness. A wide range of disorders can cause such signs with different pathophysiological processes.

The pulmonary artery and its branches are the final destination for any substance greater than 10 microns reaching the venous circulation which could be thrombi, air, amniotic fluid, fat, injected foreign materials, and tumor. It is known that malignancy is a risk factor for thromboembolism and carries a 4-fold risk of thrombosis event than normal population.

Microscopic pulmonary tumor embolism is the presence of multiple aggregates of tumor cell in the small pulmonary arteries, arterioles, and septal capillaries. This syndrome could happen with a number of malignancies including carcinoma of the breast, stomach, pancreas, liver, and prostate.

We present a case of pulmonary tumor embolic microangiopathy (PTEM) caused by occult adenocarcinoma in a lady without any history of malignancy.

2. Case Report

A twenty-nine year-old female patient, unemployed, smoker, and married had no children. She was in her usual state of health till 3 weeks prior to presentation, when she started to complain of breathlessness with exertion and progressed over weeks to be on minimal effort interfering with her usual daily activity. She had orthopnea, chest tightness, and pain which was retrosternal, stitching in character, aggravated with coughing, with no specific radiation, and not associated with sweating, nausea, or vomiting. She was evaluated in a private clinic and diagnosed as having pulmonary hypertension and received sildenafil without any subsequent improvement in her condition.

She gave a past history of unintended weight loss of about 13 kg during last 3 months. In addition, she had night fever, night sweats responding to antipyretics.

Four months back, the patient had nausea and vomiting and diagnosed to have *H. pylori* infection, which was treated by standard triple therapy. There was also a history of itchy erythematous skin rash which was managed with topical corticosteroid during that time.

She was investigated for infertility 4 years ago, where she was diagnosed to have polycystic ovary syndrome (PCOS) and fallopian tube obstruction.

There was no previous history of recent travel or immobilization, pulmonary emboli, congenital heart disease, or chronic lung disease. She had a parrot in her house.

TABLE 1

	Patient's tumor markers	Normal values upper limit
CA 125	82	0.042 IU/mL
CA 15.3	12	0.027 IU/mL
CA 19.9	13.2	0.037 IU/mL
CEA	89.79	0–5 ug/L
Alpha fetoprotein	1.91	1.09–8.04 ng/mL

There was neither history of contraceptive pill use nor family history of similar attack.

The patient's vital signs revealed blood pressure of 129/73 mmHg, heart rate of 100 beat/minute, respiratory rate of 28 breath/min, oxygen saturation on room air of 87%, and temperature of 36.8°.

She looked distressed, tachypneic, orthopneic, and cyanosed with congested neck veins. Chest examination showed bilaterally diminished air entry with fine basal crepitations up to midlung zones. Auscultation of the heart revealed normal first and second heart sounds with no additional sounds or audible murmur. There was mild epigastric tenderness on abdominal examination. Her extremities showed neither edema, nor clinical evidence of DVT which was confirmed later by venous Doppler study. She was conscious, alert, and oriented to time, place, and person.

Laboratory work-up showed normal liver, renal function tests, and electrolytes as well. CBC revealed anemia with normal leucocytes and eosinophilic counts.

ECG displayed sinus tachycardia. Echocardiography showed severe pulmonary hypertension with estimated pulmonary artery pressure of 78 mmHg, mild to moderate tricuspid regurgitation, septal wall flattening due to right ventricular pressure overload, and normal LV systolic function with ejection fraction of >55%.

Pulmonary function test (PFT) result was moderate restrictive defect with mild reduction of gas diffusion, while the tumor markers results are shown in Table 1.

Chest X-ray (Figure 1) revealed bilateral prominent interstitial reticulonodular infiltrate, with no focal pulmonary lesion detected.

Afterward, high resolution CT of the chest (Figure 2) was done and showed bilateral diffuse ground glass density of the lungs, with centrilobular nodular densities and mild reticulations. However, no volume loss, honeycombing formation, or pleural effusion was seen. Similarly, no significant axillary, hilar, or mediastinal lymph nodes were seen either. Small pericardial effusion was noted. CT Chest PE Study excluded any evidence of pulmonary embolism.

The patient had worsening reticulonodular infiltrations on subsequent chest X-rays, and she became more tachypneic and hypoxic despite the high flow oxygen delivered.

The plan was to obtain an open lung biopsy by thoracic surgeon trying to identify the cause of rapidly worsening interstitial lung disease.

Biopsy result showed (Figure 3) predominantly moderately differentiated adenocarcinoma tumor emboli within vessels (black arrow heads) with no solid tumor mass present.

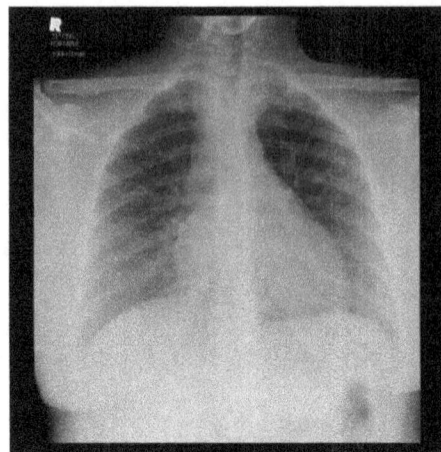

FIGURE 1

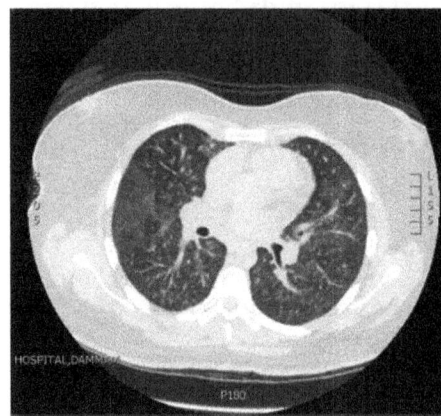

FIGURE 2

Immunohistochemical staining was done later trying to identify the primary origin of the tumor and returned as positive for CK7, CK20, CK19, Villin, CEA, and CDx2, focally positive for HER2neu, and negative for ER, PR, GCDFP-15, and TTF-1, supporting a primary GI and pancreaticobiliary origin.

After few days the patient had refractory hypoxemia and developed cardiac arrest, CPR was done but failed, and the patient was declared dead. Autopsy was not done due to family refusal.

3. Discussion

The pulmonary tumor thromboembolism syndrome had been portrayed by Kane and Hawkins in 1975 [1].

The incidence of pulmonary tumor thromboembolism depends on the type of malignancy. It is worth noting that, in diagnosed cancer patients, the accurate identification of tumor embolism is made in less than 6% cases [2].

Pulmonary tumor embolism syndrome (also known as pulmonary tumor embolic microangiopathy "PTEM") has been reported to present 3% to 26% of postmortem examination of cancer patients [3].

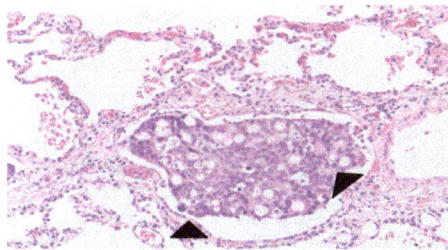

FIGURE 3

The presence of isolated or clusters of tumor cells in the pulmonary arterial circulation is the pathological picture of PTEM [4]. In fact pulmonary tumor emboli (PTEM) are not metastases; they lack the lung specific adhesion molecules and lung specific growth factor.

The incarcerated tumor cells within pulmonary capillaries may activate the coagulation cascade. The occlusion is primarily due to both the tumor cells and the associated clot, but reactive concentric hypertrophy and intimal fibrosis of the pulmonary vessels also contribute [5]. Such histopathological picture is the main reason to term this syndrome as pulmonary tumor embolism microangiopathy (PTEM).

This description is typical to our patient pathology report of the open lung biopsy and explains the restrictive pattern of her PFT.

Not only cancer related factors can affect blood coagulopathy but also a list of known factors including reduced mobility, surgery, chemotherapy, and the use of central venous catheters for chemotherapy and also amplify the risk [6]. Considering our patient's condition, It is obvious that the tumor cells are the main cause of hypoxemia and the embolic event, as she was active and mobilizing few days before her presentation.

Dyspnea, orthopnea, and respiratory failure are frequent complications of malignancy and are often noted near death. Common causes of respiratory failure in patients with cancer are

(i) pleural effusion,

(ii) infection,

(iii) ARDS,

(iv) lymphangitic carcinomatosis,

(v) acute cor pulmonale,

(vi) chemotherapy or radiotherapy related restrictive lung disorder,

(vii) thromboembolism,

(viii) primary or secondary involvement mainly endobronchial,

(ix) PTEM.

Nevertheless, survival appears to be poor after the onset of symptoms, probably because pulmonary tumor emboli are often associated with concomitant lymphangitic or metastatic carcinoma [7].

PTEM is rapidly progressing and fatal disorder, as almost all reported cases died within a week from onset, and the same had happened in the current case.

It may be important to diagnose PTEM before development of pulmonary hypertension with early immunehistopathology identification, which may lead to a clinically preferable outcome. Kayatani et al. reported a case of antemortem diagnosis of PTEM which was identified prior to the development of pulmonary hypertension which responded to chemotherapy [8].

Yanagitani et al. also recorded a case of adenocarcinoma of the lung with pulmonary thromboembolism with positive epidermal growth factor receptor (EGFR) which responded well to gefitinib both the embolism and the primary tumor with its metastasis [9].

Our patient was diagnosed after development of severe pulmonary hypertension and her immune-histochemical staining was negative for EGFR, ER, and PR which added to her dismal outcome.

Several ancillary studies may be helpful in distinguishing pulmonary tumor emboli from thromboemboli. For example, ventilation-perfusion lung scans, pulmonary angiography, right heart catheterization and sampling from pulmonary capillaries after wedging, FDG-PET (18F-2-deoxy-2-flouro-D-glucose (FDG) position emission tomography), and lung biopsy were investigated in similar cases [10].

From these investigations, lung biopsy is the gold standard diagnostic test for PTEM.

Another important investigation is echocardiography which differentiates between pulmonary embolism and lymphangitis carcinomatosis [7].

Treatment of PTEM should be directed to the primary tumor. Conventional pulmonary embolism therapies like anticoagulation, thrombolysis, inferior vena, and cava filter placement seem to be ineffective. The main therapeutic options are either surgical resections of the primary tumor, for example, atrial myxoma and renal cell carcinoma, or targeted chemotherapy in case of positive immunohistochemistry [11].

4. Conclusion

Pulmonary tumor embolic microangiopathy is a rare and potentially fatal disorder in either diagnosed or undiagnosed cancer patients.

Intensivists should consider tumor embolism along with pulmonary venous thromboembolism as a cause of PE in cancer patients having dyspnea with unremarkable chest X-ray findings.

Early diagnosis may initiate timely appropriate chemotherapy treatment that results in improved outcome of PTEM patients.

References

[1] R. D. Kane, H. K. Hawkins, J. A. Miller, and P. S. Noce, "Microscopic pulmonary tumor emboli associated with dyspnea," *Cancer*, vol. 36, no. 4, pp. 1473–1482, 1975.

[2] S. Z. Goldhaber, E. Dricker, J. E. Buring et al., "Clinical suspicion of autopsy-proven thrombotic and tumor pulmonary embolism in cancer patients," *The American Heart Journal*, vol. 114, no. 6, pp. 1432–1435, 1987.

[3] N. G. Keenan, A. G. Nicholson, and P. J. Oldershaw, "Fatal acute pulmonary hypertension caused by pulmonary tumour thrombotic microangiopathy," *International Journal of Cardiology*, vol. 124, no. 1, pp. e11–e13, 2008.

[4] S. Mehrishi, A. Awan, A. Mehrishi, and A. Fein, "Pulmonary tumor microembolism," *Hospital Physician*, vol. 40, no. 1, pp. 23–30, 2004.

[5] S. Z. Goldhaber, "Pulmonary embolism," in *Braunwald's Heart Disease: A Textbook of Cardiovascular Medicine*, P. Libby, R. O. Bonow, D. L. Mann, and D. P. Zipes, Eds., p. 1876, W. B. Saunders, Maryland Heights, Mo, USA, 8th edition, 2007.

[6] A. Fennerty, "Venous thromboembolic disease and cancer," *Postgraduate Medical Journal*, vol. 82, no. 972, pp. 642–648, 2006.

[7] A. G. Bassiri, B. Haghighi, R. L. Doyle, G. J. Berry, and N. W. Rizk, "Pulmonary tumor embolism," *The American Journal of Respiratory and Critical Care Medicine*, vol. 155, no. 6, pp. 2089–2095, 1997.

[8] H. Kayatani, K. Matsuo, Y. Ueda et al., "Pulmonary tumor thrombotic microangiopathy diagnosed antemortem and treated with combination chemotherapy," *Internal Medicine*, vol. 51, no. 19, pp. 2767–2770, 2012.

[9] N. Yanagitani, A. Horiike, K. Kudo, F. Ohyanagi, M. Nishio, and T. Horai, "A case of adenocarcinoma of the lung with a pulmonary thromboembolism which improved with gefitinib," *Nihon Kokyūki Gakkai Zasshi*, vol. 49, no. 4, pp. 282–286, 2011.

[10] R. G. Masson, J. Krikorian, P. Lukl, G. L. Evans, and J. McGrath, "Pulmonary microvascular cytology in the diagnosis of lymphangitic carcinomatosis," *The New England Journal of Medicine*, vol. 321, no. 2, pp. 71–76, 1989.

[11] R. L. Seagle, A.-M. Nomeir, L. E. Watts, S. A. Mills, and W. E. Means, "Left atrial myxoma and atrial septal defect with recurrent pulmonary emboli," *Southern Medical Journal*, vol. 78, no. 8, pp. 992–994, 1985.

5

Ventricular Tachycardia from a Central Line Fracture Fragment Embolus: A Rare Complication of a Commonly Used Procedure—A Case Report and Review of the Relevant Literature

Saptarshi Biswas and Patrick McNerney

Department of Trauma and Acute Care Surgery, Allegheny Health Network, Pittsburgh, PA, USA

Correspondence should be addressed to Saptarshi Biswas; saptarshibiswas@comcast.net

Academic Editor: Claudius Diez

A 22-year-old male admitted with multiple gunshot wounds (GSW) had central line placed initially for hemodynamic monitoring and later for long term antibiotics and total parenteral nutrition (TPN). On postoperative day 4 he presented with bouts of nonsustained ventricular tachycardia; the cause was unknown initially and later attributed to a catheter fragment accidentally severed and lodged in the right heart. Percutaneous retrieval technique was used to successfully extract the catheter fragment and complete recovery was achieved.

1. Introduction

Central catheters are widely used throughout the United States for conditions and/or treatments that require frequent intravenous access [1], to permit hemodynamic monitoring by measurement of central venous pressure, to provide long term administration of intravenous antibiotics, or to provide reliable access to provide parenteral nutrition and blood products [2].

However, despite the widespread use both catheter related infections and mechanical complications remain significantly high [3]. Complications can happen during insertion of the catheter and/or during maintenance of the line [3]. Inadvertent arterial puncture resulting in bleeding, venous thrombosis, pneumothorax, and cardiovascular side effects can all occur during insertion [4]. Central line catheter fracture/fragmentation and catheter migration are some of the rare reported mechanical complications.

We report the case of an accidental fracture of an internal jugular central line during manipulation, subsequent migration and presentation as ventricular tachyarrhythmia,

and later successful retrieval by interventional percutaneous methods.

2. Case Report

A 20-year-old male was brought in by the EMS as an activated level 1 trauma. The patient had sustained multiple gunshot wounds to the abdomen.

On arrival the patient was alert and oriented to time and place. The patient was also complaining of abdominal pain. Primary survey revealed a patent airway, bilateral air entry on auscultation, questions answered appropriately, and movement of all his extremities. There was one wound on either side of the mid anterior abdomen as well as on the left suprapubic region and left buttock. However within a span of few minutes the patient became progressively more lethargic and obtunded. The decision was made to emergently intubate the patient and transfer to the OR. Volume resuscitation was started, with 1 liter of normal saline (NS) being given and massive transfusion activated. Initial labs showed WBC $9.19 \times 10^3/\mu L$, Hgb 10.3 g/dL, Hct 31.1%, Plt 102×10^3/microliter,

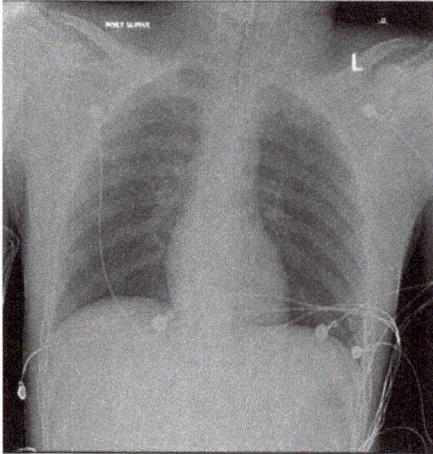

FIGURE 1: Chest X-ray post-op.

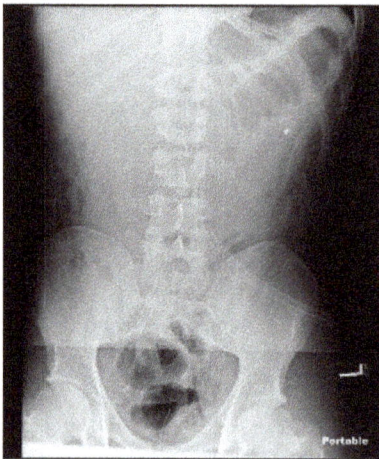

FIGURE 2: Post-op abdomen X-ray showing bullet fragment in left upper quadrant.

Na 146 mEq/L, K 4.5 mEq/L, Cl 102 mEq/L, CO_2 19 mEq/L, BUN 10 mg/dL, Cr 1.4 mEq/L, ALT 272 IU/L, AST 185 IU/L, ALP 51 IU/L, and TPR 0.6 ng/mL. Pre-op blood gases showed a pH of 6.8, $paCO_2$ of 56 mm Hg, and HCO_3 of 9.3 mmol/L.

An exploratory laparotomy was performed emergently. Injuries to the right colic artery, 1st jejunal branch of mesentery, and 3rd portion of the duodenum were found as well as two "through and through" injuries to the small bowel and a complete transection of the descending colon that involved "fecal spillage." The two small bowel injuries were resected and the devitalized tissue surrounding the descending colon transection was also excised. Considering the physiological status of the patient intraoperatively a damage control surgery was performed, the bowel ends were stapled, obvious bleeders were addressed, contamination was controlled, and the was abdomen packed. The abdomen was left open and covered by an Abthera wound vacuum. Post-op chest and abdominal X-rays were taken, seen in Figures 1 and 2, and the patient was transferred to the ICU for further resuscitation and stabilization of hemodynamics.

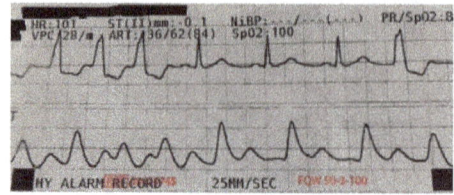

FIGURE 3: EKG strip showing ventricular tachycardia.

The patient was returned to the OR 3 days later. An exploratory laparotomy was performed along with one jejunojejunal anastomosis, one side to side ileocolic anastomosis, both hands sewn, closure of the mesenteric rents, and closure of the abdominal fascia. The skin was closed with staples. The patient tolerated the surgery well. The patient was reprepped and draped. A right subclavian central line was placed on second attempt after the first attempt resulted in the catheter being bunched up in the vein with brief period of arrhythmia. The patient experienced a brief period of hypotension and a chest X-ray was ordered which did not show any hemothorax or pneumothorax. The right IJ was guide wired by pulling the line back, clamping it with a hemostat and dividing it, and then going down the central lumen with a guide wire. A Mahurkar catheter was placed into the right IJ vein. Both the subclavian and the IJ dialysis lines were secured and sterile dressings applied prior to transferring the patient.

The patient developed nonsustained runs of ventricular tachycardia 3 days after the second operation, visible in Figure 3. The EKG on admission was sinus tachycardia. Cardiology was consulted. The electrolytes were checked and with the exception of magnesium which was 1.1 mEq/L, the rest of the electrolytes were within normal range. The magnesium was replaced. The ventricular tachycardia persisted despite electrolyte replenishment and amiodarone drip was started. The amiodarone was changed to lidocaine but the patient continued to have runs of ventricular tachycardia. Four days post-op the source of the patient's arrhythmia remained a mystery until a chest X-ray revealed a piece of what was suspected to be a fractured central catheter, seen in Figure 4. The catheter fragment had lodged itself within the inferior vena cava and the right atrium. All lines and tubes connected to the patient including the EKG leads were disconnected to make sure it is not superimposed image causing confusion. A Chest CT imaging was performed which confirmed the suspicions produced by the chest X-ray, shown in Figure 5.

Interventional radiology was consulted and plans for immediate retrieval were made. A fluoroscopy guided percutaneous intervention resulted in retrieval of the 10 cm catheter fragment via a triple loops snare, demonstrated in Figures 6 and 7. The removed catheter fragment was briefly inspected and can be seen in Figure 8. The procedure was performed without any complications and the patient was found to tolerate it well. Repeat chest imaging confirmed successful removal of the catheter fragment, as seen in Figure 9. No further ventricular tachycardia was observed during several

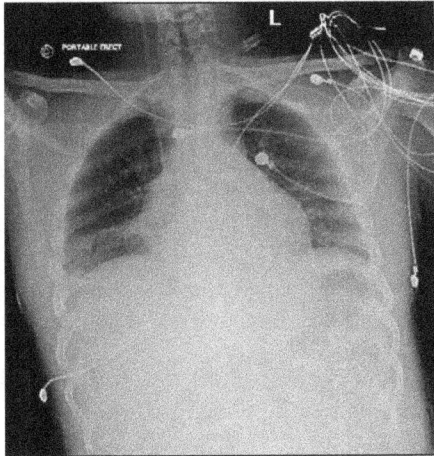

FIGURE 4: Chest X-ray AP view showing catheter projected over right atrium and superior IVC.

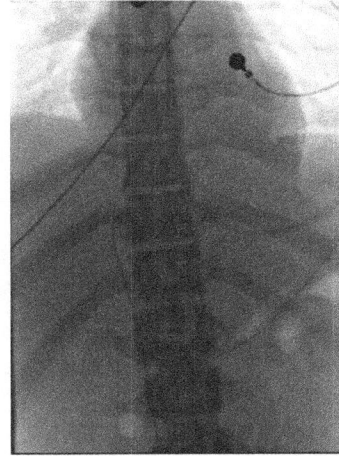

FIGURE 5: Confirmatory CT of radiopaque catheter, 10 cm, tubing extending from retrohepatic IVC through the right atrium into the low SVC.

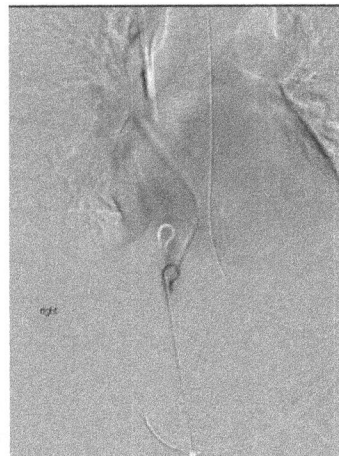

FIGURE 6: Triple loops snare used to retrieve catheter fragment.

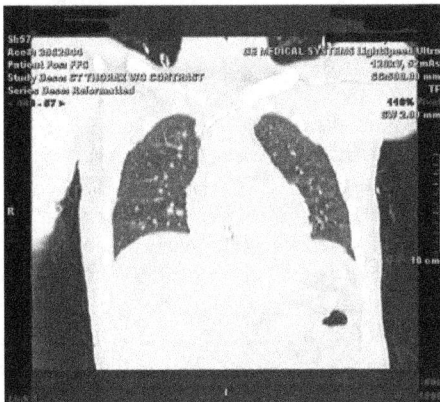

FIGURE 7: Another view of the catheter fragment retrieval procedure.

days of continued monitoring while the patient was in the hospital recovering from his other injuries.

3. Discussion

Central catheters are used in situations requiring prolonged intravenous access such as parenteral nutrition, antibiotic infusion, chemotherapy infusion, hemodialysis, or infusion of drugs known to cause phlebitis when infused directly into peripheral veins [5, 6]. Hemorrhage at the insertion site, pneumothorax, pneumohemothorax, and venous thrombosis are some of the frequent adverse events encountered from central catheter use [4]. On rare occasions severe complications like fracture/fragmentation and embolization can occur.

Surov et al. [7] had done a comprehensive review of all articles published in English literature between 1985 and 2007 [7]. He noted that Pinch-off Syndrome accounted for the majority (40.9%) and was the most common cause for catheter fragmentation [7]. Other causes sited were catheter

injury during extraction (17.7%), catheter disconnection (10.7%), catheter rupture (11.6%), and unknown cause (19.1%) [7]. The catheter fracture rate was highest among central catheters inserted from peripheral veins [6]. Fracture may occur during insertion secondary to high syringe pressure or due to removal or traction on the catheter-hub junction. Loughran and Borzatta reported an incidence of 9.7% in a series of 322 applications [8]. Mortality rate was reported as 1.8% by Surov et al. in their series of 215 cases of catheter embolization [7]. The mortality depends on the duration as well as the site of embolization. Richardson et al. [9] noted that the embolized fragment lodged in the right atrium carried the highest mortality while the lowest was recorded in those in the pulmonary artery [9].

Catheter fracture has an estimated rate of occurrence of 0.1%, making it much rarer than other complications associated with central catheter use [10]. Fractured catheters have been found to have a high 71% morbidity and a 38% mortality rate [10]. Fractured catheters are reported to have travelled throughout the venous system before eventually lodging

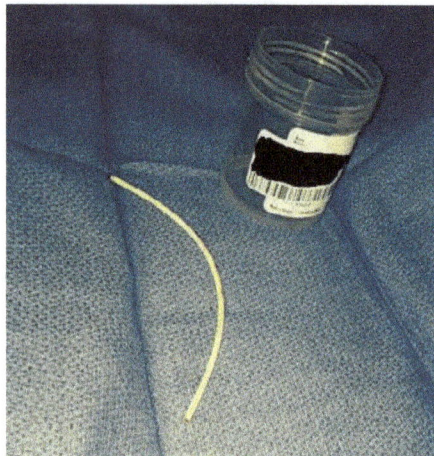

FIGURE 8: Embolized catheter fragment.

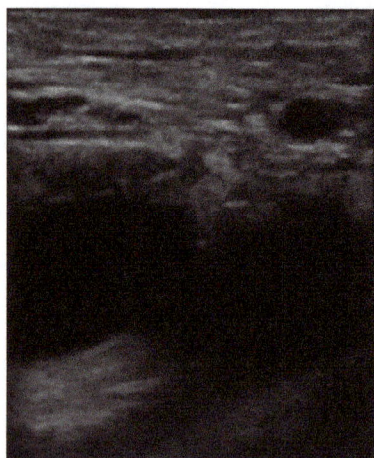

FIGURE 9: Follow-up image of IVC showing wide patency after removal of catheter fragment.

themselves somewhere. The lodged fragment can potentially obstruct blood flow or alter normal organ function. Common sites of deposition of fractured catheters are the central veins, pulmonary artery system, or within the right side of the heart [11].

Central catheter fractures can result from a multitude of situations including shearing of the catheter during insertion due to contact with the introducer needle, increased intra-catheter pressure often due to bolus infusion, patient body movement resulting in fracture of the external portion of the line seen specially in infants, mechanical forces between the first rib and clavicle, and catheter fatigue due to prolonged exposure to motion of the tricuspid valve and/or right ventricle [10]. A fractured catheter can result in pulmonary embolism, cardiac arrhythmia, myocardial ischemia, valvular perforation, abscess formation, septicemia, cardiac arrest, or even sudden death and will often present with symptoms associated with those conditions [2, 5].

Catheter fatigue from use for a prolonged period of time can result in in situ fracture, as well as fragmentation and

distal embolization [12]. The catheter fragment often migrates distally and finally lodges in the vena cava, right atrium, right ventricle, pulmonary artery, or its branches [10]. Interestingly the length, weight, and the material stiffness often determine the final lodgment site [10]. There have been reports of that vigorous vomiting, sneezing, or coughing has resulted in catheter tip migration [10]. Retained foreign bodies can act as a nidus for subsequent thrombus formation with resultant embolism. Endocarditis, secondary superadded infections of the thrombus, mycotic aneurysm, and pulmonary abscesses are some of the well recorded infectious complications of the process.

In some unusual situations the patient may remain asymptomatic, potentially for an extended period of time, sometimes even a number of years [4]. A case reported by Thanigaraj et al. describes a patient that was found to have a pulmonary embolism as a result of catheter fragmentation 11 years after the initial removal of the catheter [13]. Deep et al. also describe a case of an asymptomatic 80-year-old male patient, found to have an accidentally cut external portion of the central catheter with hair trimming shears, causing it to embolize [10].

Other cases have mentioned a more acute or subacute presentation. Gowda et al. report on a 34-year-old female that presented with shortness of breath and palpitations that were exacerbated when lying in the left lateral position [1]. An outpatient Holter monitor showed ventricular tachycardia that would occur when the patient was in the aforementioned position [1]. This presentation is similar to that of the patient mentioned in this case report, with the exception of this case report's patient's tachycardia not being induced by position. Chest radiograph confirmed that a catheter fragment was responsible for the symptoms after having lodged itself in the right ventricle [1]. A case described by Faircloth and Benjamin involves a less common presentation; an 8-year-old male patient that presented with shoulder pain was found via chest radiograph to have a catheter fragment embolus in his left main pulmonary artery [11]. In another male pediatric patient, aged 17, the patient complained of a cough and what he described as "feeling funny"; in this case the initial chest radiograph was incorrectly read as normal [11]. Later a chest CT was performed and the catheter fragment was identified to be present in the right atrium and ventricle after being initially described by the radiologist as a "unipolar transvenous pacemaker" [11]. Eryılmaz et al. also reported on a pediatric case; it involved a 7-year-old male that presented with a fever and signs of pneumonia [14]. A CXR was initially performed and found to be negative, a chest CT was then performed, and two catheter fragments were discovered, one in the left pulmonary artery and the other at the junction of the vena cava superior and subclavian veins [14]. These various cases allow for a general understanding of the sequela that is often present in these scenarios. Similar to a previously mentioned case, our patient suffered from a cardiac arrhythmia as a result of the catheter fragmentation, more specifically a ventricular tachycardia. The patient did not have positional arrhythmias but rather nonsustained bouts of the ventricular tachycardia that occurred while lying still and with any movement. Similar to other cases the ventricular tachycardia completely resolved on removal of the catheter fragment.

Imaging not only allows for a diagnosis of central catheter fracture but also can serve as a preventative measure. "Pinch-off Sign" is a radiological sign that appears on fluoroscopy as focal catheter narrowing that presents between the first rib and the clavicle [11]. Pinch-off Sign is a finding of "Pinch-off Syndrome" which results from catheter compression between the clavicle and the first rib, a situation that is exacerbated by excessive medial insertion of the catheter [1]. The Pinch-off Sign is one of the earliest findings associated with imminent catheter fracture [11]. Pinch-off Sign has an associated fracture risk of around 40% [11]. It has been suggested that follow-up chest radiographs spaced every 4 weeks be done on patients with central catheters as a preventive measure against catheter fracture [1]. Pain with or without swelling at the catheter site and sudden difficulty of infusion via the catheter are the first and second most common presenting signs of Pinch-off Syndrome, respectively, and are also associated with imminent catheter fracture [15].

Chest radiography and chest CT appear to be the preferred radiological modes used in the diagnosis of catheter fragmentation, with chest fluoroscopy preferred for the retrieval of the catheter fragment, if retrieval is being done via percutaneous intervention [1]. CXR and CT were used to diagnose and confirm, respectively, the catheter fragmentation found in the patient discussed in our case.

The preferred procedure for removal of a catheter fragmentation is percutaneous intervention [1]. Thomas et al. first reported in 1964 a case of nonsurgical removal of an intravascular steel guide wire fragment [16]. Percutaneous retrieval of a free floating catheter fragment has now become technique of choice. Looped wire snares, hooked guide wire, and Fogarty balloon catheters are the primary tools used in the capture of the catheter by interventional radiologists or cardiologists [10]. Percutaneous intervention retrieval of catheter fragments is generally preferred due to its relatively low adverse event rate and its greater than 95% success rate [1]. The choice of device and the technique used to retrieve the foreign body are dependent on the circumstances and the dimensions of the embolized fragment [14], since Yedlicka et al. [14, 17] gooseneck snares have gained popularity in retrieving embolized fragments. Noninvasive imaging should be done to exclude the presence of thrombus which may predispose to pulmonary embolism. Adverse events related to percutaneous retrieval of catheter fragments include blood vessel damage and/or perforation, arrhythmia, MI, stroke, insertion site bleeding, and intramural hematoma [18].

Situations do exist where percutaneous intervention is not favored or is unsuccessful, especially when both ends are fixed or entrapped and thus impossible to grasp, in which case the remaining option is surgical intervention via a thoracotomy [14]. Thoracotomy is, fortunately, rarely required with some centers reporting rates as low as 2.3% of retrievals requiring thoracotomy [14]. A triple loops snare was used to retrieve the catheter fragment via percutaneous intervention in our case, with no obvious complication.

4. Conclusion

Despite widespread use, central catheters are not without risk. Common risks of catheter placement include infection, hematoma, and pneumothorax [4]. Less reported complications are catheter fracture, catheter malposition, migration, cardiac perforation, and extravasation breakage [1]. Despite its rarity catheter fracture is a serious event carrying a high morbidity and mortality rate [10]. Ventricular tachycardia triggered by fragment embolism is rarely reported. Awareness of the possibility of such complication can lead to early identification and immediate management of these potentially life threatening complications, for example, septicemia, pulmonary embolism, abscess formation, arrhythmias, perforation of the great vessels or the heart, and even sudden death [13, 19].

Centrally placed catheters should be manipulated with extreme caution. Any implanted catheter should be removed after completion of the treatment and the integrity of the system should be checked on a regular basis [20]. Some authors [2] recommend early heparinization to prevent thrombus formation around catheter fragment and use of intravenous antibiotics to prevent sepsis until the time for intervention [2]. Once fractured the preferred method of retrieval is percutaneous intervention, often using a looped wire snare [10]. Thoracotomy is a less desirable method of retrieval but is at times a necessity [14].

Acknowledgments

The trauma surgeons, physician assistants, and surgical ICU nurses are acknowledged for their contribution to the clinical management of the patient, as well as the interventional radiology team for their prompt intervention.

References

[1] M. R. Gowda, R. M. Gowda, I. A. Khan et al., "Positional ventricular tachycardia from a fractured mediport catheter with right ventricular migration: a case report," *Angiology*, vol. 55, no. 5, pp. 557–560, 2004.

[2] P. B. Thapa, R. Shrestha, D. R. Singh, and S. K. Sharma, "Removal of central venous catheter fragment embolus in a young male," *Kathmandu University Medical Journal*, vol. 4, no. 15, pp. 340–341, 2006.

[3] A. H. Akmal, M. Hasan, and A. Mariam, "The incidence of complications of central venous catheters at an intensive care unit," *Annals of Thoracic Medicine*, vol. 2, no. 2, pp. 61–63, 2007.

[4] N.-D. Miao, H. Xu, L. Yang et al., "Successful removal of a peripherally inserted central catheter fragment from the heart with a vena cava filter retrieval set," *Cardiovascular System*, vol. 2, no. 1, p. 7, 2014.

[5] F. Fang, H. Zhang, and W. Yang, "An unusual peripherally inserted central catheter (PICC) fractured in vivo with embolization happened in a child: a case report," *Case Reports in Clinical Medicine*, vol. 4, no. 1, article 10, 2015.

[6] Y. Bashir, S. Bhat, F. Manzoor, N. Bashir, and A. Ahmad, "Catheter fracture-a rare complication of Peripherally Inserted Central Catheter (PICC)," *National Journal of Medical Research*, vol. 4, no. 3, pp. 262–263, 2014.

[7] A. Surov, A. Wienke, J. M. Carter et al., "Intravascular embolization of venous catheter—causes, clinical signs, and management: a systematic review," *Journal of Parenteral and Enteral Nutrition*, vol. 33, no. 6, pp. 677–685, 2009.

[8] S. C. Loughran and M. Borzatta, "Peripherally inserted central catheters: a report of 2506 catheter days," *Journal of Parenteral and Enteral Nutrition*, vol. 19, no. 2, pp. 133–136, 1995.

[9] J. D. Richardson, F. L. Grover, and J. K. Trinkle, "Intravenous catheter emboli: experience with twenty cases and collective review," *The American Journal of Surgery*, vol. 128, no. 6, pp. 722–727, 1974.

[10] S. Deep, S. Deshpande, and P. Howe, "Traumatic fracture of central venous catheter resulting in potential migration of distal fragment: a case report," *Cases Journal*, vol. 1, no. 1, article 394, 2008.

[11] J. Faircloth and B. Benjamin, *Subclavian Central Venous Catheter Fracture and Embolization*, Physicians Practice, Portland, Ore, USA, 2010.

[12] H.-P. Dinkel, M. Muhm, A. K. Exadaktylos, H. Hoppe, and J. Triller, "Emergency percutaneous retrieval of a silicone port catheter fragment in pinch-off syndrome by means of an Amplatz gooseneck snare," *Emergency Radiology*, vol. 9, no. 3, pp. 165–168, 2002.

[13] S. Thanigaraj, A. Panneerselvam, and J. Yanos, "Retrieval of an IV catheter fragment from the pulmonary artery 11 years after embolization," *Chest*, vol. 117, no. 4, pp. 1209–1211, 2000.

[14] E. Erylmaz, C. Canpolat, and A. Çeliker, "Catheter fragment embolization: a rare yet serious complication of catheter use in pediatric oncology," *The Turkish Journal of Pediatrics*, vol. 54, no. 3, pp. 294–297, 2012.

[15] J.-B. Cho, I.-Y. Park, K.-Y. Sung, J.-M. Baek, J.-H. Lee, and D.-S. Lee, "Pinch-off syndrome," *Journal of the Korean Surgical Society*, vol. 85, no. 3, pp. 139–144, 2013.

[16] J. Thomas, B. Sinclair-Smith, D. Bloomfield, and A. Davachi, "Non-surgical retrieval of a broken segment of steel spring guide from the right atrium and inferior vena cava," *Circulation*, vol. 30, no. 1, pp. 106–108, 1964.

[17] J. W. Yedlicka Jr., J. E. Carlson, D. W. Hunter, W. R. Castañeda-Zúñiga, and K. Amplatz, "Nitinol gooseneck snare for removal of foreign bodies: experimental study and clinical evaluation," *Radiology*, vol. 178, no. 3, pp. 691–693, 1991.

[18] H. V. Anderson, R. E. Shaw, R. G. Brindis et al., "A contemporary overview of percutaneous coronary interventions: the American College of Cardiology-National Cardiovascular Data Registry (ACC-NCDR)," *Journal of the American College of Cardiology*, vol. 39, no. 7, pp. 1096–1103, 2002.

[19] R. G. Fisher and R. Ferreyro, "Evaluation of current techniques for nonsurgical removal of intravascular iatrogenic foreign bodies," *American Journal of Roentgenology*, vol. 130, no. 3, pp. 541–548, 1978.

[20] C. R. Reed, C. N. Sessler, F. L. Glauser, and B. A. Phelan, "Central venous catheter infections: concepts and controversies," *Intensive Care Medicine*, vol. 21, no. 2, pp. 177–183, 1995.

6

Herpes Simplex Virus Hepatitis in an Immunocompetent Adult: A Fatal Outcome due to Liver Failure

Rachel A. Poley,[1] Jaime F. Snowdon,[2] and Daniel W. Howes[1]

[1] Department of Emergency Medicine and Department of Critical Care Medicine, Kingston General Hospital,
 Queen's University, Kingston, ON, Canada K7L 2V7
[2] Department of Pathology, Queen's University, Kingston, ON, Canada K7L 3N6

Correspondence should be addressed to Rachel A. Poley, raply@mta.ca

Academic Editors: M. Egi and K. S. Waxman

Objective. To present a case of a healthy 41-year-old female who developed fulminant hepatic failure leading to death. The cause of hepatic failure identified on postmortem exam was herpes simplex virus hepatitis. *Design.* Observation of a single patient. *Setting.* Intensive care unit of a tertiary care university teaching hospital in Canada. *Patient.* 41-year-old previously healthy female presenting with a nonspecific viral illness and systemic inflammatory response syndrome. *Intervention.* The patient was treated with intravenous fluids and broad-spectrum antibiotics. On the second day of admission, she was found to have elevated transaminases, and, over 48 hours, she progressed to fulminant liver failure with disseminated intravascular coagulopathy, refractory lactic acidosis, and shock. She progressed to respiratory failure requiring intubation and mechanical ventilation. She was started on N-acetylcysteine, a bicarbonate infusion, hemodialysis, and multiple vasopressors and inotropes. *Measurements and Main Results.* Despite treatment, the patient died roughly 70 hours after her initial presentation to hospital. Her postmortem liver biopsy revealed herpes simplex virus hepatitis as her cause of death. *Conclusions.* Herpes simplex virus must be considered in all patients presenting with liver failure of unknown cause. If suspected, prompt treatment with acyclovir should be initiated.

1. Introduction

We present the case of a previously healthy 41-year-old female who developed herpes simplex virus hepatitis leading to fulminant liver failure and death. Antemortem diagnosis of this disease is often difficult, and, as a result proper treatment is delayed. The aim of this paper is to review this rare but important cause of liver failure, its clinical presentation, and available treatment options.

2. The Case

A 41-year-old female presented ambulatory to the Emergency Department at 11:41 PM with a 3-week history of feeling generally unwell. She complained of severe myalgias, chills, and a fever two days earlier. She had been unable to go to work for the previous 4 days due to her illness. She admitted to taking ibuprofen, up to 800 mg every 2 hours for several days for her myalgias, but she and her husband denied any significant acetaminophen ingestion. She was hemodynamically unstable on presentation with a heart rate of 114 beats per minute and a blood pressure of 71/40 mm Hg. She was afebrile with a temperature of 36.4°C. Her respiratory rate was 18 breaths per minute, and her oxygen saturations were 98% on room air. She was alert and oriented with a GCS of 15 and was able to give a history of her illness. Her head and neck exam was unremarkable, and no oral lesions were documented. Her respiratory and cardiac examinations were normal. Her abdomen was soft and nontender with no organomegaly, and her skin was clear. A pelvic exam was not performed. Her past medical history was significant only for two uncomplicated pregnancies, a tubal ligation, and dysfunctional uterine bleeding. Her only medication was an oral contraceptive pill. Her social history was significant for 26 ounces of alcohol per week, mostly on weekends. There was no history of smoking, drug use, travel, or high-risk sexual behaviors.

Her investigations were significant for acute renal failure with a creatinine of 214 umol/L. Her white blood cell count was 7.2×10^9/L, hemoglobin was 130 g/L, and platelets were slightly decreased at 115×10^9/L. Her lactate was 1.5 mmol/L, and her venous blood gas showed a mild compensated metabolic acidosis with a ph of 7.32, a CO_2 of 39 mm Hg, and a HCO_3 of 20 mmol/L. Her urine b-HCG was negative. Liver function studies and liver enzymes were not performed on initial presentation.

No focus for infection was found, and she was presumed to have a viral illness with a systemic inflammatory response syndrome (SIRS). She was treated with intravenous fluid administration, and she was given broad-spectrum antibiotics to cover for any bacterial pathogen that may be causing her SIRS. The next morning a liver panel was ordered and showed significantly elevated transaminases (AST 4090 U/L, ALT 1692 U/L, ALP 123 U/L, total bilirubin 24 umol/L, INR 2.3, PT 25.9 seconds, PTT 91 seconds, platelets 85×10^9/L) with signs of liver failure and disseminated intravascular coagulopathy but a relatively normal bilirubin. She was now leukopenic with a white blood cell count of 3.6×10^9/L. Her acetaminophen level later that day was undetectable. Regardless, she was started on an N-acetylcysteine infusion as treatment for a possible late presentation of acetaminophen toxicity. Her ultrasound showed gallbladder wall thickening (5 mm) but a negative sonographic Murphy's signs; the portal vein was patent. The imaging was considered consistent with hepatitis. She was initially thought to have liver dysfunction due to prolonged hypotension on presentation resulting in hepatic ischemia. Throughout that day, the patient developed fulminant liver failure with a severe lactic acidosis and disseminated intravascular coagulopathy and required intubation. She was seen by multiple specialists throughout the course of the day and was considered for liver transplant but was deemed unsuitable. No cause for her liver failure was identified. She died later that day after developing vasopressor refractory hypotension, roughly 70 hours after presentation.

Serologic test results were available shortly after her death. She was negative for hepatitis A, B, and C viruses (hepatitis B surface antigen nonreactive and surface antibody reactive, hepatitis A IgG antibody nonreactive and IgM antibody nonreactive, hepatitis C antibody nonreactive). She was screened for multiple additional viruses including parvovirus b19, cytomegalovirus, Ebstein-Barr virus, and all of these were negative. On her postmortem liver biopsy, she had signs of severe acute liver necrosis. There was no evidence of chronic underlying liver disease. All other organ systems were spared. Tissue samples from her liver were sent for multiple tests and were negative for influenza, adenovirus, enterovirus, rhinovirus, parainfluenza virus, metapneumovirus, corona virus, and respiratory syncytial virus. Her polymerase chain reaction (PCR) testing was negative for cytomegalovirus virus and varicella zoster but positive for herpes simplex virus (HSV) type 1. Viral culture of her liver sample was positive for HSV type 1. Liver

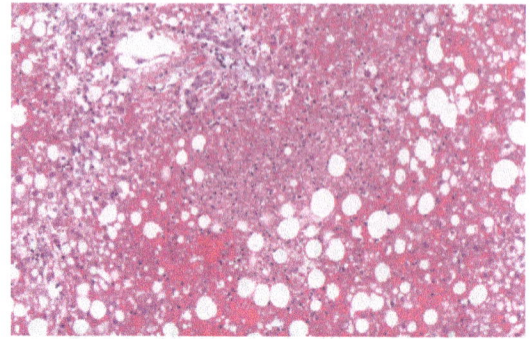

FIGURE 1: Zones of hepatocyte necrosis surrounded by hemorrhage without significant inflammation. (100x magnification; Hematoxylin-Phloxine-Saffron (HPS) stain.)

histology revealed diffuse acute liver necrosis with few inflammatory changes (Figure 1). Multiple viral inclusion bodies with the characteristic clear halo distinctive of Cowdry type A inclusions were seen in her hepatocytes (Figure 2). Immunostaining was positive for HSV antibodies (Figure 3). There was no evidence of disseminated HSV. Her cause of death was determined to be herpes simplex viral hepatitis causing fulminant liver failure.

Our Institutional Research Ethics Board has approved this case report, and the need for informed consent has been waived.

3. Discussion

Herpes simplex virus (HSV) is extremely common throughout North America and the world. It is estimated that up to 80% of adults contract HSV throughout their lifetime [1] and that most infections are asymptomatic or produce only mild nonspecific viral symptoms. HSV hepatitis is rare and accounts for only 1% of all acute liver failure cases and only 2% of all viral causes of acute liver failure (ALF) [1, 2]. It occurs most commonly in organ transplant patients, in the third trimester of pregnancy or in patients who are otherwise immunocompromised, but up to 25% of patients who develop HSV hepatitis are immunocompetent [3].

HSV hepatitis presents with nonspecific flu-like symptoms including fever, myalgias, and abdominal pain. Only 30–50% show characteristic herpetic skin lesions [3–7]. Laboratory investigations often show leucopenia, thrombocytopenia, and coagulopathy [3–6, 8–10]. Renal failure is not uncommon in these patients [5, 11–14], and it has been shown to occur in up to 65% of patients with HSV-related ALF [3]. Disseminated intravascular coagulopathy is frequently reported [5, 8, 9, 15, 16], and encephalopathy is a late sign of the disease. Ninety percent of patients with HSV hepatitis have a characteristic liver profile, known as "anicteric hepatitis" [6, 9, 17, 18]. Anicteric hepatitis refers to a liver profile showing a significant increase in transaminases (100–1000 fold) with a relatively normal or low bilirubin [1, 3, 6, 9, 16]. There may be a marked elevation of AST greater than ALT [6].

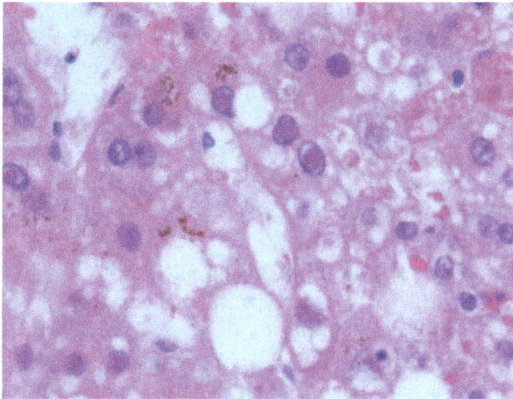

FIGURE 2: Viral inclusions are readily visible in infected hepatocytes. (600x magnification; Hematoxylin-Phloxine-Saffron (HPS) stain.)

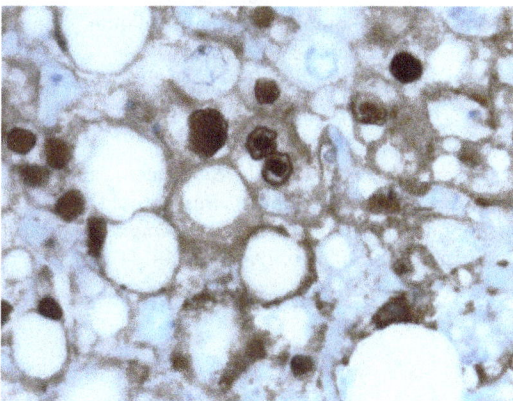

FIGURE 3: Immunohistochemistry for HSV virus highlights viral inclusions (600x magnification).

Antemortem diagnosis of HSV hepatitis is difficult and is considered in only 23–42% of cases prior to autopsy [3, 15, 19]. Investigations to aid in the diagnosis for HSV hepatitis are limited. Viral serology cultures are extremely sensitive and can be used as a screening tool but are very poorly specific. Viral PCR testing may be useful but is often not rapidly available. Although not always possible due to coagulopathy, the gold standard for diagnosis is liver biopsy. Cowdry type A inclusions, nuclei with large eosinophilic ground glass-like inclusions surrounded by a clear halo, are pathognomonic for HSV hepatitis [8, 15]. Histology shows extensive areas of hepatocyte necrosis with adjacent congestion but minimal inflammatory infiltrates [20]. Immunohistochemical staining can be done to confirm the diagnosis of HSV, and the presence of viral antigens can be demonstrated by immunoperoxidase staining and by identifying monoclonal antibodies against HSV antigens [20].

HSV hepatitis leads to ALF in 74% of cases, and, in these cases, the mortality rate reaches up to 90% [1, 3, 6, 19, 21]. Antiviral treatment with acyclovir has been used successfully [3, 5–7, 14, 17, 19, 22–25]. The extent of disease at the initiation of acyclovir plays a large role in its effectiveness,

but outcomes probably improve with earlier initiation of therapy [3, 8, 15, 22]. Many authors recommend empiric treatment with acyclovir in patients with ALF of unknown origin [1, 3, 6, 8]. High urgency liver transplant should also be considered early in the course of the disease as it has shown to improve outcomes [3, 8, 22, 23].

Physicians should consider HSV hepatitis in patients with fulminant liver failure of unknown cause. A thorough examination, including examination of the oropharynx and a complete pelvic exam, may provide clues to the diagnosis. If possible, liver biopsy is the gold standard for diagnosis. In any patient presenting with flu-like illness and anicteric hepatitis, HSV should be suspected and early treatment with acyclovir should be strongly considered.

References

[1] C. Riediger, P. Sauer, E. Matevossian, M. W. Müller, P. Büchler, and H. Friess, "Herpes simplex virus sepsis and acute liver failure," *Clinical Transplantation*, vol. 23, no. 21, pp. 37–41, 2009.

[2] F. V. Schiødt, T. J. Davern, A. O. Shakil, B. McGuire, G. Samuel, and W. M. Lee, "Viral hepatitis-related acute liver failure," *American Journal of Gastroenterology*, vol. 98, no. 2, pp. 448–453, 2003.

[3] J. P. Norvell, A. T. Blei, B. D. Jovanovic, and J. Levitsky, "Herpes simplex virus hepatitis: an analysis of the published literature and institutional cases," *Liver Transplantation*, vol. 13, no. 10, pp. 1428–1434, 2007.

[4] J. Polson and W. M. Lee, "AASLD position paper: the management of acute liver failure," *Hepatology*, vol. 41, no. 5, pp. 1179–1197, 2005.

[5] M. Velasco, E. Llamas, M. Guijarro-Rojas, and M. Ruiz-Yagüe, "Fulminant herpes hepatitis in a healthy adult: a treatable disorder," *Journal of Clinical Gastroenterology*, vol. 28, no. 4, pp. 386–389, 1999.

[6] D. J. Peters, W. H. Greene, F. Ruggiero, and T. J. McGarrity, "Herpes simplex-induced fulminant hepatitis in adults a call for empiric therapy," *Digestive Diseases and Sciences*, vol. 45, no. 12, pp. 2399–2404, 2000.

[7] R. W. Farr, S. Short, and D. Weissman, "Fulminant hepatitis during herpes simplex virus infection in apparently immuno-competent adults: report of two cases and review of the literature," *Clinical Infectious Diseases*, vol. 24, no. 6, pp. 1191–1194, 1997.

[8] A. D. Pinna, J. Rakela, A. J. Demetris, and J. J. Fung, "Five cases of fulminant hepatitis due to herpes simplex virus in adults," *Digestive Diseases and Sciences*, vol. 47, no. 4, pp. 750–754, 2002.

[9] G. L. Goyert, S. F. Bottoms, and R. J. Sokol, "Anicteric presentation of fatal herpetic hepatitis in pregnancy," *Obstetrics and Gynecology*, vol. 65, no. 4, pp. 585–588, 1985.

[10] A. H. Kang and C. R. Graves, "Herpes simplex hepatitis in pregnancy: a case report and review of the literature," *Obstetrical and Gynecological Survey*, vol. 54, no. 7, pp. 463–468, 1999.

[11] Y. Miyazaki, S. Akizuki, H. Sakaoka, S. Yamamoto, and H. Terao, "Disseminated infection of herpes simplex virus with fulminant hepatitis in a healthy adult. A case report," *APMIS*, vol. 99, no. 11, pp. 1001–1007, 1991.

[12] A. Manoux, F. Ferchal, and L. Bars, "Lethal herpetic hepatitis in a healthy adult," *Gastroenterologie Clinique et Biologique*, vol. 7, no. 4, pp. 340–345, 1983.

[13] Z. D. Goodman, K. G. Ishak, and I. A. Sesterhenn, "Herpes simplex hepatitis in apparently immunocompetent adults," *American Journal of Clinical Pathology*, vol. 85, no. 6, pp. 694–699, 1986.

[14] T. Czartoski, C. Liu, D. M. Koelle, S. Schmechel, A. Kalus, and A. Wald, "Fulminant, acyclovir-resistant, herpes simplex virus type 2 hepatitis in an immunocompetent woman," *Journal of Clinical Microbiology*, vol. 44, no. 4, pp. 1584–1586, 2006.

[15] S. Sharma and M. Mosunjac, "Herpes simplex hepatitis in adults: a search for muco-cutaneous clues," *Journal of Clinical Gastroenterology*, vol. 38, no. 8, pp. 697–704, 2004.

[16] L. Abbo, M. L. Alcaide, J. R. Pano, P. G. Robinson, and R. E. Campo, "Fulminant hepatitis from herpes simplex virus type 2 in an immunocompetent adult," *Transplant Infectious Disease*, vol. 9, no. 4, pp. 323–326, 2007.

[17] D. V. Glorioso, P. J. Molloy, D. H. Van Thiel, and R. J. Kania, "Successful empiric treatment of HSV hepatitis in pregnancy. Case report and review of the literature," *Digestive Diseases and Sciences*, vol. 41, no. 6, pp. 1273–1275, 1996.

[18] S. M. Jacques and F. Qureshi, "Herpes simplex virus hepatitis in pregnancy: a clinicopathologic study of three cases," *Human Pathology*, vol. 23, no. 2, pp. 183–187, 1992.

[19] P. Mudido, G. S. Marshall, R. S. Howell, D. S. Schmid, S. Steger, and G. Adams, "Disseminated herpes simplex virus infection during pregnancy: a case report," *Journal of Reproductive Medicine for the Obstetrician and Gynecologist*, vol. 38, no. 12, pp. 964–968, 1993.

[20] P. Ichai, A. M. Roque Afonso, M. Sebagh et al., "Herpes simplex virus-associated acute liver failure: a difficult diagnosis with a poor prognosis," *Liver Transplantation*, vol. 11, no. 12, pp. 1550–1555, 2005.

[21] C. G. Fink, S. J. Read, J. Hopkin, T. Peto, S. Gould, and J. B. Kurtz, "Acute herpes hepatitis in pregnancy," *Journal of Clinical Pathology*, vol. 46, no. 10, pp. 968–971, 1993.

[22] M. Montalbano, G. I. Slapak-Green, and G. W. Neff, "Fulminant hepatic failure from herpes simplex virus: post liver transplantation acyclovir therapy and literature review," *Transplantation Proceedings*, vol. 37, no. 10, pp. 4393–4396, 2005.

[23] C. J. Shanley, D. K. Braun, K. Brown et al., "Fulminant hepatic failure secondary to herpes simplex virus hepatitis. Successful outcome after orthotopic liver transplantation," *Transplantation*, vol. 59, no. 1, pp. 145–149, 1995.

[24] T. J. Joseph and P. J. Vogt, "Disseminated herpes with hepatoadrenal necrosis in an adult," *American Journal of Medicine*, vol. 56, no. 5, pp. 735–739, 1974.

[25] L. Özokcu, L. M. de Bruijckere, J. Jansen, and M. D. van den Berge, "Herpes simplex virus-induced hepatitis: rare in immunocompetent patients," *Nederlands Tijdschrift voor Geneeskunde*, vol. 153, no. 29, pp. 1444–1447, 2009.

7

Traumatic Injury Causing Intraperitoneal Hemorrhage of an Occult Pheochromocytoma

Arpit Amin, Saptarshi Biswas, and Francis Baccay

Department of Surgery, New York Medical College, Westchester Medical Center, Valhalla, NY 10595, USA

Correspondence should be addressed to Saptarshi Biswas, saptarshibiswas@comcast.net

Academic Editors: C. D. Roosens, M. R. Suchyta, and C. Zauner

Pheochromocytoma is a rare catecholamine-secreting tumor derived from chromaffin cells. The diagnosis is usually suggested by classic history in a symptomatic patient, presence of a strong family history in a patient, or discovery of an incidental mass on imaging in an asymptomatic patient. Traumatic hemorrhage into an occult pheochromocytoma presenting as hypovolemic shock is a rare presentation of pheochromocytoma. We report a case of a 48-year-old female, who presented in hypovolemic shock due to unilateral adrenal hemorrhage secondary to a fall from horse. Computed tomographic imaging revealed that the source of the hypovolemic shock was hemorrhagic right adrenal mass with active extravasation. The patient underwent emergent selective arterial embolization of right superior adrenal artery and a small adrenal branch from the right renal artery to control the hemorrhage. The patient subsequently progressed to sepsis and MODS, needing multiple surgical procedures and a protracted recovery in the ICU. In the ICU, the patient suffered from rapid cyclic fluctuation of her systolic blood pressure and was subsequently diagnosed with pheochromocytoma secondary to traumatic hemorrhage. We discuss this rare case along with the presentation and diagnostic workup of this critically ill patient with a previously undiagnosed pheochromocytoma.

1. Introduction

Pheochromocytoma is a rare catecholamine-secreting tumor derived from chromaffin cells. The diagnosis is usually suggested by classic symptoms of headaches, paroxysmal or essential hypertension, sweating, and tachycardia in a symptomatic patient. We present an unusual case of a 48-year-old female with blunt trauma presenting with intraperitoneal hemorrhage due to actively bleeding unilateral right-sided adrenal mass.

2. Case Presentation

A 48-year-old female sustained a fall while riding her horse. The patient was evaluated at a community level 2 trauma center. The patient was transferred to our institution once the initial trauma evaluation revealed perihepatic hematoma, left internal carotid artery dissection, and bilateral pulmonary contusions. En route, the patient became hemodynamically unstable requiring crystalloids and packed red blood cell transfusion.

Vital signs on arrival were T 95.5, HR 140, BP 107/65, and O2 sat 99% on assist-controlled ventilation. Repeat imaging at our institution revealed a heterogeneously enhancing mass with active extravasation suggesting hemorrhagic adrenal mass rather than inferior hepatic lobe hematoma (Figures 1(a) and 1(b)). The patient underwent emergent angiography with selective arterial embolization of right superior adrenal artery and a small adrenal branch from the right renal artery to control the hemorrhage (Figure 2).

The patient was admitted to trauma intensive care unit for further resuscitation and stabilization. Profound hypovolemic shock led to myocardial infarction and acute kidney injury prior to control of her hemorrhage. Peritoneal signs were revealed on clinical examination on hospital day 2 leading to emergent exploratory laparotomy. Extended right hemicolectomy was performed for ischemic colitis and the abdomen was temporarily left open. Subsequently, on reexploration, an ileocolic side-to-side anastomosis was performed and abdominal wall closure was performed using component separation. On hospital day 24, patient developed an episode of melena resulting in another episode of

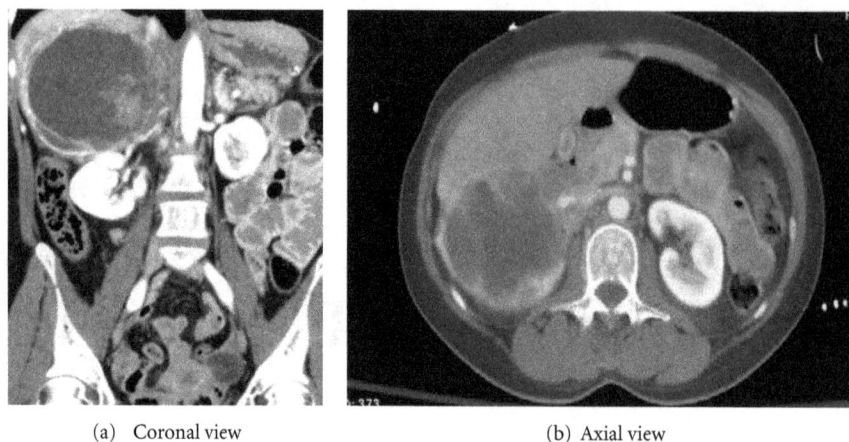

(a) Coronal view   (b) Axial view

FIGURE 1: Two views of 11.4 cm∗1.4 cm∗1.7 cm adrenal mass actively extravasating right adrenal mass.

hypovolemic shock requiring vasopressors. Nasogastric tube lavage ruled out any upper GI bleeding. Patient underwent sigmoidoscopy and exploratory laparotomy. These procedures did not reveal any source of lower GI bleeding or any evidence of anastomotic bleeding. The patient's blood pressure became stable on hospital day 28 with no further vasopressor requirement.

On hospital day 30, the patient developed rapid cyclic fluctuations in systolic blood pressure from 50 to 240. The patient denied any symptoms while these fluctuations in blood pressure were noted. The cyclic fluctuation was finally controlled after an interval of 15 minutes with the use of labetalol. 24-hour urine catecholamines were sent and found to be as follows: normetanephrine 3195 μg (normal range: 88–649), metanephrine 5238 μg (normal range: 182–739), norepinephrine 27 μg (normal range: 15–100), epinephrine 16 μg (normal range: 9–21), and vanillylmandellic acid 8.4 μg (normal range: <6.0). Diagnosis of functional pheochromocytoma was made.

A detailed history was performed to elucidate prior history of hypertension and any symptoms related to pheochromocytoma. The patient did not have any past history of hypertension or cancer in her family. Detailed physical examination did not reveal any evidence of atypical cutaneous findings like café-au-lait spots or axillary freckling. Further laboratory evaluation showed low corrected calcium (8.3 mg/dL, normal range 8.6–10.2 mg/dL), low phosphate (1.8 mg/dL, normal range 2.3–4.7 mg/dL), high PTH 67.9 pg/mL (normal range 7–53.0 pg/mL), low Vitamin D (25-OH) 19 ng/mL (normal range 30–80 ng/mL), and normal Vitamin D (1,25-OH$_2$) 22 pg/mL (normal range 18–72 pg/mL). The patient underwent a sestamibi scan, which revealed no parathyroid pathology. Thyroid ultrasound revealed 0.3 cm∗0.3 cm∗0.3 cm hypoechoic nodule in the right lobe and 0.5 cm∗0.4 cm∗0.4 cm hypoechoic nodule in the left lobe. CEA and calcitonin levels were within normal limits. Having ruled out multiple endocrine neoplasia syndrome in this patient, we proceeded to control the patient's symptoms with a nonselective α-blocker. Thereafter,

the patient was put on a long-acting β-blocker for planned resection of pheochromocytoma.

MRI of the abdomen was obtained for preoperative planning and showed 10.3 cm∗9.9 cm∗11.4 cm right adrenal mass with solid components anteriorly and cystic components posteriorly (Figure 3). There was no evidence of inferior vena cava involvement.

Exploratory laparotomy was performed and the right adrenal mass was located after extensive lysis of adhesions. The right triangular ligament and the right posterior segment of the liver were involved (segment 7). As a result, intraoperative decision was made to perform right adrenalectomy along with segment 7 hepatic resection. The mass was sent for pathology. The patient tolerated the procedure well and was discharged home on fifth post-operative day.

Pathology revealed 13.0 cm∗12.5 cm∗4.5 cm size right adrenal mass consistent with a diagnosis of pheochromocytoma. Approximately, 90% of the tumor showed necrosis with hemorrhage, fibrosis, and hyalinization with a peripheral viable rim of the tumor (Figure 4). No vascular invasion was found. Focal rim of benign hepatocytes was identified. Immunohistochemically, the tumor stained positive for CD56, chromogranin, synaptophysin, and neuron-specific enolase (Figure 5).

3. Discussion

Our patient sustained a traumatic fall leading to adrenal gland hemorrhage causing hypovolemic shock and subsequently manifested symptoms of pheochromocytoma once the patient's hemorrhage was controlled with embolization. There have been multiple case reports in the literature describing hemorrhagic shock due to spontaneous rupture of adrenal pheochromocytoma [1]. However, the mechanism of blunt trauma causing hemorrhagic shock and subsequent, delayed activation of a "latent" pheochromocytoma once the hemorrhagic shock is controlled is a unique and rare presentation of pheochromocytoma.

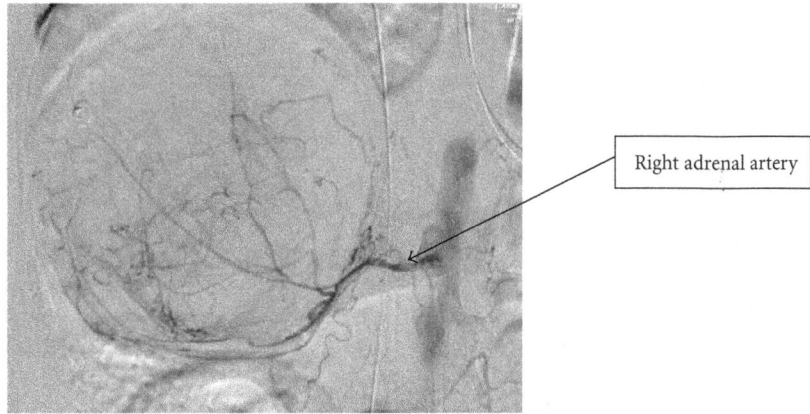

(a) Right adrenal hypervascular mass perfused by right adrenal artery originating directly from the aorta

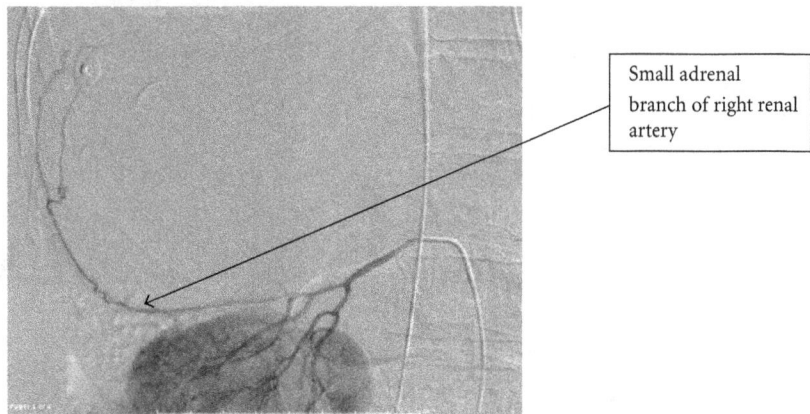

(b) Right hypervascular adrenal mass partially perfused by small adrenal branch originating from the right renal artery

FIGURE 2: Angiogram of right adrenal mass.

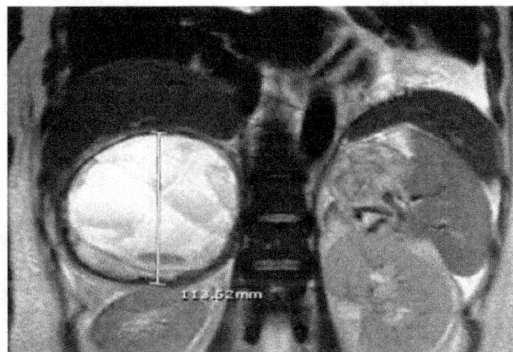

FIGURE 3: MRI abdomen (T2-weighted) of right adrenal mass.

The prevalence of pheochromocytoma is about 0.2% based on autopsy studies and the mean age at diagnosis of pheochromocytoma is about 40 years [2]. Pheochromocytoma is traditionally described by the "rule of tens"— 10% are bilateral, 10% are extra-adrenal, 10% are hereditary, and 10% are malignant [3]. Pheochromocytomas are catecholamine-secreting, well-vascularized tumors that arise from chromaffin cells derived from the neural crest cells.

The clinical presentation of pheochromocytoma is highly variable. The classic triad of symptoms consisting of episodic palpitations, headaches, and profuse sweating in the presence of hypertension, either persistent or paroxysmal, usually raises the suspicion of pheochromocytoma [2]. This classic presentation occurs in only 85%–90% of cases and the diagnosis is fairly straightforward [4]. However, the atypical presentation of pheochromocytoma makes it challenging from the diagnostic and therapeutic point of view. For instance,

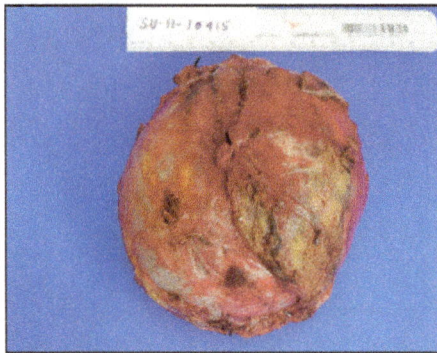

(a)

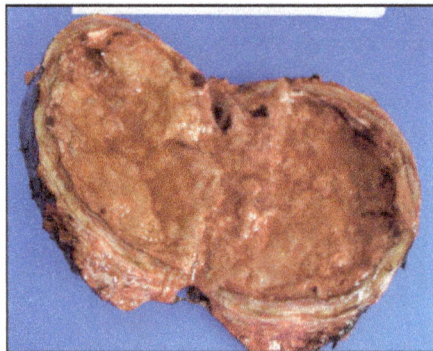

(b)

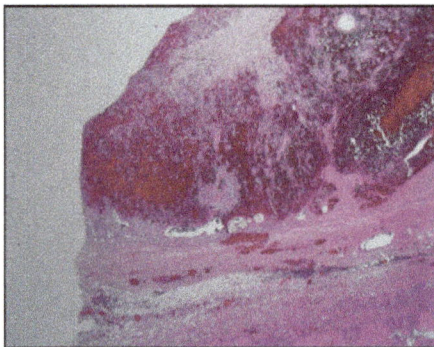

(c)

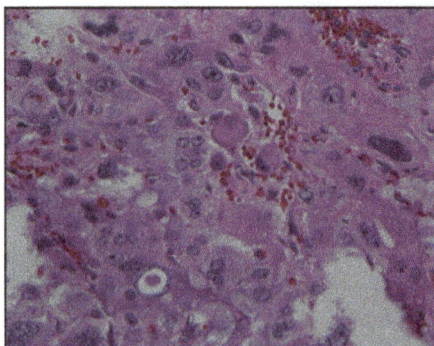

(d)

FIGURE 4: (a) and (b) Enlarged cystic adrenal mass filled with tan red necrotic material. (c) Hemorrhagic and fibrotic components within adrenal medulla mass (H & E; 100X). (d) Tumor cells are large with abundant pink to mauve cytoplasm and arranged in nests with capillaries in between (H & E; 400X).

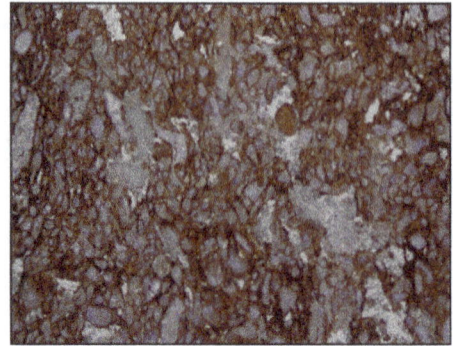

(a)

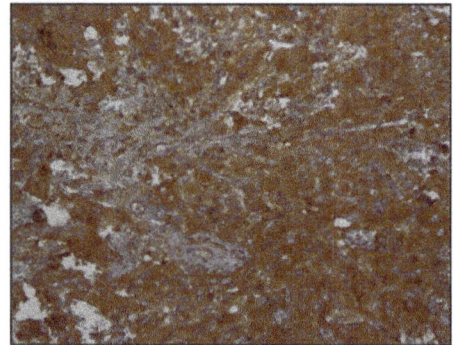

(b)

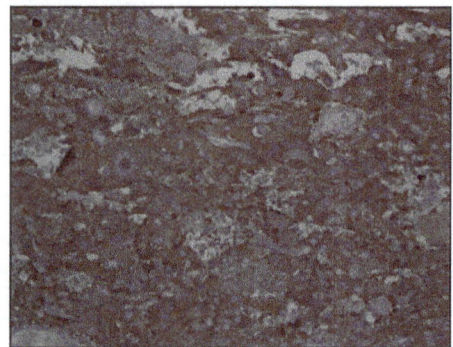

(c)

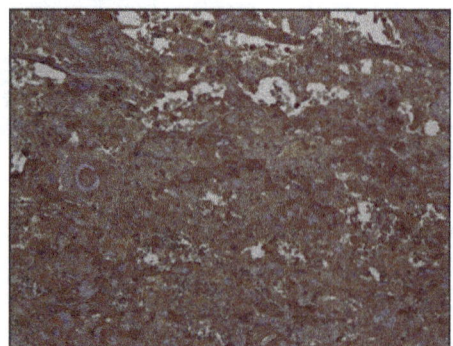

(d)

FIGURE 5: Membranous staining for CD56 (a) and cytoplasmic staining for neuron-specific enolase (b), synaptophysin (c), and chromogranin (d) in tumor cells (H & E; 200X).

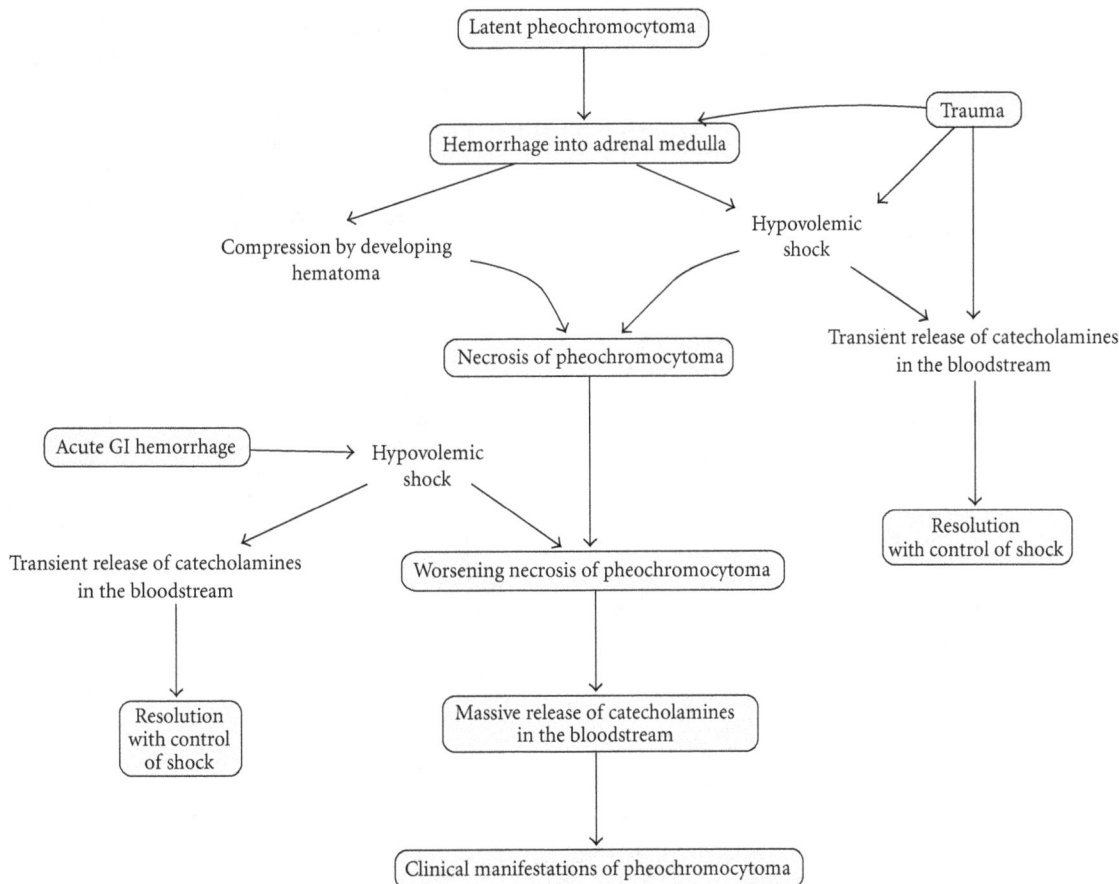

FIGURE 6: Pathophysiology of activation of "latent" pheochromocytoma.

there are cases reported in the literature of atypical presentations of pheochromocytoma in the form of cardiogenic shock due to dilated cardiomyopathy and hemorrhagic shock due to spontaneous intraperitoneal hemorrhage [1, 3, 5].

Once clinical presentation raises suspicion for pheochromocytoma, the diagnosis can be made with help of biochemical assays that determine levels of catecholamines and metanephrines in the plasma and the urine. Plasma metanephrines have been found to have the highest sensitivity while 24-hour urine vanillylmandellic acid has been found to have the highest specificity for the diagnosis of pheochromocytoma [6]. It should be noted that the false positives for these biochemical test may occur in the presence of acute traumatic injury or in presence of critical illness. The patient in our case was critically ill when the clinical manifestations of her "latent" pheochromocytoma occurred. In order to rule out false positives, sequential 24-hour urine catecholamine levels and plasma catecholamine levels were obtained once the patient was more stable and were found to be persistently elevated.

Following biochemical confirmation, CT scan with iodinated contrast or MRI (T2-weighted) imaging with gadolinium contrast can be utilized to determine the location and extent of pheochromocytoma [2]. In our case, CT scan with IV contrast was performed in the acute trauma setting and the finding of actively extravasating hemorrhagic component of adrenal mass was noted. Once the diagnosis

of pheochromocytoma was established, MRI scan (T2-weighted) was performed for preoperative planning and demonstrated cystic as well as solid changes. The findings of necrosis on pathology and hemorrhagic as well as cystic components on imaging are not uncommon for pheochromocytoma [4].

About 25% of patients with pheochromocytoma have an associated hereditary syndrome. As a result, once a diagnosis of pheochromocytoma is made, it is important to rule out any evidence of hereditary syndromes like multiple endocrine neoplasia type 2, neurofibromatosis type 1, and von Hippel-Landau syndrome in the patient. Our patient did not have any clinical manifestations associated with hereditary syndromes and laboratory testing was performed to rule out presence of these hereditary syndromes before offering definitive surgical management of pheochromocytoma.

Treatment of a patient diagnosed with pheochromocytoma involves medical optimization with alpha-adrenergic blockade and hydration followed by adequate beta-blockade. Once medical optimization is satisfactory, transperitoneal or retroperitoneal approach can be utilized to complete surgical removal of pheochromocytoma.

The pathophysiologic mechanism of activation of a "latent" pheochromocytoma in the setting of trauma in our patient can be postulated as shown in Figure 6.

In reviewing the literature we came across one reported case of latent pheochromocytoma diagnosed in the setting of blunt trauma. In the case reported by May and colleagues, the patient presented with traumatic hemorrhagic shock requiring embolization followed immediately by massive catecholamine surge resulting in persistent hypertension, which was found to be refractory to treatment with nitroprusside and esmolol and subsequently led the authors to pursue emergent adrenelectomy to help alleviate the patient's symptoms [7]. This emergent approach was successful in their case.

Our management of latent pheochromocytoma diagnosed in the setting of acute traumatic hemorrhagic shock was different. In the acute trauma setting, it should be noted that hemodynamically unstable patient with actively hemorrhaging adrenal mass will most likely undergo embolization at most trauma centers with interventional radiology capability. Once the acute hemorrhage has been controlled, latent pheochromocytoma has a potential to become activated. In our case, this occurred after the patient suffered another episode of hypovolemic shock due to gastrointestinal bleeding. In the case reported by May and colleagues, it occurred immediately after the source of hemorrhage was controlled. Regardless of the presentation, we recommend controlling the hypertensive paroxysm in the acute trauma setting with intravenous labetalol. The review of the literature regarding the management of spontaneous hemorrhagic pheochromocytoma reveals that emergent surgical management is associated with a higher mortality rate compared to elective surgical management [5, 8]. Based on this data, we favored the sequential approach of medically optimizing the patient with alpha-blockade followed by beta-blockade and thereafter proceeding with an elective open transperitoneal unilateral adrenelectomy. The open approach was favored over the laparoscopic approach in this case due to patient's recent history of exploratory laparotomy and proximity of the mass to the liver on pre-operative MRI.

Acknowledgments

For the pathologic images submitted in this paper, the authors would like to acknowledge the contribution of S. Jain and Y. Yusuf, Department of Pathology, New York Medical College, Westchester Medical Center, Valhalla, NY 10595.

References

[1] J. A. Bittencourt, M. A. Averbeck, and H. J. Schmitz, "Hemorrhagic shock due to spontaneous rupture of adrenal pheochromocytoma," *International Brazilian Journal of Urology*, vol. 29, no. 5, pp. 428–430, 2003.

[2] H. P. Neumann, A. F. Fauci, D. L. Kasper et al., "Pheochromocytoma," in *Harrison's Principles of Internal Medicine*, pp. 2269–2275, McGraw-Hill, New York, NY, USA, 17th edition, 2005.

[3] J. S. Hanna, P. J. Spencer, C. Savopoulou, E. Kwasnik, and R. Askari, "Spontaneous adrenal pheochromocytoma rupture complicated by intraperitoneal hemorrhage and shock," *World Journal of Emergency Surgery*, vol. 6, pp. 27–34, 2011.

[4] P. B. O'Neal, F. D. Moore, A. Gawande, N. Cho, J. Moalem, and D. Ruan, "Hemorrhagic shock as presentation of pheochromocytoma: report of a sequential management strategy," *Endocrine Practice*, vol. 18, no. 4, pp. e81–e84, 2012.

[5] J. Steppan, J. Shields, and R. Lebron, "Pheochromocytoma presenting as acute heart failure leading to cardiogenic shock and multiorgan failure," *Case Reports in Medicine*, vol. 2011, Article ID 596354, 4 pages, 2011.

[6] J. W. Lenders, K. Pacak, M. M. Walther et al., "Biochemical diagnosis of pheochromocytoma: which test is best?" *Journal of the American Medical Association*, vol. 287, no. 11, pp. 1427–1434, 2002.

[7] E. E. May, A. L. Beal, and G. J. Beilman, "Traumatic hemorrhage of occult pheochromocytoma: a case report and review of the literature," *American Surgeon*, vol. 66, no. 8, pp. 720–724, 2000.

[8] T. Kobayashi, A. Iwai, R. Takahashi, Y. Ide, K. Nishizawa, and K. Mitsumori, "Spontaneous rupture of adrenal pheochromocytoma: review and analysis of prognostic factors," *Journal of Surgical Oncology*, vol. 90, no. 1, pp. 31–35, 2005.

8

Nicardipine-Induced Acute Pulmonary Edema: A Rare but Severe Complication of Tocolysis

Claire Serena,[1,2] Emmanuelle Begot,[2] Jérôme Cros,[1] Charles Hodler,[1,2] Anne Laure Fedou,[2] Nathalie Nathan-Denizot,[1] and Marc Clavel[2]

[1] Service d'Anesthésie-Réanimation, Hôpital Mère Enfant, 08 avenue Dominique Larrey, 87000 Limoges, France
[2] Service de Réanimation Polyvalente, CIC 0801, CHU Dupuytren, 02 avenue Martin Luther King, 87000 Limoges, France

Correspondence should be addressed to Marc Clavel; marc.clavel@chu-limoges.fr

Academic Editor: Chiara Lazzeri

We report four cases of acute pulmonary edema that occurred during treatment by intravenous tocolysis using nicardipine in pregnancy patients with no previous heart problems. Clinical severity justified hospitalization in intensive care unit (ICU) each time. Acute dyspnea has begun at an average of 63 hours after initiation of treatment. For all patients, the first diagnosis suspected was pulmonary embolism. The patients' condition improved rapidly with appropriate diuretic treatment and by modifying the tocolysis. The use of intravenous nicardipine is widely used for tocolysis in France even if its prescription does not have a marketing authorization. The pathophysiological mechanisms of this complication remain unclear. The main reported risk factors are spontaneous preterm labor, multiple pregnancy, concomitant obstetrical disease, association with beta-agonists, and fetal lung maturation corticotherapy. A better knowledge of this rare but serious adverse event should improve the management of patients. Nifedipine or atosiban, the efficiency of which tocolysis was also studied, could be an alternative.

1. Introduction

In industrialized countries, prematurity is the main cause of perinatal morbidity and mortality and is a major public health issue in obstetrics. Its incidence varies across the country from 5 to 11% [1]. About 75% of premature births are due to spontaneous premature labor [2] which is also the most frequent cause of hospitalization [3]. Tocolytics are used to inhibit uterine contractions so that a fetal lung maturation corticotherapy can be administrated. Whether to prescribe a tocolysis as well as the choice of the molecule to use is still discussed. Massive use of β_2-adrenergic agonists in premature labor treatments induced adverse effects and sometimes severe complications especially acute pulmonary edemas (APE) [4, 5]. Other therapeutic classes are thus more and more preferred. Even if they are prescribed without marketing authorization, calcium channel blockers from the dihydropyridine group, that is, nicardipine (Loxen) and nifedipine (Adalat), have become the first line tocolytic treatments in many French centers [6–9]. After several years

of use, rare observations of APE induced by nicardipine are described.

We are reporting four additional observations of APE (from January 2009 to December 2013) occurring in patients hospitalized for premature labor after nicardipine administration. Clinical severity justified hospitalization in intensive care unit (ICU) each time. The objective of this work is to better explain to the physician this rare but classic complication and so to improve its management by preventing inappropriate treatments and especially useless further investigation.

2. Case Reports

2.1. Case 1. A 31 year-old patient, nullipara, without relevant history and with a single pregnancy, was hospitalized for premature labor at 33 weeks of amenorrhea + 1 day associated with preeclampsia. Her blood pressure had been checked twice a week by a nurse since the 22nd week of amenorrhea as she presented with pregnancy-induced hypertension (PIH).

At admission she also presented with a proteinuria higher than 0.3 g/24 h. First she was treated with nicardipine (Loxen) 20 mg × 3/days per os (PO), and 48 hours later as contractions persisted, calcium channel blockers dosage was increased (intravenous (IV) nicardipine, 3.5 mg/h injected with an automatic syringe). Fetal lung maturation corticotherapy was started (two intramuscular (IM) injections of betamethasone 12 mg (Celestene) performed 24 h apart). About 12 hours after tocolytics increase, the patient exhibited a sudden dyspnea with oxygen desaturation at 86% associated with dry cough but without clear signs of acute respiratory distress. She was transferred to ICU for clinical suspicion of pulmonary embolism. Hypoxemia improved under 3 L/min nasal oxygen therapy (SaO_2 = 96%). Lung examination disclosed crepitant rales at both bases. Arterial blood gas disclosed an uncompensated respiratory alkalosis (pH = 7.50, arterial carbon dioxide tension [$PaCO_2$] = 28.2 mmHg, bicarbonates = 21.7 mmol/L, base excess = −1.1 mmol/L, and arterial oxygen tension [PaO_2] = 107 mmHg) and an increased BNP at 2,474 ng/L. Electrocardiogram (ECG) was normal. A bilateral alveolar-interstitial syndrome was revealed by the chest X-ray. Transthoracic echocardiography (TTE) evidenced a nondilated left ventricle (LV) with a usual systolic function (LV ejection fraction (LVEG) = 70–75%), increased left filling pressures (E/E' = 13), and moderately dilated right cavities with pulmonary hypertension (systolic pulmonary artery pressure (SPAP) estimated at 48 mmHg) without paradoxical septum and a noncompliant superior vena cava (SVC) of limited size. Pleural ultrasound showed bilateral pleural effusions measuring around 2 cm. Acute pulmonary edema was diagnosed in light of the X-ray and ultrasound data. Nicardipine was stopped and replaced by atosiban (Tractocile) at a dosage of 8 mL/h IV with an automatic syringe (dilution = 1 ampule, i.e., 37.5 mg in 48 mL).

Following a symptomatic treatment, the disease improved quickly; the 24 h diuresis was equal to 3,050 mL after an IV injection of 80 mg furosemide (Lasilix). Pulmonary disorders disclosed at examination disappeared after 24 h and the chest X-ray was normal again. However the patient still needed oxygen therapy for 36 hours. She was discharged from the ICU at D2 still under furosemide 20 mg/day. At 34 weeks of amenorrhea, that is, D6, emergency cesarean section was decided because of an acute fetal distress with heart rhythm disorders. The newborn was a boy weighing 1,890 grams with an Apgar score of 10/10/10 at 1, 5, and 10 minutes, respectively. No incident occurred after the delivery and the control cardiac and nephrologic assessment performed at 4 months did not disclose any disorder.

2.2. Case 2. A 28-year-old patient, G3P1, with a spontaneous monochorionic diamniotic twin pregnancy was hospitalized for premature labor at 26 weeks of amenorrhea + 1 day. She successively received a tocolytic treatment with nicardipine (Loxen) IV with an automatic syringe, then atosiban (Tractocile) IV with an automatic syringe, and finally nifedipine (Adalat) PO and salbutamol PO. She also received a fetal lung maturation corticotherapy with betamethasone (Celestene; two IM injections of 12 mg 24 h apart). At D4, because of uterine contraction recurrence, a

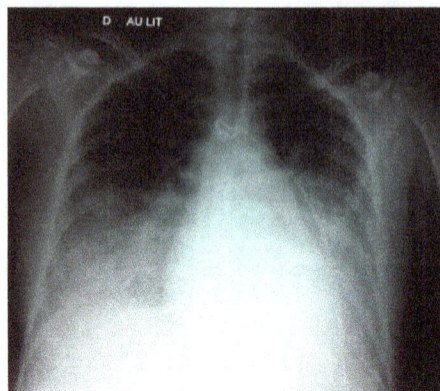

FIGURE 1: Chest X-ray face-on in prone position (Case 2).

treatment with nicardipine IV with an automatic syringe at 3 and then 4 mg/h was initiated again. The patient suffered from severe back pain radiating toward the nape, associated with polypnea and desaturation (94% under 15 L/min oxygen in a nonrebreather (NRB) mask). She also presented with photophobia, headaches, and visual disorders induced by nicardipine. Clinical observation revealed no sensory motor deficiency and quick tendon reflexes. Nicardipine therapy was stopped and replaced by atosiban (Tractocile) IV with an automatic syringe. A first TTE disclosed a 70% LVEF, a grade 2 mitral insufficiency, and an aspect similar to an acute cor pulmonale especially a paradoxical septum. In light of the acute respiratory distress with suspected pulmonary embolism, the patient was transferred to ICU. Hemodynamics parameters was stable and there was a jugular turgidity without lower limb edema. The patient still suffered from hypoxia with 90% saturation under 15 L/min oxygen in a NRB mask. A polypnea with supraclavicular indrawing was noted. Examination showed hypoventilation of both bases. Arterial blood gas disclosed an uncompensated respiratory alkalosis (pH = 7.47, $PaCO_2$ = 31.2 mmHg, bicarbonates = 22.3 mmol/L, and base excess = −0.9 mmol/L) with hypoxia (PaO_2 = 59 mmHg under 15 L/min oxygen in a NRB mask) and an increased BNP at 3,686 ng/L. The ECG presented a regular sinus rhythm without conduction or repolarization disorders. Chest X-ray evidenced an alveolar-interstitial infiltrate of both bases (Figure 1). A new TTE confirmed that there was no LV systolic dysfunction but a moderate mitral insufficiency (grade 2); it also revealed increased LV filling pressures (E/E' = 15) and pulmonary hypertension (SPAP estimated at 55 mmHg). The aspect of the acute cor pulmonale was not confirmed. Pleural ultrasound revealed two pleural effusions.

We thus assumed that it was an APE induced by the high doses of nicardipine. The patient was treated with diuretics (furosemide Lasilix, 80 mg as bolus then 250 mg/24 h) to which she responded (diuresis of 3,520 mL in 20 h) and with noninvasive ventilation sessions which were not very efficient. As the uterine contractions persisted under atosiban and as a chorioamnionitis was suspected, the patient was intubated and mechanically ventilated to perform an emergency delivery by C-section at 26 weeks of amenorrhea + 5 days. The newborns were two girls weighing 933 and 763 grams hospitalized in neonatal ICU. The patient was extubated 24 hours later as she exhibited respiratory improvement thanks to the diuretics. The patient was discharged at D3 from the ICU still under diuretic treatment. Control echocardiography performed 2 months later was normal.

2.3. Case 3. A 28-year-old patient, G2P0, with history of spontaneous miscarriage one year ago (without curettage) was followed in a level 1 maternity for a single pregnancy complicated with an incompetent cervix due to recurrent uterine contractions. She was hospitalized at 29 weeks of amenorrhea + 5 days as uterine contractions were frequent and efficient resulting in cervix dilatation. Premature labor was thus suspected. A tocolytic treatment was started with nicardipine (Loxen) IV with an automatic syringe at doses which rapidly increased up to 4 mg/h. Dyspnea progressively appeared with sensation of thoracic oppression and palpitations. The sensation became more intense during the night of the 5th hospitalization day. The patient presented with febricula at 38.5° and a desaturation at 89% so that nasal oxygen therapy was initiated. At the same time, uterine contractions became more and more intense and fetal lung maturation corticotherapy with betamethasone (Celestene, two IM injections of 12 mg 24 h apart) was started. Laboratory tests revealed an inflammatory syndrome (hyperleukocytosis = 19,000 white blood cells/mm^3, CRP at 70 mg/L). BNP equaled 660 ng/L with normal troponin. The ECG presented a regular sinus rhythm without any relevant disorder. The TTE disclosed a maintained LVEF with no dilatation of the right cavities. LV filling pressures were normal. SPAP was estimated at 35 + 10 mmHg. As a new desaturation episode occurred, the patient was transferred in ICU. She was still dyspneic with saturation at 89% under oxygen therapy at 6 L/min in a face mask and tended to have high blood pressure. Lung examination disclosed crepitant rales on both lungs especially on the bases. There was no cyanosis or sign of acute respiratory distress. Arterial blood gas revealed an uncompensated respiratory alkalosis (pH = 7.48, PaCO$_2$ = 26.7 mmHg, bicarbonates = 19.9 mmol/L, and base excess = −3 mmol/L) associated with hypoxemia (PaO$_2$ = 73 mmHg under 6 L/min oxygen). The remaining laboratory tests were normal. Chest X-ray showed bilateral alveolar-interstitial infiltrate in a butterfly distribution without noticeable pneumonia focus (Figure 2). APE induced by tocolysis with nicardipine was diagnosed. The patient was treated with diuretics (furosemide Lasilix, 40 mg PO) and oxygen therapy. Tocolytic treatment was replaced by suppository salbutamol associated with phloroglucinol (Spasfon). The diuretic-induced water and sodium depletion (diuresis of 1,460 mL within 12 h) allowed for a clear improvement of ventilation: polypnea and crepitant rales in the lung disappeared. Under nasal oxygen therapy at 3 L/min, the patient was eupneic with an improved hematosis (PaO$_2$ = 187 mmHg). She was discharged from the ICU at D2 still under furosemide 20 mg/day. She gave birth at 35 weeks of amenorrhea + 7 days by vaginal delivery and underwent at 4 months a control TTE that was normal.

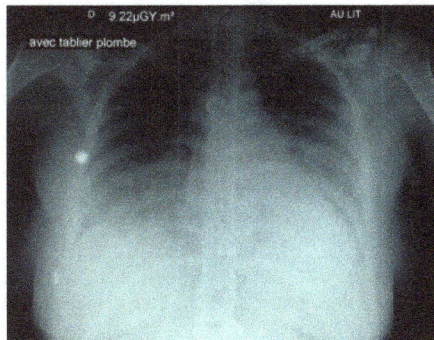

FIGURE 2: Chest X-ray face-on in prone position (Case 3).

2.4. Case 4. A 35-year-old patient, primipara, presented with a single pregnancy after *in vitro* fertilization due to altered tubes. She had a history of smoking, which was weaned, substituted hypothyroidism, and a previous *in vitro* fertilization which resulted in an ectopic pregnancy. She was hospitalized in a level 1 maternity for premature labor occurring at 34 weeks of amenorrhea. She received nicardipine (Loxen) which she tolerated well (IV with an automatic syringe at 4 mg/h), associated with suppository salbutamol. Betamethasone was administered (Celestene, two IM injections of 12 mg 24 h apart) for fetal lung maturation. Forty-eight hours after nicardipine administration, the patient suddenly exhibited dyspnea associated with a sensation of thoracic oppression and dry cough with apyrexia. Arterial blood gas disclosed a "shunt" effect (PaO$_2$ = 69 mmHg and PaCO$_2$ = 27 mmHg). As pulmonary embolism was suspected, a treatment with heparin IV with an automatic syringe, preceded by a bolus, was initiated. The patient was then transferred to the emergency department without relevant complication. Under nicardipine, patient hemodynamics was stable so the treatment was stopped. The patient was apyretic. Regarding ventilation, the patient was eupneic under high flow oxygen therapy (saturation at 100% under 15 L/min in a NRB mask). Arterial blood gas disclosed a compensated metabolic acidosis (pH = 7.42, PaCO$_2$ = 29.7 mmHg, bicarbonates = 19.3 mmol/L, and base excess = −4.3 mmol/L) with an impaired hematosis (PaO$_2$ at 107 mmHg under 15 L/min oxygen). Anemia at 10.3 g/dL and hyperlactatemia at 3.16 mmol/L were also noticed. The ECG presented a regular sinus rhythm without any relevant disorder. Chest X-ray evidenced bilateral diffuse infiltrative lesions. TTE showed normal size of the LV with a LVEF estimated at 70%. The presence of a minimal mitral insufficiency was noticed and LV filling pressures were normal. SPAP was estimated at 19 + 10 mmHg. Pulmonary embolism diagnosis was ruled out thanks to a thoracic angioscan. It however disclosed a slight bilateral pleural effusion associated with large nonsystematized bilateral alveolar opacities (Figure 3). In light of the tests, APE induced by nicardipine was diagnosed and the patient was transferred to the ICU. Thanks to a symptomatic treatment (oxygen therapy at 6 L/min in face mask) and diuretics (iterative bolus of furosemide for a total dose of 180 mg), the health of the patient rapidly

TABLE 1: Clinical and paraclinical characteristics in our series.

	Age	Term	Pregnancy	ECG	BNP (ng/L)	Troponin	TTE LVEG	TTE LVFP	TTE PH	N-APE time
Case 1	31	33 WA + 1 d	G1P0	N	2474	ND	70%	↑	Yes	60 h
Case 2	28	26 WA + 1 d	G3P1, TwP	N	3686	ND	>60%	↑	Yes	24 h
Case 3	28	29 WA + 5 d	G2P0	N	660	N	N	N	Yes	≈96 h
Case 4	35	34 WA	G2P0, IVF	N	ND	N	70%	N	No	≈72 h

WA: weeks of amenorrhea; ECG: electrocardiography; TTE: thoracic echocardiography; LVEG: LV ejection fraction; LVFP: LV filling pressures; PH: pulmonary hypertension; N-APE time: time between treatment initiation and acute pulmonary edema occurrence; TwP: twin pregnancy; IVF: *in vitro* fertilization; N: normal; ND: not done.

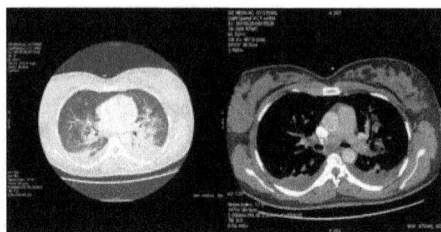

FIGURE 3: Thoracic angioscan (Case 4).

improved. The 24 h diuresis equaled 4,210 mL which allowed for the water and sodium balance to become negative again (−2,928 mL). At discharge, patient was eupneic in ambient air but discrete crepitant rales persisted at both lung bases. She was discharged from the ICU at D2 still under furosemide 40 mg/day. After her delivery, the cardiologic assessment was strictly normal.

Patients' characteristics are reported in Table 1.

3. Discussion

Premature labour diagnosis was defined in association with uterine contractions (regular and effective) and cervix changes occurring at 22 weeks of amenorrhea and 36 weeks of amenorrhea + 6 D. Without any medical intervention, they lead to premature delivery. All patients had undergone a vaginal palpation and a systematic cervical ultrasound. A 30-minute fetal monitoring was performed on admission and then once a day. Obstetric ultrasound was also performed. The occurrence of uterine contractions which are essential for the labor to begin is regulated by the increase of intracellular calcium concentration in myometrial cells. Calcium channel blockers (CCBs) from dihydropyridine family, that is, nicardipine (Loxen) and nifedipine (Adalat), fix themselves on α_{1c} subunit of the L-type voltage-gated calcium channels. This way, they block the opening of the channel and prevent the calcium to enter into the cell which explains their tocolytic mechanism [1] (Figure 4). CCBs also inhibit the activating effect of some substances such as α_1-adrenergic receptors, angiotensin II, and endothelin-1 that usually lead to the contraction of smooth muscle fibers [6]. These molecules are arterial vasodilators that decrease the afterload and lead to an increased cardiac flow [2, 10].

Adverse effects linked to β_2-adrenergic agonists, especially APE during pregnancy, resulted in the use of CCBs as tocolytic treatment [11, 12]. In obstetrics, the most studied molecule is nifedipine. Its tocolytic efficacy has been widely evidenced by several randomized trials [13–20]. Several meta-analyses confirm that it is equally efficient as β_2-adrenergic agonists and better tolerated with a decrease in neonatal morbidity [10, 21–24]. These results have led to recommend the use of CCBs as tocolytics in the CNGOF (*Collège National des Gynécologues et Obstétriciens Français*) Clinical Practice Guidelines in 2002 [25]. Clinical studies on nicardipine are rare in the literature. But paradoxically, even if there is no scientific proof of its superiority, nicardipine is more used than nifedipine in French centers because of its IV administration [8]. A first open randomized prospective study by Jannet et al., conducted on 90 patients, compared nicardipine with IV salbutamol; it did not find any difference of tocolytic efficacy but it did find less adverse effects in nicardipine group [26]. Recently, a prospective randomized study conducted on 48 patients with the same molecules confirmed the equal efficacy with a statistically significant difference regarding the adverse effects in favor of nicardipine (8% for nicardipine versus 47% for salbutamol, $P = 0.02$) [27].

CCBs thus appear as preferred tocolytics with a better tolerance than the β_2-adrenergic agonists even if they do not have a marketing authorization [28]. Since they have been used for this indication, minor adverse effects have progressively been described: tachycardia, low blood pressure, palpitations, flushes, headaches, constipation, nausea, and dizziness linked with the vasodilator effect [2].

APE during pregnancy occurs in 0.08–0.5% of the cases regardless of the etiology [29]. Out of 900 patients with a tocolytic indication, nicardipine was used in 742 patients between January 2009 and December 2013 in our hospital (55 births a week). We report here 4 cases of APE in patients who needed to be transferred in ICU regarding the severity of their condition. The incidence of this complication remains low which confirms already published data [30]. In our series, only one patient gave birth to twins whereas most cases in the literature report twin pregnancies [30–33]. No patient had cardiovascular history. The mean time of APE occurrence is 63 hours after nicardipine therapy initiation (Table 1). This mean time is comparable with the published case reports [30–34]. The initial symptoms are not very specific, dyspnea and oxygen desaturation for all cases. Dry cough, signs of acute

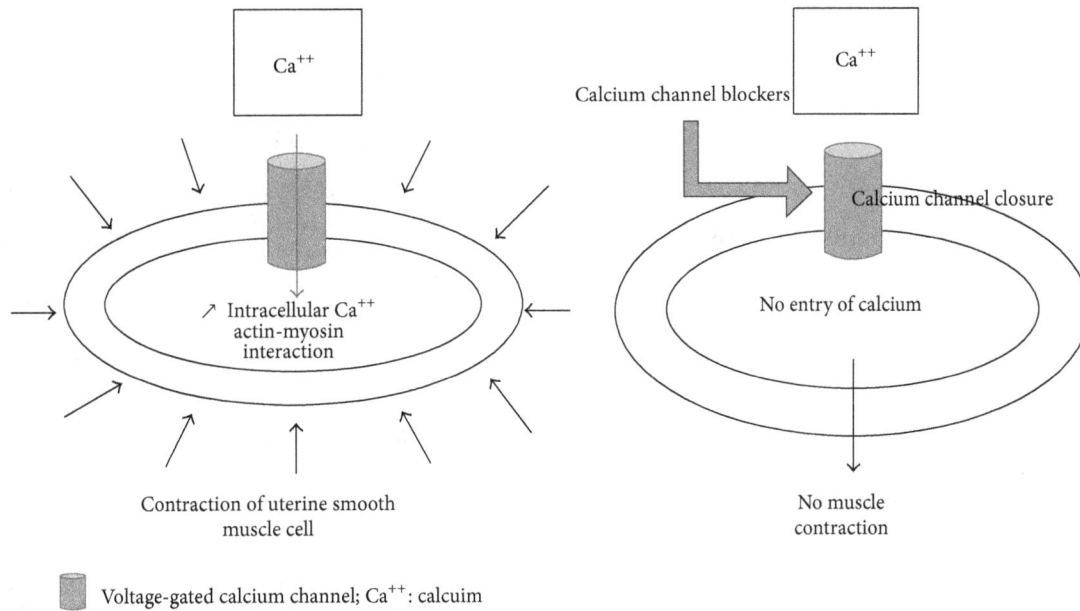

FIGURE 4: Mode of action of calcium channel blockers.

TABLE 2: Tocolytic treatment modalities and APE risk factors.

	Max flow N (mg/h)	Total dose (mg)	Salbutamol associated	CorticoT	Tachycardia	Other RFs associated
Case 1	3.5	162	No	Yes	No	Preeclampsia
Case 2	4	96	Yes	Yes	Yes	Chorioamnionitis, TwP
Case 3	6	576	No	Yes	Yes	No
Case 4	4	288	Yes	Yes	No	Smoking

N: nicardipine; CorticoT: corticotherapy; RF: risk factors; TwP: twin pregnancy.

respiratory distress, thoracic oppression, and palpitations are also found. 50% of our patients had tachycardia. Pulmonary examination disclosed crepitant rales in 50% of cases (Cases 1 and 3). Characteristic crepitant rales can be absent at the beginning but the diagnostic must not be ruled out as they can appear later.

For all 4 patients, the first diagnosis mentioned was pulmonary embolism. One patient even received a heparin bolus with a prescription of heparin at efficient continuous IV doses before she underwent a thoracic angioscan. The normal ECG and troponin rate, when it is performed (50% of cases), rapidly rule out an ischemic origin (Table 1). To our knowledge, only one case of myocardial infarction during tocolytic treatment with nifedipine has been reported in the literature [35]. Laboratory tests revealed an increased BNP each time it was measured (3/4) but a normal result should not rule out the diagnosis as a false negative is possible in case of "flash" APE [36]. Despite the guidelines for pregnant women of the European Society of Cardiology, D-dimer assay which is usually very frequent was not performed in our patients [37]. If a negative result had been obtained, it could have prevented a useless thoracic angioscan. Chest X-ray contributed to APE diagnosis in each case. Regarding echocardiography data, all patients have a maintained LV

systolic function. 50% of cases have increased LV filling pressures, and pulmonary hypertension is noted in 75% of cases (Table 1). Tocolytic treatment modalities are reported in Table 2.

The patients receive high doses of nicardipine. However, water and sodium intake linked to nicardipine remains low: a 0.5 mg/mL dilution is used. The maximal volume received equals 1,150 mL over 4 days for the patient who received the highest cumulative dose of nicardipine. In Vaast and Janower series, physiologic saline solution intake due to nicardipine administration reached 1500 mL per day during 4 days [31, 34]. It is always difficult to calculate a precise water balance outside the ICU so we cannot confirm that none of our patients presented blood volume overload out of the nicardipine intake. Our patients presented associated risk factors; a half received tocolytics associated with salbutamol and had a concomitant obstetrical disease; all received a fetal lung maturation corticotherapy which favors sodium and water retention (Table 2). Other published case reports on nicardipine-induced APE are reported in Table 3. APE occurring during a tocolytic treatment with nifedipine or atosiban seem rather rare [38–40].

The pathophysiology of APE during tocolytic treatment with nicardipine is still unclear. The mechanism of action of

TABLE 3: Published case reports on APE occurring during a tocolytic treatment with nicardipine.

Authors	N	Premature labor term	Nicardipine maximal flow rate	Associated treatments	Patients characteristics
Vaast et al. [31]	5 cases	29.2 WA (mean)	6 mg/h	IM corticosteroids	2 TwP, 1 TrP, GDM, and cardiovascular history
Bal et al. [49]	1 case	27 WA	2 mg/h	IM corticosteroids	No history
Chapuis et al. [32]	1 case	30 WA + 2 days	2.2 mg/h	IM corticosteroids and IV salbutamol	TwP and 2 abortions
Janower et al. [34]	3 cases	29 WA (mean)	4 mg/h	IM corticosteroids and IV salbutamol	GDM
Philippe et al. [33]	3 cases	31 WA (mean)	MD	IM corticosteroids and IV atosiban	Smoking and 1 TwP
Akerman et al. [30]	4 cases	29 WA (mean)	MD	IM corticosteroids, sup. salbutamol, and IV atosiban	3 TwP and IDD

N: number of cases; WA: weeks of amenorrhea; IM: intramuscular; IV: intravenous; TwP: twin pregnancy; TrP: triplet pregnancy; MD: missing data; GDM: gestational diabetes mellitus; sup.: suppository; IDD: insulin dependent diabetes.

CCBs does not interact with the determining factors usually at the origin of APE. Maternal physiological adaptation during pregnancy makes the women prone to sodium and water retention. Pregnancy also induces an increase of cardiac flow due to heart rate and systolic ejection volume increase [41]. CCBs from the dihydropyridine family have cardiovascular effects that maximize these physiological adaptations. Their antihypertension action induces a reflex sympathetic stimulation which causes an increase of tachycardia in pregnant women [42, 43]. Nicardipine-induced APE could be an APE due to altered diastolic compliance [44, 45]. Moreover, the sympathetic stimulation activates the renin-angiotensin-aldosterone system which increases sodium and water retention. Finally, in obstetrics, other risk factors are clearly identified: multiple pregnancy, spontaneous premature labor, tocolytic association, fetal lung maturation corticotherapy, preeclampsia or HELLP syndrome, overhydration with physiologic saline solution, valvular heart diseases, and finally infectious environment especially chorioamnionitis [2, 30].

Treatment of nicardipine-induced APE includes discontinuation of the involved medication and a symptomatic treatment associating oxygen therapy with diuretics. With an adapted treatment, the condition improved quickly in our 4 cases; this is comparable to the other cases described in the literature. Some authors suggested using noninvasive ventilation in case of severe hypoxemia in order to postpone orotracheal intubation [46, 47].

4. Conclusion

Nicardipine used as tocolytic is more and more frequent in France even if its prescription does not have a marketing authorization. Our series agrees with the 17 cases that have been published since 2004. However pathophysiological mechanisms causing nicardipine-induced APE are still unclear. In the literature, the main reported risk factors for nicardipine-induced APE are spontaneous premature labor, multiple pregnancy, cardiovascular history, concomitant obstetrical disease, in association with other tocolytics,

and fetal lung maturation corticotherapy. This complication remains rare but it is advised to use with caution IV nicardipine as a tocolytic in patients with APE risk factors and to avoid association with β_2-adrenergic agonists. A better knowledge of this serious adverse event should allow for an improvement of the diagnostic and therapeutic management in order to avoid useless or even dangerous examination or treatments. Other tocolytics can be used instead such as nifedipine or oxytocin antagonists [48].

Acknowledgment

The authors thank Sarah Demai (CIC 1435) for her help in the preparation of the paper.

References

[1] R. Gáspár and J. Hajagos-Tóth, "Calcium channel blockers as tocolytics: principles of their actions, adverse effects and therapeutic combinations," *Pharmaceuticals*, vol. 6, no. 6, pp. 689–699, 2013.

[2] S. G. Oei, "Calcium channel blockers for tocolysis: a review of their role and safety following reports of serious adverse events," *European Journal of Obstetrics Gynecology and Reproductive Biology*, vol. 126, no. 2, pp. 137–145, 2006.

[3] D. A. Savitz, C. A. Blackmore, and J. M. Thorp, "Epidemiologic characteristics of preterm delivery: etiologic heterogeneity," *American Journal of Obstetrics and Gynecology*, vol. 164, no. 2, pp. 467–471, 1991.

[4] G. J. Clesham, J. Scott, C. M. Oakley et al., "β Adrenergic agonists and pulmonary oedema in preterm labour," *British Medical Journal*, vol. 308, no. 6923, pp. 260–262, 1994.

[5] A. Samet, F. Bayoumeu, D. Longrois, and M. C. Laxenaire, "Acute pulmonary edema associated with the use of beta2-mimetic tocolytic agents," *Annales Françaises d'Anesthésie et de Réanimation*, vol. 19, pp. 35–38, 2000.

[6] V. Tsatsaris and B. Carbonne, "Tocolysis with calcium-channel-blockers," *Journal de Gynécologie Obstétrique et Biologie de la Reproduction*, vol. 30, pp. 246–251, 2001.

[7] C. Vayssière, "Special management for threatened preterm delivery in multiple pregnancies," *Journal de Gynécologie Obstétrique et Biologie de la Reproduction*, vol. 31, no. 5, pp. S114–S123, 2002.

[8] V. Tsatsaris, F. Goffinet, B. Carbonne, G. Abitayeh, and D. Cabrol, "Tocolysis by first intention with nifedipine," *Gynecologie Obstetrique Fertilite*, vol. 33, no. 4, pp. 263–265, 2005.

[9] Y. Bekkari, J. Lucas, T. Beillat, A. Chéret, and M. Dreyfus, "Tocolysis with nifedipine: its use in current practice," *Gynécologie Obstétrique & Fertilité*, vol. 33, no. 7-8, pp. 483–487, 2005.

[10] V. Tsatsaris, D. Papatsonis, F. Goffinet, G. Dekker, and B. Carbonne, "Tocolysis with nifedipine or beta-adrenergic agonists: a meta-analysis," *Obstetrics and Gynecology*, vol. 97, no. 5, pp. 840–847, 2001.

[11] A. de La Chapelle, S. Benoit, M. Bouregba, M. Durand-Reville, and M. Raucoules-Aimé, "The treatment of severe pulmonary edema induced by beta adrenergic agonist tocolytic therapy with continuous positive airway pressure delivered by face mask," *Anesthesia & Analgesia*, vol. 94, no. 6, pp. 1593–1594, 2002.

[12] R. J. Pisani and E. C. Rosenow III, "Pulmonary edema associated with tocolytic therapy," *Annals of Internal Medicine*, vol. 110, no. 9, pp. 714–718, 1989.

[13] J. E. Ferguson II, D. C. Dyson, T. Schutz, and D. K. Stevenson, "A comparison of tocolysis with nifedipine or ritodrine: analysis of efficacy and maternal, fetal, and neonatal outcome," *American Journal of Obstetrics and Gynecology*, vol. 163, no. 1, pp. 105–111, 1990.

[14] W. R. Meyer, H. W. Randall, and W. L. Graves, "Nifedipine versus ritodrine for suppressing preterm labor," *Journal of Reproductive Medicine for the Obstetrician and Gynecologist*, vol. 35, no. 6, pp. 649–653, 1990.

[15] L. A. Bracero, E. Leikin, N. Kirshenbaum, and N. Tejani, "Comparison of nifedipine and ritodrine for the treatment of preterm labor," *The American Journal of Perinatology*, vol. 8, no. 6, pp. 365–369, 1991.

[16] M. Kupferminc, J. B. Lessing, Y. Yaron, and M. R. Peyser, "Nifedipine versus ritodrine for suppression of preterm labour," *British Journal of Obstetrics and Gynaecology*, vol. 100, no. 12, pp. 1090–1094, 1993.

[17] C. S. Smith and M. B. Woodland, "Clinical comparison of oral nifedipine and subcutaneous terbutaline for initial tocolysis," *The American Journal of Perinatology*, vol. 10, no. 4, pp. 280–284, 1993.

[18] D. N. M. Papatsonis, H. P. van Geijn, H. J. Adèr, F. M. Lange, O. P. Bleker, and G. A. Dekker, "Nifedipine and ritodrine in the management of preterm labor: a randomized multicenter trial," *Obstetrics and Gynecology*, vol. 90, no. 2, pp. 230–234, 1997.

[19] J. A. García-Velasco and A. González González, "A prospective, randomized trial of nifedipine vs. ritodrine in threatened preterm labor," *Journal of the International Federation of Gynaecology and Obstetrics International Federation of Gynaecology and Obstetrics*, vol. 61, pp. 239–244, 1998.

[20] C. A. Koks, H. A. Brölmann, M. J. de Kleine, and P. A. Manger, "A randomized comparison of nifedipine and ritodrine for suppression of preterm labor," *European Journal of Obstetrics & Gynecology and Reproductive Biology*, vol. 77, pp. 171–176, 1998.

[21] S. G. Oei, B. W. J. Mol, M. J. K. De Kleine, and H. A. M. Brölmann, "Nifedipine versus ritodrine for suppression of preterm labor: a meta-analysis," *Acta Obstetricia et Gynecologica Scandinavica*, vol. 78, no. 9, pp. 783–788, 1999.

[22] J. F. King, V. J. Flenady, D. N. Papatsonis, G. A. Dekker, and B. Carbonne, "Calcium channel blockers for inhibiting preterm labour," *Cochrane Database of Systematic Reviews*, no. 1, Article ID CD002255, 2003.

[23] A. Conde-Agudelo, R. Romero, and J. P. Kusanovic, "Nifedipine in the management of preterm labor: a systematic review and metaanalysis," *American Journal of Obstetrics and Gynecology*, vol. 204, no. 2, pp. 134.e1–134.e20, 2011.

[24] D. M. Haas, D. M. Caldwell, P. Kirkpatrick, J. J. McIntosh, and N. J. Welton, "Tocolytic therapy for preterm delivery: systematic review and network meta-analysis," *The British Medical Journal*, vol. 345, no. 7879, Article ID e6226, 2012.

[25] B. Carbonne and V. Tsatsaris, "Which tocolytic drugs in case of preterm labor?" *Journal de Gynécologie Obstétrique et Biologie de la Reproduction*, vol. 31, pp. 5S96–5S104, 2002.

[26] D. Jannet, A. Abankwa, B. Guyard, B. Carbonne, L. Marpeau, and J. Milliez, "Nicardipine versus salbutamol in the treatment of premature labor. A prospective randomized study," *European Journal of Obstetrics Gynecology and Reproductive Biology*, vol. 73, no. 1, pp. 11–16, 1997.

[27] K. Trabelsi, H. H. Taib, H. Amouri et al., "Nicardipine versus salbutamol in the treatment of premature labor: comparison of their efficacy and side effects," *Tunisie Medicale*, vol. 86, no. 1, pp. 43–48, 2008.

[28] P. Rozenberg, "Licensed or non-licensed tocolysis?" *Gynécologie, Obstétrique & Fertilité*, vol. 33, no. 4, p. 259, 2005 (French).

[29] A. C. Sciscione, T. Ivester, M. Largoza, J. Manley, P. Shlossman, and G. H. C. Colmorgen, "Acute pulmonary edema in pregnancy," *Obstetrics and Gynecology*, vol. 101, no. 3, pp. 511–515, 2003.

[30] G. Akerman, A. Mignon, V. Tsatsaris, S. Jacqmin, D. Cabrol, and F. Goffinet, "Pulmonary edema during calcium-channel blockers therapy: Role of predisposing or pharmacologic factors?" *Journal de Gynecologie Obstetrique et Biologie de la Reproduction*, vol. 36, no. 4, pp. 389–392, 2007.

[31] P. Vaast, S. Dubreucq-Fossaert, V. Houfflin-Debarge et al., "Acute pulmonary oedema during nicardipine therapy for premature labour; report of five cases," *European Journal of Obstetrics & Gynecology and Reproductive Biology*, vol. 113, no. 1, pp. 98–99, 2004.

[32] C. Chapuis, E. Menthonnex, G. Debaty et al., "Acute pulmonary edema during nicardipine and salbutamol therapy for preterm labor in twin pregnancy," *Journal de Gynecologie Obstetrique et Biologie de la Reproduction*, vol. 34, no. 5, pp. 493–496, 2005.

[33] H.-J. Philippe, A. Le Trong, H. Pigeau et al., "Acute pulmonary edema occurred during tocolytic treatment using nicardipine in a twin pregnancy. Report of three cases," *Journal de Gynécologie Obstétrique et Biologie de la Reproduction*, vol. 38, no. 1, pp. 89–93, 2009.

[34] S. Janower, B. Carbonne, V. Lejeune, D. Apfelbaum, F. Boccara, and A. Cohen, "Acute pulmonary edema during preterm labor: Role of nicardipine tocolysis (three cases)," *Journal de Gynecologie Obstetrique et Biologie de la Reproduction*, vol. 34, no. 8, pp. 807–812, 2005.

[35] S. G. Oei, S. K. Oei, and H. A. Brölmann, "Myocardial infarction during nifedipine therapy for preterm labor," *The New England Journal of Medicine*, vol. 340, no. 2, p. 154, 1999.

[36] C. Mueller, A. Scholer, K. Laule-Kilian et al., "Use of B-type natriuretic peptide in the evaluation and management of acute

dyspnea," *The New England Journal of Medicine*, vol. 350, no. 7, pp. 647–654, 2004.

[37] A. Torbicki, A. Perrier, S. Konstantinides et al., "Guidelines on the diagnosis and management of acute pulmonary embolism: the Task Force for the Diagnosis and Management of Acute Pulmonary Embolism of the European Society of Cardiology (ESC)," *European Heart Journal*, vol. 29, no. 18, pp. 2276–2315, 2008.

[38] O. M. Abbas, A. H. Nassar, N. A. Kanj, and I. M. Usta, "Acute pulmonary edema during tocolytic therapy with nifedipine," *The American Journal of Obstetrics and Gynecology*, vol. 195, no. 4, pp. e3–e4, 2006.

[39] M. S. Kutuk, M. T. Ozgun, S. Uludag, M. Dolanbay, and A. Yildirim, "Acute pulmonary failure due to pulmonary edema during tocolytic therapy with nifedipine," *Archives of Gynecology and Obstetrics*, vol. 288, no. 4, pp. 953–954, 2013.

[40] L. H. M. Seinen, S. O. Simons, M. A. van der Drift, J. van Dillen, F. P. H. A. Vandenbussche, and F. K. Lotgering, "Maternal pulmonary oedema due to the use of atosiban in cases of multiple gestation," *Nederlands Tijdschrift voor Geneeskunde*, vol. 157, no. 1, Article ID A5316, 2013.

[41] S. Hunter and S. C. Robson, "Adaptation of the maternal heart in pregnancy," *British Heart Journal*, vol. 68, no. 6, pp. 540–543, 1992.

[42] D. R. Abernethy and J. B. Schwartz, "Calcium-antagonist drugs," *The New England Journal of Medicine*, vol. 341, no. 19, pp. 1447–1457, 1999.

[43] D. J. Triggle, "Calcium, calcium channels, and calcium channel antagonists," *Canadian Journal of Physiology and Pharmacology*, vol. 68, no. 11, pp. 1474–1481, 1990.

[44] L. B. Ware and M. A. Matthay, "Acute pulmonary edema," *The New England Journal of Medicine*, vol. 353, no. 26, pp. 2788–2796, 2005.

[45] M. Jessup and S. Brozena, "Medical progress: heart failure," *The New England Journal of Medicine*, vol. 348, no. 20, pp. 2007–2018, 2003.

[46] S. Perbet, J. Constantin, F. Bolandard et al., "Non-invasive ventilation for pulmonary edema associated with tocolytic agents during labour for a twin pregnancy," *Canadian Journal of Anesthesia*, vol. 55, no. 11, pp. 769–773, 2008.

[47] N. Fujita, K. Tachibana, M. Takeuchi, and K. Kinouchi, "Successful perioperative use of noninvasive positive pressure ventilation in a pregnant woman with acute pulmonary edema," *Masui*, vol. 63, pp. 557–560, 2014.

[48] Royal College of Obstetricians and Gynaecologists, *Tocolytic Drugs for the Women in Preterm Labour. Clinical Guideline No. 1(B)*, 2002.

[49] L. Bal, S. Thierry, E. Brocas, M. Adam, A. van de Louw, and A. Tenaillon, "Pulmonary edema induced by calcium-channel blockade for tocolysis," *Anesthesia and Analgesia*, vol. 99, no. 3, pp. 910–911, 2004.

9

Fatal Multiorgan Failure Associated with Disseminated Herpes Simplex Virus-1 Infection: A Case Report

Michael Glas,[1] Sigrun Smola,[2] Thorsten Pfuhl,[2] Juliane Pokorny,[3] Rainer M. Bohle,[3] Arno Bücker,[4] Jörn Kamradt,[5] and Thomas Volk[1]

[1] Department of Anesthesiology, Intensive Care and Pain Therapy, Saarland University Hospital, Kirrberger Straße, D-66421 Homburg, Germany
[2] Institute of Virology, Saarland University Hospital, D-66421 Homburg, Germany
[3] Institute of Pathology, Saarland University Hospital, D-66421 Homburg, Germany
[4] Department of Diagnostic and Interventional Radiology, Saarland University Hospital, D-66421 Homburg, Germany
[5] Department of Urology and Pediatric Urology, Saarland University Hospital, D-66421 Homburg, Germany

Correspondence should be addressed to Michael Glas, michael.glas@uks.eu

Academic Editors: M. Egi, Z. Molnar, and K. S. Waxman

Herpes simplex virus type 1 (HSV-1) infections cause typical dermal and mucosal lesions in children and adults. Also complications to the peripheral and central nervous system, pneumonia or hepatitis are well known. However, dissemination to viscera in adults is rare and predominantly observed in immunocompromised patients. Here we describe the case of a 70-year-old male admitted with macrohematuria and signs of acute infection and finally deceasing in a septic shock with multi organ failure 17 days after admission to intensive care unit. No bacterial or fungal infection could be detected during his stay, but only two days before death the patient showed signs of rectal, orolabial and genital herpes infection. The presence of HSV-1 was detected in swabs taken from the lesions, oropharyngeal fluid as well as in plasma. Post-mortem polymerase chain reaction analyses confirmed a disseminated infection with HSV-1 involving various organs and tissues but excluding the central nervous system. Autopsy revealed a predominantly retroperitoneal diffuse large B-cell lymphoma as the suspected origin of immunosuppression underlying herpes simplex dissemination.

1. Introduction

Newly acquired or reactivated infections of HSV-1 cause a typical vesicular rush with orolabial ulcerations, gingivostomatitis, keratitis, and also genital/perianal affections in children and adults. Complications to the peripheral and central nervous system (meningitis, encephalitis), pneumonia, or hepatitis are well known [1–3]. Viraemia and dissemination to viscera in adults are rare and can predominantly be seen in immunocompromised individuals like patients with hemato-oncologic malignancies, transplant recipients, or due to immunosuppressive medication [4, 5]. Here we describe a case of fulminant septic shock in a patient associated with a disseminated infection with HSV-1.

2. Case Presentation

A 70-year-old male patient was initially admitted to a primary hospital with fever, productive cough, fatigue, reduced vigilance, and macrohematuria. His past medical history included obesity (body mass index 38.1 kg/m²), arterial hypertension, obstructive sleep apnea, benign prostate hyperplasia, complete atrioventricular block (implanted dual chamber pacemaker), chronic heart failure, and atrial fibrillation. For the latter, the patient was orally anticoagulated with phenprocoumon. Due to chronic backache, he received lumbar injections at regular intervals. A few weeks prior to the present admission, he travelled to Tunisia and Turkey.

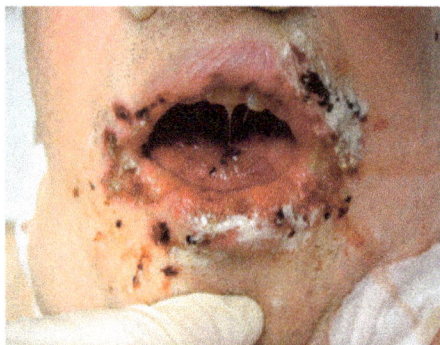

FIGURE 1: Orolabial vesicles and ulcers. Appearance of orolabial vesicles and ulcers on day 17 of ICU treatment, two days before death (percutaneous tracheotomy was performed on day 7).

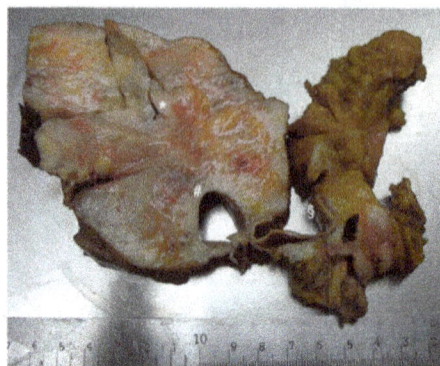

FIGURE 2: Autopsy revealed a massive retroperitoneal lymphoma. Giant retroperitoneal lymphoma masses enclosing abdominal aorta [§], inferior vena cava [#] and leading to stenosis of the right ureter [∗]. Tissue was formalin fixed.

HIV and hepatitis B/C virus serology results were negative. Blood chemistry showed elevated C-reactive protein (219 mg/L), leukocytosis (14.2 per nL), an increase in procalcitonin (0.507 ng/mL), an international normalized ratio of 5.2, and an increased creatinine (5.0 mg/dL). Searching for a septic focus an abdominal computed tomography (CT) showed massive bilateral hydronephrosis with ureteral compression by a retroperitoneal space-occupying lesion suspected to be a hematoma causing urinary retention and urosepsis.

For technical reasons, only the left ureter was stented with a double-j catheter. Calculated antibiotic treatment with Meropenem/Ciprofloxacin was initiated, and the patient was subsequently transferred to our hospital. Shortly after relieving the right ureter his state rapidly deteriorated. Body temperature increased to 39.9°C. His oxygenation index (136) necessitated invasive ventilation (fraction of inspired oxygen 0.6, positive end-expiratory pressure 12 mbar), and his hemodynamic status had to be supported by norepinephrine (up to 1.0 µg/kg/min). On day five, he became anuric necessitating continuous venovenous hemodialysis. Surgical exploration of the right retroperitoneal space was performed to exclude an infected hematoma and revealed no relevant bleeding. Microbiological analysis (blood cultures) did not show any systemic bacterial or fungal infections, merely urine culture was initially positive for candida albicans. Elevated transaminases and increased international normalized ratio, despite substitution of prothrombin complex, indicated the beginning of liver failure. Although procalcitonin fluctuated between 2.2 and a maximum of 7.3 ng/mL, repeated blood culture results did not show bacteremia or candidemia. Reevaluating a septic focus with CT scans (cranial, thoracic, and abdominal) between intensive care unit days 8 and 16 still showed the retroperitoneal space-occupying lesion without signs of inflammation. Surgical exploration of the right retroperitoneum on day 16 did not find any correlate. On day 17, colorectal endoscopy revealed several widespread rectal ulcers (up to 25 mm in diameter)—with suspect of viral origin. On the same day (almost four weeks after admission to hospital) oral aphtous ulcers, orolabial, and genital herpetiform vesicles (Figure 1) appeared. Samples obtained from oral and genital swabs as well as oropharyngeal fluid were analyzed by (semiquantitative) real-time polymerase chain reaction (PCR, LightCycler System, Roche, Basel, Switzerland) and revealed HSV-1 DNA in all samples. In addition, HSV-1 was detected in EDTA (ethylenediaminetetraacetic acid) plasma samples indicating florid systemic infection. EDTA blood and oropharyngeal fluid were additionally positive for Epstein-Barr virus, with 2,400 copies per mL and 27,000 copies per mL, respectively. Copy numbers for cytomegalovirus, varicella-zoster virus, and BK virus (human polyoma virus 1) were below the detection limit. Antiviral therapy (acyclovir, adapted to renal failure and dialysis) was immediately initiated. Two days later the patient died of multiple organ failure and septic shock on ICU day 19 (four weeks after admission to primary hospital).

On autopsy the retroperitoneal space-occupying lesion revealed a solid tumor (21 × 18 × 9.5 cm) expanding from the renal artery to the common right iliac artery and right psoas muscle, enclosing the inferior vena cava and the abdominal aorta (see Figure 2), leading to ureter stenosis and dilatation on both sides as well as to infiltration of the bladder. Microscopic examination and immunohistochemical analyses finally showed a diffuse of large B-cell lymphoma. As there was further tumor infiltration of the mesenterial root (15 × 6 × 4.8 cm), pericardium (up to 5 × 4 × 3.2 cm), cervical lymph nodes (3 cm in diameter), right visceral pleura (inferior and middle lobe), serosa of the colon, and periadrenal fat tissue, the lymphoma was categorized as Ann-Arbor stage four. Autopsy could not provide evidence for a retroperitoneal hematoma. Semiquantitative real-time PCR of postmortem specimens showed disseminated infection with HSV-1 of a variety of organs including heart, respiratory system, liver, spleen, kidney, intestines, lymphatic nodes, and muscle except for cerebrum and cerebellum (see Tables 1 and 2). Highest numbers of genome copies could be detected in organs of the gastrointestinal tract as well as in upper and lower respiratory system.

3. Discussion

In developed countries the incidence of viral sepsis is believed to be less than 1% of septic episodes of patients admitted

TABLE 1: Results of the semiquantitative PCR performed two days before death. The c_T-value (cycle threshold) specifies the number of cycles till the beginning of exponential phase when sample fluorescence exceeds background fluorescence for the first time. Low c_T-values correlate with high copy numbers of HSV-1 DNA.

Tissue	Herpes simplex 1 DNA (qualitative)	c_T-values in RT-PCR
EDTA blood	+	36
Oropharyngeal fluid	++++	17
Trial smear test	++++	20
Perianal smear test	++	33

TABLE 2: Postmortem detection of HSV-1 DNA in various tissues. Results of the semiquantitative PCR performed after mortem detecting virus DNA in all tested tissues except for cerebrum and cerebellum (c_T-value: cycle threshold).

Tissue	Herpes simplex virus-1 DNA (qualitative)	c_T-values in RT-PCR
Spleen	++	32
Liver	++	30
Left Kidney	++	30
Retroperitoneal lymphoma	++	33
Lymph nodes	++	33
Bone marrow	+	36
Muscle	++	33
Cerebrum	—	—
Cerebellum	—	—
Oral mucosa	++++	24
Trachea	++++	23
Right main bronchus	++++	23
Right lung (lower lobe)	+++	28
Right lung (upper lobe)	++	31
Right ventricle	+++	26
Left ventricle	++	30
Stomach	+++	28
Small intestine	+++	27
Colon	++	34

to intensive care [6]. Cases of herpes simplex dissemination leading to fulminant (multi) organ failure by hepatitis [7, 8], pneumonia [9], or even sepsis [10] are well described for immunocompetent and immunocompromised individuals including patients with hematologic malignancies [11].

Although there are demographic differences, seroprevalence for HSV-1 in adults is greater than 50% in Europe and infection usually takes place in the first two decades [12, 13]. Reactivation of the latent infection can be asymptomatic (recrudescence) or symptomatic (recurrence) and is supposed to be triggered by stress, hormonal changes, and immunosuppression [13, 14].

While leukopenia has been reported in 43% of cases with HSV-associated hepatic failure, accompanied by thrombocytopenia (45%), and elevation of transaminases and bilirubin [15, 16], our patient showed leukocytosis in a range from 14.2/nL to 26.6/nL and signs of disseminated intravascular coagulation. Increased procalcitonin values correlated with the conditions of a septic inflammatory response syndrome and multiorgan failure. Although procalcitonin levels are frequently below 0.5 ng/mL in viral infections, values up to 17 ng/mL and an overlap with severe bacterial infection were described for systemic viral infections [17]. The spectrum of symptoms of the disseminated HSV infection resembles the clinical picture of a bacterial sepsis, which is reflected by analogies in inflammatory host response.

The relevance of HSV-1 detection in distinct body compartments and the impact of antiviral treatment for patients' outcome are still a matter of debate. In a recent study, Berrington et al. examined the clinical correlates of HSV-1/2 in 951 serum or plasma samples. 4% of those patients had detectable levels of HSV-1/2 in PCR analysis and were observed to have a high mortality rate [18]. In this course, a review of 13 patients' medical records identified sepsis and multiorgan failure as the most common causes of death in immunosuppressed as well as immunocompetent individuals. Moreover, the detection of HSV-1 in bronchoalveolar lavage fluid (BALF) was shown to be related to poor outcome in ICU patients by Linssen et al. [19]. HSV-1 genome was detected in 32% of BALF samples from ICU patients compared to 15% from non-ICU patients. In this study, ICU treatment and age over 50 years were significantly associated with HSV-1 in BALF. Detection of more than 10^5 genome copies/mL BALF was an independent predictor and reflected an increased mortality rate of 21% in critically ill patients. In contrast, Scheithauer et al. reported 191 patients with pulmonary diseases suspected to be of viral origin with 32.5% of the respiratory specimens tested positive for HSV-1 by PCR [20]. In this context, no significant differences with respect to incidence of renal insufficiency, markers of inflammation, sepsis, need for catecholamines, and mortality were found between HSV-1-positive and -negative individuals except for days of mechanical ventilation. It is of note that treatment with acyclovir did not significantly influence mortality ($P = 0.26$) although viral load in plasma decreased significantly [20]. Referring to antiviral therapy no details were mentioned about the starting point of acyclovir administration.

In our patient, the primary hypothesis of an infected retroperitoneal hematoma had to be reassessed when his condition further decreased after sufficient drainage of the kidneys by ureteral catheters and while surgical retroperitoneal exploration and microbiological diagnostic finally excluded a superinfected retroperitoneal hematoma. Although PCR results revealed a florid systemic HSV infection, before mortem; antiviral therapy could not stem the tide.

In retrospect, it needs to be discussed why the lymphoma was not recognized during the surgical explorations. First, based on the diagnosis of a superinfected retroperitoneal hematoma, an extraperitoneal flank incision was chosen to minimize the risk of contaminating the peritoneal cavity. Although the retroperitoneum was inspected with this approach, the solid masses were hidden in the plenteous fatty tissue of the obese patient. Second, the surgical exploration on day 16 was misguided by the hypothesis of an inflammatory process in the retroperitoneum causing the worsening septic condition of the patient. No abscess was found, and diffuse bleeding in the retroperitoneum during surgery prohibited further extensive exploration.

Having repeatedly negative blood cultures for bacterial and fungal pathogens, we assume that the presence of a diffuse large B-cell lymphoma going along with the dissemination of HSV finally caused multiorgan failure in the present case. However, it remains unclear whether the presence of herpes simplex virus in blood only acted as an indicator for a disturbed immune function caused by a terminal malignant disease, or whether disseminated HSV infection was the origin of sepsis and multiorgan failure.

The importance of systemic HSV analysis and viral load determination in immunocompromised as well as in immunocompetent ICU patients and the necessity of prophylactic or preemptive therapy in this setting have to be clarified in future studies.

Authors' Contribution

M. Glas, S. Smola, and T. Volk wrote the paper. PCR analyses were performed by S. Smola and T. Pfuhl. J. Pokorny and R. Bohle were responsible for autopsy, macropathological, histopathological, immunohistological examinations, and collecting snap-frozen tissue specimens for postmortem virological analyses. A. Bücker and J. Kamradt helped to draft the paper.

References

[1] E. James, L. Robinson, P. D. Griffiths, and H. G. Prentice, "Acute myeloblastic leukaemia presenting with herpes simplex type-1 viraemia and pneumonia," British Journal of Haematology, vol. 93, no. 2, pp. 401–402, 1996.

[2] L. C. Olson, E. L. Buescher, M. S. Artenstein, and P. D. Parkman, "Herpesvirus infections of the human central nervous system," New England Journal of Medicine, vol. 277, no. 24, pp. 1271–1277, 1967.

[3] S. Plastiras and O. Kampessi, "Acute lymphocytic crisis following herpes simplex type 1 virus hepatitis in a nonimmunocompromised man: a case report," Journal of Medical Case Reports, vol. 3, article 7492, 2009.

[4] P. Khera, J. M. Haught, J. McSorley, and J. C. English, "Atypical presentations of herpesvirus infections in patients with chronic lymphocytic leukemia," Journal of the American Academy of Dermatology, vol. 60, no. 3, pp. 484–486, 2009.

[5] R. Zuckerman and A. Wald, "Herpes simplex virus infections in solid organ transplant recipients," American Journal of Transplantation, vol. 9, supplement 4, pp. S104–S107, 2009.

[6] J. L. Vincent, Y. Sakr, C. L. Sprung et al., "Sepsis in European intensive care units: results of the SOAP study," Critical Care Medicine, vol. 34, no. 2, pp. 344–353, 2006.

[7] R. Wesley Farr, S. Short, and D. Weissman, "Fulminant hepatitis during herpes simplex virus infection in apparently immunocompetent adults: report of two cases and review of the literature," Clinical Infectious Diseases, vol. 24, no. 6, pp. 1191–1194, 1997.

[8] R. J. Fahy, E. Crouser, and E. R. Pacht, "Herpes simplex type 2 causing fulminant hepatic failure," Southern Medical Journal, vol. 93, no. 7–12, pp. 1212–1216, 2000.

[9] T. Prellner, L. Flamholc, S. Haidl, K. Lindholm, and A. Widell, "Herpes simplex virus—the most frequently isolated pathogen in the lungs of patients with severe respiratory distress," Scandinavian Journal of Infectious Diseases, vol. 24, no. 3, pp. 283–292, 1992.

[10] G. Zahariadis, K. R. Jerome, and L. Corey, "Herpes simplex virus-associated sepsis in a previously infected immunocompetent adult," Annals of Internal Medicine, vol. 139, no. 2, pp. 153–154, 2003.

[11] S. A. Muller, E. C. Herrmann, and R. K. Winkelmann, "Herpes simplex infections in hematologic malignancies," The American Journal of Medicine, vol. 52, no. 1, pp. 102–114, 1972.

[12] R. G. Pebody, N. Andrews, D. Brown et al., "The seroepidemiology of herpes simplex virus type 1 and 2 in Europe," Sexually Transmitted Infections, vol. 80, no. 3, pp. 185–191, 2004.

[13] I. Steiner, P. G. Kennedy, and A. R. Pachner, "The neurotropic herpes viruses: herpes simplex and varicella-zoster," The Lancet Neurology, vol. 6, no. 11, pp. 1015–1028, 2007.

[14] S. A. Alleyne, S. S. Bukhari, M. Fraser, and P. Spiers, "Extensive perinephric abscess complicated by herpes simplex virus 1 reactivation," Journal of Clinical Pathology, vol. 63, no. 4, pp. 365–366, 2010.

[15] J. Sevilla, S. Fernández-Plaza, M. González-Vicent et al., "Fatal hepatic failure secondary to acute herpes simplex virus infection," Journal of Pediatric Hematology/Oncology, vol. 26, no. 10, pp. 686–688, 2004.

[16] G. Biancofiore, M. Bisà, L. M. Bindi et al., "Liver transplantation due to Herpes Simplex virus-related sepsis causing massive hepatic necrosis after thoracoscopic thymectomy," Minerva Anestesiologica, vol. 73, no. 5, pp. 319–322, 2007.

[17] M. Assicot, D. Gendrel, H. Carsin, J. Raymond, J. Guilbaud, and C. Bohuon, "High serum procalcitonin concentrations in patients with sepsis and infection," The Lancet, vol. 341, no. 8844, pp. 515–518, 1993.

[18] W. R. Berrington, K. R. Jerome, L. Cook, A. Wald, L. Corey, and C. Casper, "Clinical correlates of herpes simplex virus viremia among hospitalized adults," Clinical Infectious Diseases, vol. 49, no. 9, pp. 1295–1301, 2009.

[19] C. F. Linssen, J. A. Jacobs, F. F. Stelma et al., "Herpes simplex virus load in bronchoalveolar lavage fluid is related to poor outcome in critically ill patients," Intensive care medicine, vol. 34, no. 12, pp. 2202–2209, 2008.

[20] S. Scheithauer, A. K. Manemann, S. Krüger et al., "Impact of herpes simplex virus detection in respiratory specimens of patients with suspected viral pneumonia," Infection, vol. 38, no. 5, pp. 401–405, 2010.

10

Early Angiographic Resolution of Cerebral Vasospasm with High Dose Intravenous Milrinone Therapy

F. A. Zeiler and J. Silvaggio

Section of Neurosurgery, Department of Surgery, University of Manitoba, Winnipeg, MB, Canada R3A 1R9

Correspondence should be addressed to F. A. Zeiler; umzeiler@cc.umanitoba.ca

Academic Editor: Kurt Lenz

Background. Treatment of symptomatic delayed cerebral ischemia (DCI) after subarachnoid hemorrhage (SAH) is difficult. Recent studies suggest intravenous (IV) high dose milrinone as a potential therapy. The timing to angiographic response with this is unclear. *Methods.* We reviewed the chart of one patient admitted for SAH who developed symptomatic DCI and was treated with high dose IV milrinone. *Results.* A 66-year-old female was admitted with a Hunt and Hess clinical grade 4, World Federation of Neurological Surgeons (WFNS) clinical grade 4, and SAH secondary to a left anterior choroidal artery aneurysm which was clipped. After bleed day 6, the patient developed symptomatic DCI. We planned for angioplasty of the proximal segments. We administered high dose IV milrinone bolus followed by continuous infusion which led to clinical improvement prior to angiography. The angiogram performed 1.5 hours after milrinone administration displayed resolution of the CT angiogram and MRI based cerebral vasospasm such that further intra-arterial therapy was aborted. She completed 6 days of continuous IV milrinone therapy, was transferred to the ward, and subsequently rehabilitated. *Conclusions.* High dose IV milrinone therapy for symptomatic DCI after SAH can lead to rapid neurological improvement with dramatic early angiographic improvement of cerebral vasospasm.

1. Introduction

The treatment of symptomatic delayed cerebral ischemia (DCI) after aneurysmal subarachnoid hemorrhage (SAH) currently focuses on hypertensive therapy with the potential use of intra-arterial calcium channel or phosphodiesterase inhibitor (PDEI) based vasodilators [1–4]. Angioplasty is also an option for proximal large to medium vessel vasospasm resistant to medical therapy [5–7].

Recently a report has surfaced utilizing high dose intravenous (IV) PDEI based therapy with milrinone [8]. This report documented rapid neurological improvement of symptomatic DCI. Angiographic improvement has also been described with this protocol within 24 hours of administration [8]. It is unknown, despite the early symptomatic improvement, how rapid the angiographic improvement occurs with IV milrinone therapy.

Within this report, we describe a case of symptomatic DCI after SAH treated with high dose IV milrinone therapy, in isolation, leading to rapid symptomatic improvement,

and early angiographic near resolution within 1.5 hours of the initiation of therapy. This is to the author's knowledge the earliest documented angiographic response of cerebral vasospasm to high dose IV milrinone therapy.

2. Case Presentation

A 66-year-old female, with a past medical history for hypertension, presented to hospital with a 12-hour history of an acute onset severe headache and neck pain. Prior to arrival at hospital, she had progressive deterioration in her level of consciousness (LOC). Upon arrival to the emergency department, she was with GCS of 9 (motor = 5, eyes = 2, and verbal = 2). There was no witnessed seizure activity, and the patient was hemodynamically stable throughout transport. No episodes of hypotension or hypoxemia were recorded. She had a definitive airway obtained via endotracheal intubation and was sent for computed tomography (CT) of the brain.

The CT of the brain displayed a Fisher grade 4 SAH with significant clot burden in the interpeduncular, carotid,

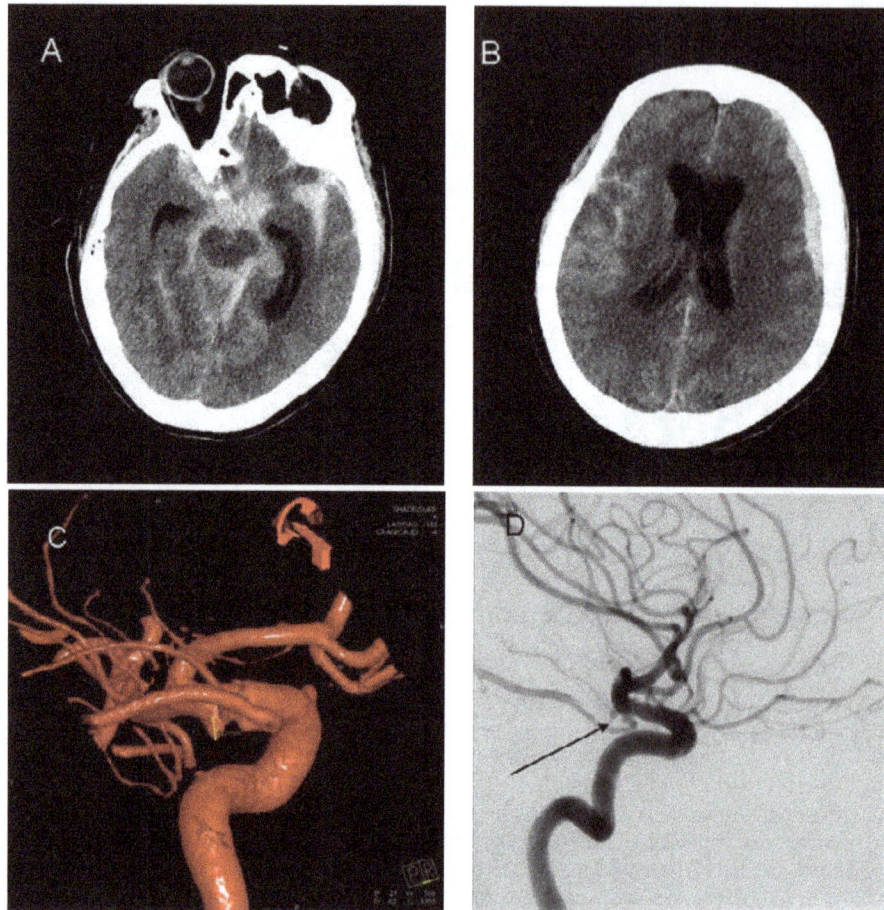

FIGURE 1: Admission CT and DSA. CT = computed tomography and DSA = digital subtraction angiogram. (A) Axial uninfused CT of the brain at the level of the mesencephalon displaying thick subarachnoid clot in the basal cisterns. (B) Axial uninfused CT of the brain at the level of the lateral ventricles displaying hydrocephalus, a small left acute subdural hematoma and diffuse SAH. (C) Lateral projection of left internal carotid artery injection via DSA displaying a small anterior choroidal artery aneurysm (black arrow). (D) Three-dimensional reconstruction of DSA displaying anterior choroidal artery aneurysm on the inferior portion of the supraclinoid internal carotid artery.

and ambient cisterns bilaterally (Figures 1(A) and 1(B)). In addition, the imaging displayed hydrocephalus. Computed tomographic angiography (CTA) of the circle of Willis (COW) was obtained and failed to display a discrete source for the SAH. Three-dimensional reconstructions of the CTA were unclear but displayed a questionable small aneurysm in the area of the left anterior choroidal artery.

Given the Fisher CT grade 4, Hunt and Hess clinical grade 4 (with a GCS of 9 and stuporous), and the World Federation of Neurological Surgeons (WFNS) clinical grade 4 SAH with the presence of hydrocephalus, a right frontal external ventricular drain (EVD) was placed. The EVD was left open at 20 cm above the tragus. The patient was transferred to the intensive care unit (ICU) with the plan for a 4-vessel digital subtraction angiogram (DSA), in order to better delineate the suspected anterior choroidal artery aneurysm. The patient improved to a GCS of 9T (motor = 6, eyes = 3, and verbal = T) after EVD placement.

The DSA images confirmed the presence of the aneurysm (Figures 1(C) and 1(D)), and the patient was taken to the operating room for microsurgical clipping 6 hours after admission to hospital.

Intraoperatively the procedure went without complication, with the exception of the need to sacrifice one large sylvian vein. Postoperative CT of brain displayed small subfrontal hypodensity consistent with venous infarct. The patient was clinically unaffected by this.

Postoperatively the patient returned to the ICU where she remained ventilator dependent on pressure support of 20 with a positive end expiratory pressure (PEEP) of 8 cm H_2O and a fractional inspired oxygen (FiO$_2$) requirement of 50%. Chest X-ray displayed pulmonary edema. She had mild tropinemia, with no significant electrocardiogram (ECG) changes. A transthoracic echocardiogram displayed biventricular failure (right worse than left) and global hypokinesis, with an ejection fraction (EF) of 40%, all consistent with catecholamine related subendocardial ischemia. She remained on minimal sedation for comfort during her ICU stay, with a fentanyl infusion at 25 mcg/hr. This was not changed at any point during her ICU admission. Nimodipine

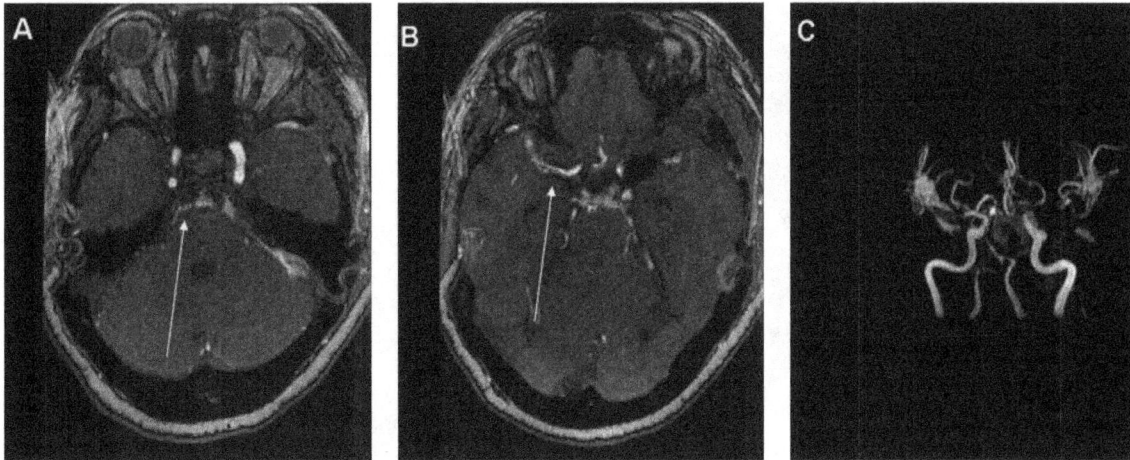

FIGURE 2: Postbleed day 5 MRI with TOF angiography. MRI = magnetic resonance imaging and TOF = time of flight. (A) Axial TOF sequence at the level of the pons displaying severe basilar artery spasm (white arrow). (B) Axial TOF sequence at the level of the mesencephalon displaying severe right middle cerebral artery vasospasm (white arrow). (C) Three-dimensional TOF reconstruction of the circle of Willis displaying severe spasm of the basilar artery trunk and the middle cerebral arteries bilaterally. The vasospasm is severe enough to prevent TOF signal from identifying the distal basilar and the left proximal middle cerebral artery.

was administered only once, at a dose of 60 mg, and resulted in a decrease in MABP from 85 mm Hg to 55 mm Hg. Given this response to nimodipine and the echo results, it was elected to not administer any further doses.

Over the following 5 days after bleed, she remained ventilator dependent secondary to her pulmonary edema. We consistently recorded central venous pressure (CVP) between 12 and 15 mm Hg. Mean arterial blood pressure (MABP) was maintained spontaneously between 80 and 90 mm Hg.

On postbleed day 5, she had a brief episode of right arm weakness lasting for 30 seconds, with return to baseline. There was no documented loss of consciousness. She remained able to obey commands both during and after this brief event. Uninfused CT of the brain failed to display any new abnormality. Electroencephalogram was conducted, with no seizure activity noted. Subsequently magnetic resonance imaging (MRI) of the brain was completed displaying signs of moderate to severe angiographic vasospasm of the basilar trunk, bilateral supraclinoid internal carotid arteries (ICA), and bilateral M1 segments of the middle cerebral artery (MCA) via time of flight (TOF) imaging (Figure 2). Given only the presence of angiographic cerebral vasospasm via TOF MRI in the absence of clinical manifestations, it was elected to monitor the patient clinically.

On postbleed day 6, the patient became drowsy and unresponsive in the early afternoon. No changes in her hemodynamics were noted during this time, with MABP recorded between 80 and 90 mm Hg. An urgent CTA of the COW was ordered confirming the results from the MRI-TOF obtained the previous evening (Figure 3). Given the significant proximal vasospasm, it was elected to arrange for angioplasty while the patient was optimized medically for the presumed diagnosis of symptomatic DCI secondary to cerebral vasospasm.

In the presence of significant subendocardial ischemia and pulmonary edema requiring ventilatory support, it was elected to avoid hypertensive therapy and trial of a high dose PDEI based therapy with IV milrinone following the previously described protocol from the Montreal Neurological Institute [8]. A 5 mg IV milrinone load over 10 minutes was given (0.1 mg/kg load; weight 55 kg), followed by continuous IV infusion of 0.75 mcg/kg/min. No hypotension or arrhythmia was encountered. The MABP during and after load was maintained at 80 to 95 mm Hg spontaneously.

Within 30 minutes of the IV milrinone load, the patient began to open her eyes spontaneously. Within 40 minutes of the infusion, the patient began to intermittently follow commands with all extremities. The patient was subsequently taken to the angiography suite for planned angioplasty approximately 1.5 hours after IV milrinone bolus.

The DSA prior to the planned angioplasty displayed significant angiographic resolution of the vasospasm in the basilar and bilateral ICA/MCA territories. Some mild residual spasm was noted at the basilar apex and the right proximal middle cerebral artery (Figure 4). Given the improvement and lack of obvious target of angioplasty, the procedure was aborted and the patient returned to the ICU. It was noted at this time that the patient was back to baseline neurologically.

The patient was maintained on 0.75 mcg/kg/min of IV milrinone for 72 hours, after which we tapered the infusion by 0.25 mcg/kg/min every 24 hours. No complications of the milrinone therapy were encountered. The MABP was maintained spontaneously between 85 and 95 mm Hg while being on the IV milrinone therapy. We were also subsequently able to liberate the patient from the ventilator 2 days after the attempted angioplasty procedure.

Continued improvement occurred during the following 1.5-week ward stay, with an eventual transfer to our stroke rehabilitation unit for ongoing therapy.

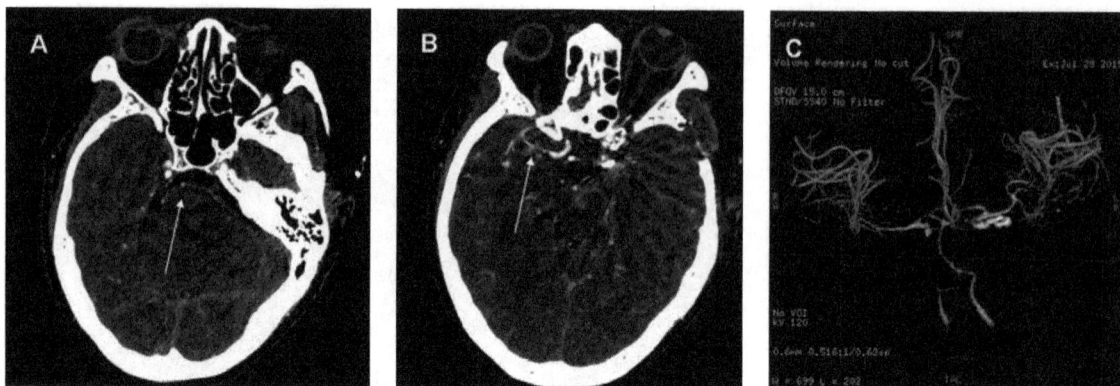

FIGURE 3: Postbleed day 6 CTA of the COW. CTA = computed tomographic angiography and COW = circle of Willis. (A) Axial CTA image at the level of the pons displaying severe spasm of the basilar artery (white arrow). (B) Axial CTA image at the level of the mesencephalon displaying severe spasm of the right proximal middle cerebral artery (white arrow). (C) Three-dimensional reconstruction of the CTA displaying the COW. Of note is the severe spasm of the basilar artery trunk and the right middle cerebral artery and bilateral proximal anterior cerebral arteries.

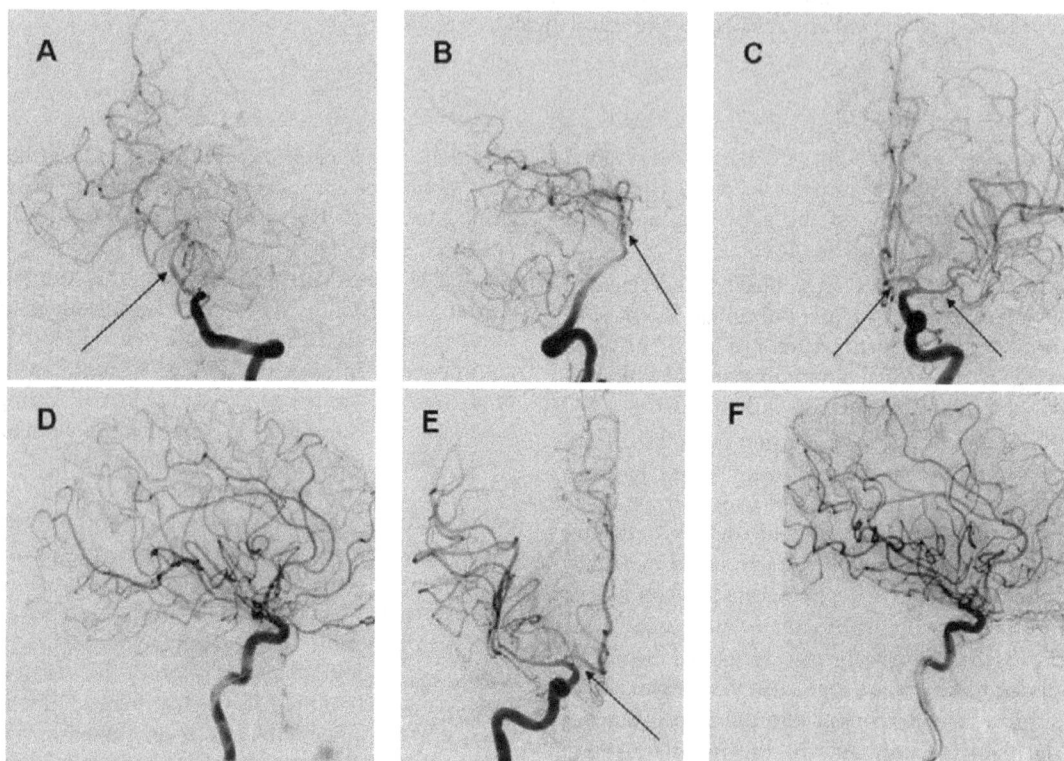

FIGURE 4: DSA performed 1.5 hours after milrinone administration. DSA = digital subtraction angiogram. (A) AP projection of a left vertebral artery injection displaying good opacification of the basilar artery trunk (black arrow). (B) Lateral projection of left vertebral artery injection displaying good opacification of the basilar artery trunk. (C) AP projection of a left internal carotid artery injection displaying resolution of all left sided vasospasm and normal appearing proximal anterior and middle cerebral arteries (black arrows). (D) Lateral projection of left internal carotid artery injection displaying no distal MCA vasospasm. (E) AP projection of right internal carotid artery injection displaying improvement in proximal middle cerebral artery spasm, with mild residual stenosis (black arrow). (F) Lateral projection of a right internal cerebral artery injection displaying no distal small vessel vasospasm.

3. Discussion

A few important points can be gathered from our case. First, IV based PDEI therapy with milrinone led to significant cerebral vasodilation of the proximal large vessel territories. Second, utilizing a high dose IV bolus of milrinone, followed by a continuous infusion, appears to have a dramatic early effect on the angiographic appearance of cerebral vasospasm in our case. With the DSA occurring within approximately 1.5 hours of the IV milrinone load, it can be seen that the effect on the cerebral vasculature is rapid. To our knowledge, this is the earliest documented DSA response to high dose IV milrinone therapy currently in the literature. Third, the symptoms of DCI resolved quite rapidly with the administration of IV milrinone and appeared to be sustained. This mirrors the effects previously described [8]. Fourth, there were no recorded side effects of the milrinone therapy during both bolus and infusion. This also mirrors the previously described reports of milrinone therapy for DCI after SAH [8]. Fifth, our particular patient had a constellation of complications for which milrinone was an ideal solution. The presence of subendocardial ischemia, with biventricular failure, and pulmonary edema requiring ventilation all improved dramatically after milrinone administration. This allowed us to liberate her from the ventilator and improved our ability to follow her neurological exam. Finally, we were able to avoid the potential complications of high dose vasopressor usage that are seen during hypertensive therapy for DCI.

Despite the interesting effects seen in our case, there are significant limitations that need acknowledgment. First, this is a single case that in no way proves that this therapy can or should be utilized as a first line treatment for symptomatic DCI after SAH. The current standard therapy is hypertensive management and should remain so until further prospective study of milrinone therapy has been conducted. Second, the positive results seen in this case cannot be extrapolated to all cases of DCI after SAH given that this is only a single case. The results however are mirrored in previously reported experiences with the described milrinone protocol [8]. Third, we compared premilrinone MRI-TOF and CTA to postmilrinone DSA. Given that these imaging modalities are very different, it is hard to say with 100% certainty that the angiographic response seen during DSA was in fact as dramatic as described. The premilrinone CTA and MRI-TOF may have overrepresented the degree of cerebral vasospasm. However, given the degree of spasm seen on the CTA and MRI-TOF, we would expect the DSA to have displayed at least some significant degree of vasospasm if the milrinone had not been effective. Fourth, one could argue that the clinical effect seen is not a cerebral vasodilatory effect but merely a cardiac index driven effect of the milrinone in the setting of subendocardial ischemia. Unfortunately we did not have a Swan-Ganz catheter or noninvasive biotransmittance cardiac monitor in order to make comments on the cardiac index both pre- and postmilrinone administration. However, the MABP remained completely unchanged during the pre- and postmilrinone administration phases of this patient's care. Thus, an improved cardiac index leading to improved CBF, in the absence of changes in the MABP, as the sole reason for neurological improvement is hard to argue. Similarly, the angiographic response seen cannot be justified with this argument. Fifth, despite no complications in our case, these high doses of milrinone should be utilized with caution. The risk for substantial hypotension and arrhythmia is very real. Finally, there currently is no data to suggest that milrinone based vasodilatory therapy in the setting of DCI after SAH has any impact on patient outcome, despite our positive outcome in this case.

Despite all of the limitations, we believe this case provides an interesting example of the early angiographic and clinical impact that high dose IV milrinone therapy can have in the setting of symptomatic DCI after SAH. At this point in time, this therapy is not standard of care in this setting and requires significant evaluation in a prospective fashion prior to widespread implementation. Future prospective study should include comparison to hypertensive therapy in a randomized controlled fashion as a frontline therapy for symptomatic DCI after SAH with the outcome measures including angiographic response, clinical response, radiological outcome (i.e., presence of strokes during follow-up), and the impact of therapy on clinical outcome.

4. Conclusions

High dose IV milrinone therapy for symptomatic DCI after SAH can lead to rapid neurological improvement with dramatic early angiographic improvement of cerebral vasospasm. Further prospective study of this therapy is requirement prior to widespread implementation in this setting.

References

[1] M. N. Diringer, T. P. Bleck, J. C. Hemphill III et al., "Critical care management of patients following aneurysmal subarachnoid hemorrhage: recommendations from the Neurocritical Care Society's Multidisciplinary Consensus Conference," *Neurocritical Care*, vol. 15, no. 2, pp. 211–240, 2011.

[2] R. Meyer, S. Deem, N. David Yanez, M. Souter, A. Lam, and M. M. Treggiari, "Current practices of triple-H prophylaxis and therapy in patients with subarachnoid hemorrhage," *Neurocritical Care*, vol. 14, no. 1, pp. 24–36, 2011.

[3] G. Dabus and R. G. Nogueira, "Current options for the management of aneurysmal subarachnoid hemorrhage-induced cerebral vasospasm: a comprehensive review of the literature," *Interventional Neurology*, vol. 2, no. 1, pp. 30–51, 2013.

[4] C. D. Baggott and B. Aagaard-Kienitz, "Cerebral vasospasm," *Neurosurgery Clinics of North America*, vol. 25, no. 3, pp. 497–528, 2014.

[5] M. Hollingworth, P. R. Chen, A. J. Goddard, A. Coulthard, M. Söderman, and K. R. Bulsara, "Results of an international survey on the investigation and endovascular management of cerebral vasospasm and delayed cerebral ischemia," *World Neurosurgery*, vol. 83, no. 6, pp. 1120.e1–1126.e1, 2015.

[6] A. M. Bauer and P. A. Rasmussen, "Treatment of intracranial vasospasm following subarachnoid hemorrhage," *Frontiers in Neurology*, vol. 5, article 72, 2014.

[7] A. S. Pandey, A. E. Elias, N. Chaudhary, B. G. Thompson, and J. J. Gemmete, "Endovascular treatment of cerebral vasospasm: vasodilators and angioplasty," *Neuroimaging Clinics of North America*, vol. 23, no. 4, pp. 593–604, 2013.

[8] M. Lannes, J. Teitelbaum, M. del Pilar Cortés, M. Cardoso, and M. Angle, "Milrinone and homeostasis to treat cerebral vasospasm associated with subarachnoid hemorrhage: the montreal neurological hospital protocol," *Neurocritical Care*, vol. 16, no. 3, pp. 354–362, 2012.

11

Extracorporeal Life Support in a Severe Blunt Chest Trauma with Cardiac Rupture

Launey Yoann,[1,2] **Flecher Erwan,**[2,3] **Nesseler Nicolas,**[1,2]
Malledant Yannick,[1,2] **and Seguin Philippe**[1,2]

[1] *Anesthesiology, Critical Care and Emergencies, Rennes University Hospital, 35000 Rennes, France*
[2] *Anesthesiology, Critical Care, Emergencies, and SAMU (Service d'Aide Médicale Urgente), Rennes 1 University,*
Inserm U991, Centre Hospitalier Universitaire (CHU) Pontchaillou, 35000 Rennes, France
[3] *Department of Cardiovascular and Thoracic Surgery, Rennes University Hospital, 35000 Rennes, France*

Correspondence should be addressed to Launey Yoann; yoann.launey@chu-rennes.fr

Academic Editors: K. Chergui, Y. Durandy, and Z. Molnar

This report presents a case of severe blunt chest trauma secondary to a horse riding accident with resultant free-wall rupture of the left ventricle in association with severe lung contusion. We describe the initial surgical and medical management of the cardiac rupture which was associated with a massive haemoptysis due to severe lung trauma. Extra corporeal membrane oxygenation (ECMO) support was initiated and allowed both the acute heart and lung failure to recover. We discuss the successful use and pitfalls of ECMO techniques which are sparsely described in such severe combined cardiac and thoracic trauma.

1. Introduction

Traumatic cardiac rupture rarely complicates blunt chest trauma but is almost always fatal due to sudden and massive bleeding. A rare proportion of victims who reach the hospital alive benefits from emergency cardiac surgery. However, heart rupture is often associated with severe heart failure in the postoperative period often resulting in death [1]. Extra corporeal life support (ECLS) has been utilized for the last 15 years, and its indications are now rapidly spreading [2]. With permission from our local Institutional Review Board, we are publishing an original case report of heart and lung traumatic injuries requiring urgent surgery and ECLS implantation during the surgical procedure and the postoperative course.

2. Case Report

A 37-year-old woman was admitted to our emergency department for thoracic blunt trauma caused by chest trampling after a fall from a horse. Her medical history includes a Guillain-Barré syndrome without sequelae and a previous traumatic brain injury responsible of rare mnesic disorders. At the initial evaluation, the patient was conscious without any motor deficit. Clinical examination revealed severe hypoxia with pulse oximetry (SpO_2) at 89% increasing to 98% breathing under O_2 at 15 liters/min, a tachycardia of 120 bpm without hypotension (arterial blood pressure = 110/78 mmHg). The patient was complaining, however, of dorsal and left-sided chest pain. At admission, the respiratory status promptly deteriorated with increased hypoxemia. Initial chest X-ray revealed a left pneumothorax with bilateral lung contusions. Despite chest tube insertion, respiratory failure worsened, and trachea was intubated with immediate bradycardia, ventricular fibrillation, and finally asystole. Cardiopulmonary resuscitation with chest compression associated with intravenous (iv) adrenaline (total amount = 2.6 mg) was necessary for recovery of an effective circulatory activity. FAST-ultrasound scan identified pericardial tamponade and a small intraperitoneal effusion. The initial blood tests revealed an acute fibrinolysis (prothrombin rate < 10%, fibrinogen < 0.1 g/L, and D-dimers > 45 μg/mL with normal platelet count) and an anemia with hemoglobin level of 74 g/L. Under mechanical ventilation, arterial blood analysis revealed acidosis with a pH of 6.99, $PaCO_2$ of 57 mmHg, bicarbonate of 16 mmol/l, and PaO_2/FiO_2 ratio of 114 mmHg.

As blood transfusion was initiated the patient was transferred to the operating room. A massive hemopericardium was first evacuated through median sternotomy, revealing active bleeding from a left free-wall ventricle rupture with a myocardial tear measuring 3 cm wide, located close to the circumflex coronary artery. In order to repair the ventricular rupture, emergent extracorporeal circulation was established between the ascending aorta and the right atrium after systemic anticoagulation with 20,000 units (300 ui/kg) iv of heparin. Two strips of felt were then placed lengthwise on the epicardial surface and were used to support the closure of the rupture from outside the myocardium, using multiple horizontal mattress sutures of 2/0 polyesters (Figures 1 and 2). Surgical glue was then added to obtain perfect haemostasis. After weaning from cardiopulmonary bypass, significant lung haemorrhage from the left lower lobe (confirmed with preoperative bronchial endoscopy) was found to be responsible for massive haemoptysis and severe preoperative hypoxemia (SpO_2 = 80%). Via median sternotomy, the lung contusion was evident, with significant left lower lobe destruction responsible for the intrabronchial bleeding. At that time, the platelet count was 92 giga/L, prothrombin ratio (PT) was 52%, activated partial thromboplastin time (APTT) ratio was increased by 2.1 times normal (71 versus 34 for control), and the fibrinogen was 2.31 g/L. As it was deemed technically impossible to perform the lobar resection for haemostasis through the sternotomy and taking into account the hemodynamic and respiratory instability, the surgeon decided to first establish venoarterial extracorporeal membrane oxygenation (ECMO) between the right femoral vein and artery with heparin-coated cannulas. Following this, a standard posterolateral left thoracotomy was performed and permitted the performance of a left-lower lobectomy with immediate resolution of the intrabronchial bleeding. During pre- and postoperative periods, a total of 17 units of packed red blood cells, 8 fresh frozen plasma units, 2 platelets units, and 6 g of fibrinogen were administered. During the immediate postoperative period, the ECMO support was maintained, and the patient was transferred to our intensive care unit (ICU). A full-body scan was performed to evaluate other potential concurrent injuries and revealed a peritoneal effusion and a splenic contrast leak. The decision was made to perform an emergency laparotomy and splenectomy on the same day, still under ECMO support. No other intra-abdominal injury was found. Inotropic support (dobutamine) was used during both surgical procedures and ceased in the early stage of ICU recovery. The ECMO support was continued due to persistence of left heart failure.

Thereafter, the ventricular function slowly improved. Initially severe myocardium dysfunction was observed (left ventricular ejection fraction (LVEF) of 25%, as measured by transoesophageal echography) with associated grade 3/4 mitral regurgitation caused by ischemic restriction of the posterior mitral valve leaflet. At day 8, the LVEF was found to be 50% associated with 2/4 mitral regurgitation allowing ECMO removal. During this period, acute renal failure with anuria required continuous venovenous hemofiltration

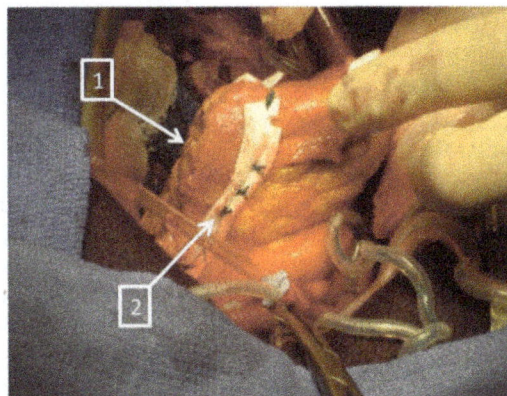

FIGURE 1: Arrows entitled (1) show the left-ventricle rupture stitched during cardiac surgery with the ECMO device. Arrows entitled (2) depicts two strips of felt placed lengthwise on the epicardial surface and used to support the closure of the rupture from outside the myocardium, using horizontal mattress sutures of 2/0 polyester.

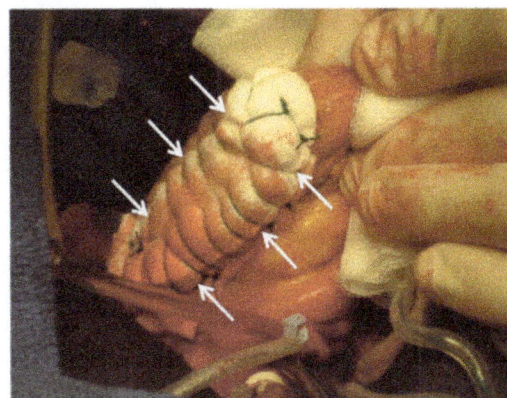

FIGURE 2: Arrows delimit the insertion of the felt patch used for the closure of the left-ventricle rupture.

for three weeks, at which point a complete renal recovery was made. The weaning of sedative medication commenced on day 4, and neurological evaluation revealed slight psychomotor weakness and behaviour disturbances. Mechanical ventilation weaning was delayed on day 18 due to *Enterobacter cloacae* pneumonia. This was treated by cefepime and amikacin administration for 8 and 3 days, respectively. A ruptured pseudoaneurysm developed on the insertion site of ECMO cannula required emergent surgery on day 26. The evolution was then complicated by acute respiratory failure of multifactorial origins (including muscular weakness, bronchitis, and pulmonary oedema) requiring a repeated mechanical ventilation period of 8 days (from day 30 to day 37), to achieve a definitive weaning at day 37.

The patient was transferred to the cardiology ward on day 40 and discharged from hospital on day 50 with a complete neurologic recovery and good cardiac function. Her medication included aspirin, a beta-blocker, and an ACE-inhibitor. At 3-month followup, the clinical condition was satisfactory without any dyspnea (class I NYHA), and Doppler-echocardiographic control showed a left-ventricle ejection fraction of 60% with lateral hypokinesis and residual grade 2/4 mitral regurgitation.

3. Discussion

Cardiac rupture is rarely observed mainly because most patients die prior to reach the hospital as it was highlighted in an autopsy study performed on patients with blunt chest trauma [3]. Nevertheless, in a recent retrospective study focusing on blunt chest trauma, cardiac rupture incidence was found in only 1/2400 patients, but with a very high mortality rate of 89.2% [4]. Traumatic free-wall heart rupture management is a difficult medical and surgical challenge. Survival depends on the rapidity of the patient transfer to a cardiac surgery center. Active bleeding, frequently associated with tamponade, makes the blood pressure initially unstable. Secondary myocardial contusion and myocardial stunning complicate the surgical repair and result in an uncertain postoperative recovery. In the present case, the circumflex coronary artery was located adjacent to the ventricular rupture, and the repair resulted in the occlusion of one of the obtuse marginal coronary arteries as has previously been reported [5]. Myocardial contusion and iatrogenic lateral infarction due to the repair resulted in postoperative left ventricular failure. In our case, the clinical situation deteriorated further due to massive hemoptysis which contributed to hemodynamic disturbances and poor oxygenation. Left lung surgery was impossible through the sternotomy, and the patient required to be repositioned to perform the standard posterolateral left thoracotomy. In this case, venoarterial ECMO support seemed the most appropriated strategy to manage the pitfalls of LV dysfunction and hypoxia prior to the lobectomy being performed. The ECMO was used during the lung resection to facilitate the surgery in terms of ventilation and oxygenation and to support associated unstable blood pressure. Furthermore, ECMO support allowed the maintenance of normothermia, as well as rapid and massive administration of fluids and blood products into the circuit of the pump as needed. In the postoperative course, ECMO support allowed maintaining good systemic perfusion and decreasing the doses of vasopressor drugs despite severe cardiac dysfunction. The ECMO partially unloaded the left ventricle with a view to optimizing myocardium recovery and to limit pulmonary injury. The patient transport for CT-scan and even abdominal surgery was realized under ECMO support without bleeding complication or thrombosis. ECMO pretreated heparinized tubing often allows a lower level of anticoagulation, especially when the pump speed is high.

In cases of cardiac injuries, few data exist on the management of free-wall cardiac rupture. The diagnosis is based on clinical status associated with a systematic echocardiographic assessment in the context of trauma [6]. Surgical treatment is mandatory, but no guidelines are defined. The use of ECMO support has already been described in a right ventricular rupture due to blast injury [7] or to manage severe combined pulmonary and myocardial contusion [8]. Indeed, myocardial contusion in chest trauma may require high dose of vasoactive drugs and time to recover. Surgical

sutures through an injured myocardium are fragile and may lacerate the muscle if the wall tension is too high. Partial unloading of the left ventricle using ECMO might play a role in those fragile surgical repairs. Moreover, such temporary mechanical circulatory support supplies the transiently low native cardiac output and allows decreasing the dose of vasoactive drugs while maintaining good organs perfusion and function.

To conclude, the present case highlights that ECMO support is a helpful and useful tool to manage the surgical treatment of cardiac ruptured and/or lung injuries induced by trauma and is also of benefit in the postoperative recovery.

Authors' Contribution

All authors helped in writing the paper and approved the final paper. Flecher Erwan helped with the figures and photos preparation.

Acknowledgments

The authors specially thank Doctor Eric Slimani for his careful review of this paper.

References

[1] G. Orliaguet, M. Ferjani, and B. Riou, "The heart in blunt trauma," *Anesthesiology*, vol. 95, no. 2, pp. 544–548, 2001.

[2] R. H. Bartlett, "Extracorporeal life support: history and new directions," *ASAIO Journal*, vol. 51, no. 5, pp. 487–489, 2005.

[3] R. Fedakar, N. Türkmen, D. Durak, and U. N. Gündoğmuş, "Fatal traumatic heart wounds: review of 160 autopsy cases," *The Israel Medical Association Journal*, vol. 7, pp. 498–501, 2005.

[4] P. G. R. Teixeira, C. Georgiou, K. Inaba et al., "Blunt cardiac trauma: lessons learned from the medical examiner," *Journal of Trauma*, vol. 67, no. 6, pp. 1259–1264, 2009.

[5] S. J. Canovas, E. Lim, F. Hornero, and J. Montero, "Surgery for left ventricular free wall rupture: patch glue repair without extracorporeal circulation," *European Journal of Cardio-Thoracic Surgery*, vol. 23, no. 4, pp. 639–641, 2003.

[6] W. A. Schiavone, B. K. Ghumrawi, D. R. Catalano et al., "The use of echocardiography in the emergency management of nonpenetrating traumatic cardiac rupture," *Annals of Emergency Medicine*, vol. 20, no. 11, pp. 1248–1250, 1991.

[7] E. Barreda, E. Flecher, S. Aubert, and P. Leprince, "Extracorporeal life support in right ventricular rupture secondary to blast injury," *Interactive Cardiovascular and Thoracic Surgery*, vol. 6, no. 1, pp. 87–88, 2007.

[8] P. T. Masiakos, E. F. Hirsch, and F. H. Millham, "Management of severe combined pulmonary and myocardial contusion with extracorporeal membrane oxygenation," *The Journal of Trauma*, vol. 54, no. 5, pp. 1012–1015, 2003.

12

Cardiac and Pulmonary Ultrasound for Diagnosing TRALI

J. I. Alonso-Fernández, J. R. Prieto-Recio, C. García-Bernardo, I. García-Saiz, J. Rico-Feijoo, and C. Aldecoa

Anesthesiology and Postoperative Critical Care Department, Río Hortega University Hospital, 47009 Valladolid, Spain

Correspondence should be addressed to C. Aldecoa; caldecoaal@saludcastillayleon.es

Academic Editor: Zsolt Molnár

Unexpected acute respiratory failure after anesthesia is a diagnostic challenge: residual neuromuscular blockade, bronchial hyperresponsiveness, laryngospasm, atelectasis, aspiration pneumonitis, and other more uncommon causes should be taken into account at diagnosis. Lung ultrasound and echocardiography are diagnostic tools that would provide the differential diagnosis. We report a suspected case of a transfusion related acute lung injury (TRALI) following administration of platelets. The usefulness of lung and cardiac ultrasound is discussed to facilitate the challenging diagnosis of the acute early postoperative respiratory failure.

1. Introduction

Respiratory failure which happens unexpectedly after anesthesia is a diagnostic challenge. Several concurrent causes in emergent surgery could explain respiratory distress and postoperative hypoxemia: residual neuromuscular blockade, bronchial hyperresponsiveness, laryngospasm, atelectasis, chemical pneumonitis, and other rarer causes such as heart failure by volume overload, ARDS due to a septic process, pulmonary embolism, or acute respiratory distress due to transfusion reactions.

2. Case Report

We report the case of a 56-year-old woman with personal history of smoking, dyslipidemia, hypertension, overweight (BMI 28), and amaurosis fugax episode whereby continued antiplatelet therapy with clopidogrel. The patient came to the emergency room for severe abdominal pain in the right lower quadrant with nausea and vomiting of 24-hour duration. The examination revealed abdominal distension, painful palpation in the right iliac fossa, and decreased bowel sounds.

The woman underwent abdominal ultrasound, which reported appendage of increased caliber with thickened wall, data compatible with uncomplicated acute appendicitis. She entered the surgery department, beginning antibiotic treatment with amoxicillin/clavulanic and deciding urgent open intervention. The preintervention clinical situation was stable from both respiratory and hemodynamic points of view. The laboratory exams and X-ray exams were also normal before the surgery.

It was decided to administer a pool of platelets, obtained by apheresis with a volume of 250 cc in 30 minutes, half an hour before intervention due to platelet dysfunction by clopidogrel. Pharmacological induction of anesthesia with propofol, fentanyl, and rocuronium was performed. Standard monitorization included SpO_2, ECG, and noninvasive arterial pressure and neuromuscular block monitoring was applied. Intubation was performed without any problems including vomiting or aspiration. After induction elevated airway pressures were evident, without bronchospasm signs in the auscultation, improving after lung recruitment maneuvers. Subsequently she remained stable from both respiratory and hemodynamic points of view during the whole intervention. The surgery lasted 60 minutes. No general peritonitis was observed. Extubation was performed when the Train of Four ratio was higher than 0.9 and the conscious was recovered. After extubation, while staying at the postanesthesia care unit fifteen minutes after the extubation, she presented with progressive dyspnea, cyanosis, and severe agitation which may

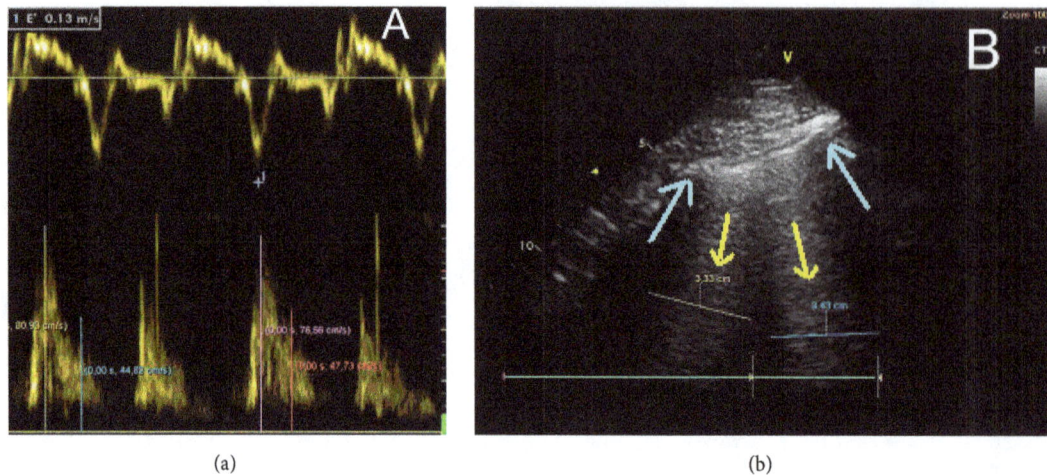

(a)   (b)

FIGURE 1: (a) Top: Doppler tissue of the lateral mitral annulus showing the value of e'. Bottom: Doppler mitral filling. Together both images show a pattern of normal mitral filling estimate normal filling pressure (value $E/e' < 8$). (b) The picture shows lung ultrasound realized with a sectorial probe in the patient's right chest, between fourth and fifth ribs in midclavicular line. Figure shows presence of vertical B lines > 3 mm (yellow arrows), indicative of pulmonary edema. Blue arrows show rib shadows.

be related to the hypoxia and necessitated the administration of high-flow oxygen. A lung auscultation showed no rales, rhonchi, or wheezing. She was moved to the Resuscitation Unit where she persisted in need of high concentrations of oxygen. The patient remained hemodynamically stable without tachycardia and in sinus rhythm. No hypothermia and shivering were observed.

She underwent an urgent echocardiogram by an expert operator showing cardiac chambers of normal size, preserved systolic function, and normal pattern of relaxation filling mitral $E/e' = 6.2$ (lateral measures) and the tissue Doppler shows a' minor compared to e' (see Figure 1). Also the presence of significant valvular and pericardial effusion was discarded. In the thoracic ultrasound the presence of B lines and areas of subpleural condensation in both hemithoraces were shown (see Figure 1). An urgent chest radiograph was requested showing the presence of bilateral pulmonary infiltrates, not present previously on admission. Noninvasive mechanical ventilation was established after the TEE and the results were observed. Arterial blood and gas analysis were repeated, confirming the existence of moderate respiratory failure ($PaO_2/FiO_2 = 84/0.6 = 140$).

Faced with the possibility of having platelet transfusion reaction, it was reported to the Hematology Department that dismissed the remaining blood components from the same donor. Procalcitonin and lactate were also requested, showing values within normal ranges. Diuretic therapy was initiated without improvement of pulmonary infiltrates in the following hours. In serial radiographs in 48 hours, the pulmonary infiltrates persisted. She remained hemodynamically stable during the next three days. The antibiotic treatment was discontinued on the third day of admission due to lack of fever and leukocytosis. From a respiratory point of view she needed noninvasive ventilation with pressure support of $15 \, cmH_2O$. The patient was discharged with supplemental oxygen by nasal cannula on the fifth day of admission in the Resuscitation Unit. X-ray and lung ultrasound at discharging were normal.

3. Discussion

TRALI is a clinical syndrome presented as acute hypoxemia and noncardiogenic pulmonary edema during or after a transfusion of blood products. There is no single definition of this process, but in 2004 the Canadian Blood Service and Hema-Quebec proposed in its consensus conference some criteria [1] that have been widely accepted. Its incidence is not well established. Thus, Silliman et al. [2] establish the existence of TRALI in 1 over 1323 blood product transfusions. Predisposition also seems to be different depending on the type of blood product infused, from highest to lowest risk: platelet transfusion of whole blood, apheresis platelets, packed red cells, and fresh frozen plasma. Its pathophysiology is not completely enlightened [3] and could be explained by a dual mechanism, with the presence of leukocyte immune antibodies or a cytokine liberation due to a preexisting lung damage and subsequent migration of neutrophils, causing that pulmonary capillary injury.

The clinical presentation includes dyspnea, tachypnea, and hypoxemia as cardinal symptoms. Fever, tachycardia, hypotension, and even hypertension may also be present. There is no laboratory test to confirm the diagnosis of TRALI.

The differential diagnosis of a patient who suddenly develops respiratory failure after a transfusion of blood products should include hemodynamic overload, anaphylactic reaction, bacterial contamination of blood products transfused, and hemolytic transfusion reaction.

In the reported case, the differential diagnosis of hemodynamic overload was performed using echocardiographic assessment, including both systolic function as noninvasive estimation of filling pressure by E/e'.

Transthoracic two-dimensional echocardiography has become an essential tool for the confirmation of ARDS, after following the redefinition of Berlin. The morphological study will allow us to analyze the size, morphology, and global and segmental contraction. It allows discarding dilated cardiomyopathy, hypertrophic cardiomyopathy, ventricular dysfunction, or acute stress cardiomyopathy. Application of Doppler will allow us to assess valvular dysfunction and a more detailed assessment of the hemodynamic status and diastolic function [4]. The "early mitral flow peak velocity to early diastolic mitral annulus displacement velocity" (E/e') ratio correlates closely with left ventricular end-diastolic pressures (LVEDP). The mitral filling pattern with E/e' is a method to estimate the right ventricular filling. Values above 15 have been correlated with high pulmonary wedge pressure and values below 9 have been correlated with normal one [5]. Adding pulmonary venous flow to E/e' ratio may facilitate LVEDP assessment. To improve the accuracy of E/e' to assess the left ventricular pressure and discard a pseudonormal pattern, the use of the values of tissue Doppler has been proposed. When the relationship in e'/a' is higher than 1, a normal pattern is present. However, the assessment of pulmonary venous flow using a transthoracic approach is difficult.

The morphology and function of the right ventricle can also rule out the presence of acute or chronic cor pulmonale. Overall, the information provided by echocardiography allowed excluding cardiogenic pulmonary edema as the primary cause of respiratory failure.

Lung ultrasound is a supplement to the information provided by echocardiography. The pulmonary ultrasound is able to define numerous causes that alter pulmonary function [6]. In the ultrasound technique, lung, ribs, spine, and lung air act as barriers to ultrasounds, causing artifacts that we recognize and interpret for a correct diagnosis. The altered lung presents a change in the air/intrathoracic liquid ratio, with this liquid being either alveolar or interstitial edema or also blood, mucus, pus, or increased cellularity. The exploration is done in the supine position, allowing easy anterolateral approach, and according to the BLUE protocol [7] 3 points in each hemithorax are enough to draw conclusions. Firstly, the presence of pleural sliding sign rules out pneumothorax as a cause of respiratory failure. The presence of B lines, vertical lines starting from the pleural line and extending in depth, with variations in size synchronized with the respiratory cycle is suggestive of an alveolar interstitial syndrome, which means cardiogenic or noncardiogenic pulmonary edema. Multiple B lines 7 mm apart are caused by thickened interlobular septa characterizing interstitial edema [8]. In contrast, B lines 3 mm or less apart are caused by "ground-glass" areas characterizing alveolar edema [9]. The presence of subpleural parenchyma with patchy consolidations and lines B is more suggestive of ARDS heart failure, as what happened in our case [10]. The learning curve for B line assessment is short [11] and this method is reproducible without any variability [12]. Thus, the information that has been given by pulmonary ultrasound outdoes chest X-ray [13]. The data supplied by echocardiography on systolic and diastolic function help to define better the origin of pulmonary disorders.

However, although this approach is useful in most cases, an area of uncertainty exists when E/e' values are between 9 and 15 and lung ultrasound does not show any data of parenchymal damage. In such cases, advanced echocardiographic methods [14] for estimating pulmonary wedge pressure, further evaluations, or invasive measurements may be needed.

The absence of rash, urticaria, or angioedema during administration of platelets and the absence of clinical and laboratory data (procalcitonin) in severe sepsis and pre-post intervention also strengthens the diagnosis of acute lung injury associated with transfusion (TRALI).

In conclusion, while managing a patient who has received some type of blood product, the presence of respiratory failure requires a differential diagnosis with TRALI. The reversal of antiplatelet effect through platelet transfusion should be individualized on urgent interventions. Echocardiography together with thoracic ultrasound facilitates the differential diagnosis of respiratory failure in the surgical critical patient.

Acknowledgment

The authors acknowledge James H. Taylor, MD, as collaborator.

References

[1] S. Kleinman, T. Caulfield, P. Chan et al., "Toward an understanding of transfusion-related acute lung injury: statement of a consensus panel," *Transfusion*, vol. 44, no. 12, pp. 1774–1789, 2004.

[2] C. C. Silliman, L. K. Boshkov, Z. Mehdizadehkashi et al., "Transfusion-related acute lung injury: epidemiology and a prospective analysis of etiologic factors," *Blood*, vol. 101, no. 2, pp. 454–462, 2003.

[3] A. P. J. Vlaar and N. P. Juffermans, "Transfusion-related acute lung injury: a clinical review," *The Lancet*, vol. 382, no. 9896, pp. 984–994, 2013.

[4] S. F. Nagueh, C. P. Appleton, T. C. Gillebert et al., "Recommendations for the evaluation of left ventricular diastolic function by echocardiography," *Journal of the American Society of Echocardiography*, vol. 22, no. 2, pp. 107–133, 2009.

[5] S. R. Ommen, R. A. Nishimura, C. P. Appleton et al., "Clinical utility of Doppler echocardiography and tissue Doppler imaging in the estimation of left ventricular filling pressures: a comparative simultaneous Doppler-catheterization study," *Circulation*, vol. 102, no. 15, pp. 1788–1794, 2000.

[6] D. Lichtenstein, "Lung ultrasound in acute respiratory failure an introduction to the BLUE-protocol," *Minerva Anestesiologica*, vol. 75, no. 5, pp. 313–317, 2009.

[7] D. A. Lichtenstein and G. A. Mezière, "Relevance of lung ultrasound in the diagnosis of acute respiratory failure: the BLUE protocol," *Chest*, vol. 134, no. 1, pp. 117–125, 2008.

[8] D. Lichtenstein, "Should lung ultrasonography be more widely used in the assessment of acute respiratory disease?" *Expert Review of Respiratory Medicine*, vol. 4, no. 5, pp. 533–538, 2010.

[9] G. Volpicelli, M. Elbarbary, M. Blaivas et al., "International evidence-based recommendations for point-of-care lung ultrasound," *Intensive Care Medicine*, vol. 38, no. 4, pp. 577–591, 2012.

[10] F. Corradi, C. Brusasco, and P. Pelosi, "Chest ultrasound in acute respiratory distress syndrome," *Current Opinion in Critical Care*, vol. 20, no. 1, pp. 98–103, 2014.

[11] V. E. Noble, L. Lamhaut, R. Capp et al., "Evaluation of a thoracic ultrasound training module for the detection of pneumothorax and pulmonary edema by prehospital physician care providers," *BMC Medical Education*, vol. 9, article 3, 2009.

[12] D. Lichtenstein, I. Goldstein, E. Mourgeon, P. Cluzel, P. Grenier, and J.-J. Rouby, "Comparative diagnostic performances of auscultation, chest radiography, and lung ultrasonography in acute respiratory distress syndrome," *Anesthesiology*, vol. 100, no. 1, pp. 9–15, 2004.

[13] P. Van der Linden, M. Lambermont, A. Dierick et al., "Recommendations in the event of a suspected transfusion-related acute lung injury (TRALI)," *Acta Clinica Belgica*, vol. 67, no. 3, pp. 201–208, 2012.

[14] F. Gonzalez-Vilchez, M. Ares, J. Ayuela, and L. Alonso, "Combined use of pulsed and color M-mode Doppler echocardiography for the estimation of pulmonary capillary wedge pressure: an empirical approach based on an analytical relation," *Journal of the American College of Cardiology*, vol. 34, no. 2, pp. 515–523, 1999.

13

Disseminated Intravascular Coagulation as a Possible Cause of Acute Coronary Stent Thrombosis: A Case Report and Literature Review

Syed Amer,[1] Ali Shafiq,[1] Waqas Qureshi,[1] Mohammed Muqeetadnan,[2] and Syed Hassan[1]

[1] *Department of Medicine, Henry Ford Hospital, Detroit, MI 48202, USA*
[2] *Department of Medicine, University of Oklahoma Health Sciences Center, Oklahoma City, OK 73104, USA*

Correspondence should be addressed to Syed Amer, drsyedamer1@gmail.com

Academic Editors: C. Diez, C. Lazzeri, C. Mammina, G. Pichler, and C. D. Roosens

Disseminated intravascular coagulation (DIC), as a cause of acute coronary stent thrombosis, has not yet been reported to our knowledge. We report a case of 64-year-old male, who presented with non-ST-segment elevation myocardial infarction (NSTEMI). Coronary angiography revealed right coronary artery (RCA) stenosis and a drug eluting stent was deployed. Fifteen hours following the intervention, the patient developed an inferior wall ST elevation myocardial infarction. Repeat cardiac catheterization showed an acute in-stent thrombosis. Following thrombectomy, another stent was placed. The patient noted to have an acute drop in platelet count following the second intervention. Two hours following repeat intervention, the patient again developed chest pain and EKG showed recurrent ST-segment elevations in leads II, III, and aVF. Prior to repeat cardiac catheterization, the patient became unresponsive and developed cardiogenic shock. The patient was resuscitated and intubated, and repeat catheterization showed complete stent thrombosis. Intracoronary tissue plasminogen activator (tPA) was given. The platelet count further dropped. Additional studies confirmed the diagnosis of DIC. No further cardiac catheterization was done at this point. The patient then later had a cardiac arrest and unfortunately cardiopulmonary resuscitation could not revive him. Amongst the etiologies of acute stent thrombosis, DIC was deemed a possible cause.

1. Introduction

Percutaneous coronary intervention (PCI) is widely performed for the treatment of obstructive coronary artery disease (CAD) with good results [1, 2]. Acute stent thrombosis is an unusual complication after PCI [3]. Among the etiologies of acute stent thrombosis, DIC has not been reported before. We describe a case of the patient who developed DIC after suffering myocardial infarction and subsequently had recurrent coronary stent thrombosis.

2. Case Description

A 64-year-old Caucasian male presented with left arm pain and numbness for 1 day. The patient was not on any medications and had no family history of coronary artery disease or sudden death. Physical examination was unremarkable

for any significant abnormalities. Electrocardiogram (ECG) showed normal sinus rhythm and T wave inversions in leads II, III, and aVF. Chest X-ray was negative for any acute process. Patient was started on aspirin 325 mg along with intravenous heparin, nitroglycerin, and eptifibitide. Initial troponin-I level was at 0.47 ng/mL which later increased to 2.28 ng/mL, and a decision was made to perform left heart catheterization. RCA angiogram showed >90% stenosis (Figure 1) and a drug eluting stent was deployed with post-stent residual 0% stenosis and Thrombolysis in Myocardial Infarction (TIMI) III flow (Figure 2). The patient was started on clopidogrel after the procedure at a loading dose of 600 mg.

The patient developed left sided chest pain 15 hours following the initial intervention and ECG revealed an ST segment elevation in leads II, III, and aVF. Repeat cardiac catheterization showed an acute thrombosis of the initially

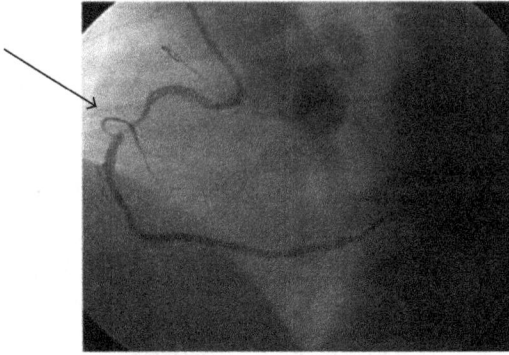

FIGURE 1: RCA angiogram showing >90% stenosis.

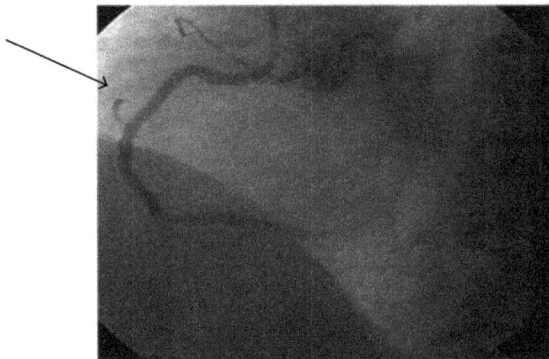

FIGURE 2: Post RCA stent residual showing 0% stenosis.

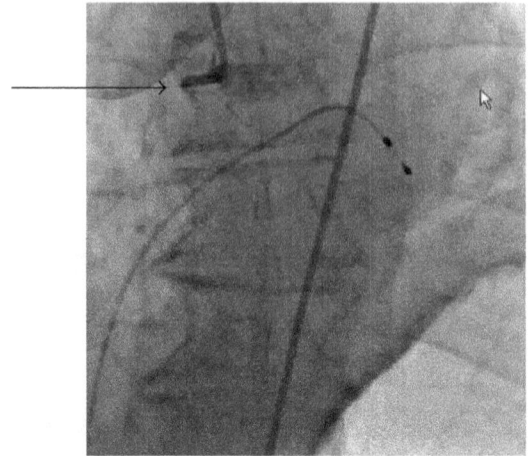

FIGURE 3: RCA revealing 100% thrombosis of the recently placed stent.

Fresh frozen plasma and blood transfusion were given. Patient's echocardiogram showed right ventricular dilatation with hypokinesis, consistent with right ventricular infarction. The patient continued to deteriorate clinically despite all aggressive therapy. There was a continuous rise in troponin I levels and persisted ST segment elevation. No further cardiac catheterization was done despite an ST elevation in inferior wall leads. The patient later had a cardiac arrest and cardiopulmonary resuscitation could not revive him.

3. Discussion

Acute coronary stent thrombosis remains a worrisome complication after PCI. There are many risk factors and causes associated with this problem. The patient in this case presented with NSTEMI, underwent PCI with stent placement, and developed recurrent acute stent thrombosis despite multiple revascularization attempts. A workup was done to determine the possible etiology for these events. A final diagnosis was not made with certainty for the cause of the thrombotic events. Amongst the differential diagnoses, DIC was also considered as a possible cause. We present a review of literature related to the definition and causes of acute stent thrombosis and discuss DIC as a possible etiological factor.

Stent thrombosis has been classified in previous studies as acute (intraprocedural or within 24 hours of the procedure), subacute (from 24 h to 30 days), late (30 days to 1 year), or very late (1 year). Acute and subacute ST were also defined as early ST. General risk factors associated with stent thrombosis include malignant disease, old age, black race, and diabetes mellitus. [4–6]. Predictors of stent thrombosis include bifurcation lesions, under sizing, uncovered dissection, and suboptimal procedural result (TIMI flow grade < 3 after PCI). None of these factors were present in our patient. Patients with low left ventricular ejection fraction, use of drug eluting stents, and total number of stents are also important predictors for early

placed stent. Thrombectomy was performed with Export catheter and another drug eluting stent was placed.

There was an acute drop in platelet count to 74,000/μL from 145,000/μL following the second intervention. Heparin-induced thrombocytopenia (HIT) was suspected. IV heparin was stopped and argatroban was started. Heparin platelet factor 4 antibodies results were 0.419 OD (mildly abnormal), which were not significant to confirm HIT. Two hours later, the patient again complained of chest pain and EKG showed recurrent ST-segment elevations in the inferior leads. Prior to repeat cardiac catheterization, the patient became unresponsive, hypotensive and developed ventricular tachycardia. The patient was cardioverted and started on vasopressors. After resuscitation a transvenous pacemaker and an intra-aortic balloon pump were placed. Repeat angiogram of the RCA revealed 100% thrombosis of the recently placed stent (Figure 3).

Intra-arterial TPA and thrombectomy were performed which allowed partial restoration of the flow. Clopidogrel was replaced with prasugrel.

Further workup showed a rise in creatinine to 2.02 mg/dL, and a drop in platelet count to 46,000/mcL and skin showed generalized petechiae. The patient started bleeding from his nasogastric tube and ultrasound of the abdomen revealed free intraperitoneal fluid. A workup for DIC was performed which showed an international normalized ratio (INR) of 7, partial thromboplastin time (PTT) of 205, D dimer: 1400, and fibrinogen of 84 mg/mL.

stent thrombosis [7]. Heparin-induced thrombocytopenia has been reported to cause acute stent thrombosis [8] and was suspected in our patient. However the heparin platelet factor 4 antibodies were 0.419 OD (mildly abnormal) which were not consistent with a diagnosis of HIT [9]. Clopidogrel and aspirin resistance have been shown to be associated with stent thrombosis [10, 11]. Our patient suffered from very early stent thrombosis despite therapy with antiplatelet agents (aspirin, clopidogrel, and eptifibitide). Prasugrel was also substituted later in the course of his management. His clinical deterioration despite use of multiple medications suggested that these were unlikely the dominant cause of the patient's cascade of events. Our patient developed DIC after his multiple coronary interventions. DIC as a cause of early stent thrombosis has never been reported and was considered as a possible cause in the absence of other etiologies.

There is no direct evidence of the association of DIC with coronary stent thrombosis. However indirect evidence suggests that DIC may have a role in these measures. DIC has been shown to be involved in the thrombosis of coronary vessels [12] and severe cardiac dysfunction as a result of the thrombotic occlusive events [13]. The body's natural anticoagulants, namely, protein C and antithrombin-III have been found to be at low levels in patients with DIC [14–16]. This predisposes the blood vessels to increased thrombosis. This has also been suggested by previous literature, for instance, protein C deficiency has been shown to cause thrombosis of the mesenteric artery [17], coronary artery, and jugular vein [18]. We reviewed a case report in which AT-III deficiency was shown to be associated with recurrent coronary in-stent thrombosis in an emergent PCI [19]. These examples are suggestive that it is a likely possibility that DIC may lead to recurrent coronary stent thrombosis in the absence of other obvious causes.

After repetitive NSTEMIs our patient developed ecchymosis, purpura, and intraperitoneal bleeding. His lab work showed severe thrombocytopenia, low fibrinogen, and elevated PT and PTT levels. The clinical scenario suggested a diagnosis of DIC. We excluded common causes of DIC such as sepsis, trauma, and malignancy. Clopidogrel has been shown to cause DIC and was considered as a possible etiological factor. We also found that acute myocardial infarction has been reported to cause DIC [20]. As our patient suffered from multiple myocardial insults, AMI was deemed the likely cause of the DIC in this scenario.

4. Conclusion

A patient undergoing acute stent thrombosis in emergent percutaneous interventions may have fatal results. We want to emphasize that DIC should be considered as one of the etiological factors in cases of acute stent thrombosis.

References

[1] P. W. Serruys, P. De Jaegere, F. Kiemeneij et al., "A comparison of balloon-expandable-stent implantation with balloon angioplasty in patients with coronary artery disease," *The New England Journal of Medicine*, vol. 331, no. 8, pp. 489–495, 1994.

[2] D. L. Fischman, M. B. Leon, D. S. Baim et al., "A randomized comparison of coronary-stent placement and balloon angioplasty in the treatment of coronary artery disease," *The New England Journal of Medicine*, vol. 331, no. 8, pp. 496–501, 1994.

[3] J. Shiraishi, Y. Kohno, T. Sawada et al., "In-hospital outcomes of primary percutaneous coronary interventions performed at hospitals with and without on-site coronary artery bypass graft surgery," *Circulation Journal*, vol. 71, no. 8, pp. 1208–1212, 2007.

[4] P. K. Kuchulakanti, W. W. Chu, R. Torguson et al., "Correlates and long-term outcomes of angiographically proven stent thrombosis with sirolimus- and paclitaxel-eluting stents," *Circulation*, vol. 113, no. 8, pp. 1108–1113, 2006.

[5] S. H. Park, G. R. Hong, H. S. Seo, and S. J. Tahk, "Stent thrombosis after successful drug-eluting stent implantation," *Korean Circulation Journal*, vol. 35, pp. 163–171, 2005.

[6] S. Kim, M. Jeong, D. Sim et al., "Very late thrombosis of a drug-eluting stent after discontinuation of dual antiplatelet therapy in a patient treated with both drug-eluting and bare-metal stents," *Korean Circulation Journal*, vol. 39, no. 5, pp. 205–208, 2009.

[7] J. W. van Werkum, A. A. Heestermans, A. C. Zomer et al., "Predictors of coronary stent thrombosis. The dutch stent thrombosis registry," *Journal of the American College of Cardiology*, vol. 53, no. 16, pp. 1399–1409, 2009.

[8] R. K. Al-Lamee, R. T. Gerber, and J. S. Kooner, "Heparin-induced thrombocytopenia (HIT) as an unusual cause of acute stent thrombosis," *European Heart Journal*, vol. 31, no. 5, article 613, 2010.

[9] T. E. Warkentin, J. I. Sheppard, J. C. Moore, C. S. Sigouin, and J. G. Kelton, "Quantitative interpretation of optical density measurements using PF4-dependent enzyme-immunoassays," *Journal of Thrombosis and Haemostasis*, vol. 6, no. 8, pp. 1304–1312, 2008.

[10] S. Kim, M. Jeong, H. Kim, S. Bae, K. Ryu, K. Cho et al., "Acute and subacute stent thrombosis in a patient with clopidogrel resistance: a case report," *Korean Circulation Journal*, vol. 39, no. 10, pp. 434–438, 2009.

[11] J. Ruef and R. Kranzhöfer, "Coronary stent thrombosis related to aspirin resistance: what are the underlying mechanisms?" *Journal of Interventional Cardiology*, vol. 19, no. 6, pp. 507–509, 2006.

[12] M. Sugiura, K. Hiraoka, and S. Ohkawa, "A clinicopathological study on cardiac lesions in 64 cases of disseminated intravascular coagulation," *Japanese Heart Journal*, vol. 18, no. 1, pp. 57–69, 1977.

[13] K. Ueda, M. Sugiura, and S. Ohkawa, "Disseminated intravascular coagulation in the aged complicated by acute myocardial infarction," *Japanese Journal of Medicine*, vol. 20, no. 3, pp. 202–210, 1981.

[14] H. Takahashi, E. Takakuwa, and N. Yoshino, "Protein C levels in disseminated intravascular coagulation and thrombotic thrombocytopenic purpura: its correlation with other coagulation parameters," *Thrombosis and Haemostasis*, vol. 54, no. 2, pp. 445–449, 1985.

[15] R. A. Marlar, J. Endres-Brooks, and C. Miller, "Serial studies of protein C and its plasma inhibitor in patients with

disseminated intravascular coagulation," *Blood*, vol. 66, no. 1, pp. 59–63, 1985.

[16] A. E. Kogan and S. M. Strukova, "Protein C decreases in experimental DIC in rats," *Thrombosis Research*, vol. 57, no. 5, pp. 825–826, 1990.

[17] A. Onwuanyi, R. Sachdeva, K. Hamiram, M. Islam, and R. Parris, "Multiple aortic thrombi associated with protein C and S deficiency," *Mayo Clinic Proceedings*, vol. 76, no. 3, pp. 319–322, 2001.

[18] O. Cakir, O. Ayyildiz, A. Oruc, and N. Eren, "A young adult with coronary artery and jugular vein thrombosis: a case report of combined protein S and protein C deficiency," *Heart and Vessels*, vol. 17, no. 2, pp. 74–76, 2002.

[19] B. Kaku, S. Katsuda, T. Taguchi, Y. Nitta, and Y. Hiraiwa, "A case of acute myocardial infarction with repetitive stent thrombosis during emergent percutaneous coronary intervention: transient decrease in antithrombin III activity and heparin resistance," *International Heart Journal*, vol. 50, no. 1, pp. 111–119, 2009.

[20] F. J. Thomson, E. W. Benbow, R. F. T. McMahon, and C. M. Cheshire, "Pulmonary infarction, myocardial infarction, and acute disseminated intravascular coagulation," *Journal of Clinical Pathology*, vol. 44, no. 12, pp. 1034–1036, 1991.

14

Severe Diltiazem Poisoning Treated with Hyperinsulinaemia-Euglycaemia and Lipid Emulsion

Nadine Monteiro,[1] Joana Silvestre,[1,2] João Gonçalves-Pereira,[1,2] Camila Tapadinhas,[1] Vitor Mendes,[1] and Pedro Póvoa[1,2]

[1] Polyvalent Intensive Care Unit, São Francisco Xavier Hospital, West Lisbon Hospital Centre, 1449-005 Lisbon, Portugal
[2] Faculty of Medical Sciences, New University of Lisbon, 1169-056 Lisbon, Portugal

Correspondence should be addressed to Nadine Monteiro; nadine_rodrigues@hotmail.com

Academic Editors: C. Diez, M. Egi, C. Lazzeri, K. Lenz, W. S. Park, and K. S. Waxman

Introduction. Calcium channel blockers (CCBs) drugs are widely used in the treatment of cardiovascular diseases. CCB poisoning is associated with significant cardiovascular toxicity and is potentially fatal. Currently, there is no specific antidote and the treatment of CCB poisoning is supportive; however, this supportive therapy is often insufficient. We present a clinical case of severe diltiazem poisoning and the therapeutic approaches that were used. *Case Report.* A 55-year-old male was admitted to the intensive care unit (ICU) after voluntary multiple drug intake, including extended release diltiazem (7200 mg). The patient developed symptoms of refractory shock to conventional therapy and required mechanical ventilation, a temporary pacemaker, and renal replacement therapy. Approximately 17 hours after drug intake, hyperinsulinaemia-euglycaemia with lipid emulsion therapy was initiated, followed by progressive haemodynamic recovery within approximately 30 minutes. The toxicological serum analysis 12 h after drug ingestion revealed a diltiazem serum level of 4778 ng/mL (therapeutic level: 40–200 ng/mL). *Conclusions.* This case report supports the therapeutic efficacy of hyperinsulinaemia-euglycaemia and lipid emulsion in the treatment of severe diltiazem poisoning.

1. Introduction

Diltiazem is a nondihydropyridine L-type calcium channel blocker (CCB) which is widely used in the treatment of cardiovascular diseases. The prescription of CCB has increased significantly in recent years, [1, 2] and concomitantly the number of cases of voluntary and involuntary poisoning.

In 2011, the *American Association of Poison Control Centers* reported 1995 deaths from exposure to toxic substances, 1689 of which were from medications (84.7%) [3]. Following analgesics and antidepressants, cardiovascular drugs were the most often involved. Of these drugs, CCB were most commonly used [3].

Calcium channel blockers overdose can cause life-threatening effects, such as bradycardia, atrioventricular (AV) block, hypotension, metabolic acidosis, and shock that is often refractory to conventional therapy.

The treatment of CCB poisoning has been limited to organ support measures. The importance of hyperinsulinaemia-euglycaemia and lipid emulsion therapy has recently

been recognised in the treatment of these patients [4–12]. Traditionally, these approaches are used as late salvage therapy in cases of CCB poisoning when other measures have failed.

We hereby present a clinical case of a patient with severe diltiazem poisoning in which hyperinsulinaemia-euglycaemia and lipid emulsion therapy contributed to haemodynamic stabilisation.

2. Clinical Case

A 55-year-old male was admitted to the emergency room (ER) with a low level of consciousness approximately two hours after voluntary multiple drug ingestion, including diltiazem (7200 mg), perindopril (150 mg), simvastatin (280 mg), and escitalopram (600 mg).

The patient presented a past history of essential arterial hypertension, ischemic cardiac disease, dyslipidaemia, and major depression.

TABLE 1: Laboratory data.

	Hospital admission	UCI admission	12 hrs after ICU admission	48 hrs after ICU admission
Red blood cells ($\times 10^{12}$/L)	4.72	3.9	3.94	4.01
Haemoglobin (g/dL)	14.0	11.5	11.7	12.1
White cell count ($\times 10^9$/L)	10.5	23.8	19.0	19.1
Platelet count ($\times 10^9$/L)	224	216	127	93
Prothrombin time (sec)	10.9	11.8	13.7	11.0
C-reactive protein (mg/dL)	0.41	0.49	11.3	9.8
Urea (mg/dL)	40	49	50	23
Creatinine (mg/dL)	1.22	1.79	2.47	1.70
Glucose (mg/dL)	225	306	275	186
Potassium (mmol/L)	3.56	4.54	3.85	4.2
Sodium (mmol/L)	135	137	137	135
Calcium (mg/dL)	8.5	6.6	9.7	8.8
Alanine transaminase (U/L)	36	49		
Aspartate transaminase (U/L)		28		
γ-glutamyltransferase (U/L)	55	119		
Total bilirubin (mg/dL)	0.37	0.88	0.44	0.46

TABLE 2: Evolution of arterial blood gases in the ICU.

	0 h (FiO$_2$: 0.3)	4 h* (FiO$_2$: 0.6)	9 h (FiO$_2$: 0.8)	10 h (FiO$_2$: 0.6)	12 h (FiO$_2$: 0.5)	48 h** (FiO$_2$: 0.4)
pH	7.241	7.242	7.195	7.263	7.35	7.396
PaCO$_2$ (mmHg)	46.1	35.5	29.3	31.1	31.4	38.8
PaO$_2$ (mmHg)	68.6	72.5	207	188	217	134
HCO^{-3} (mEq/L)	16.7	15.5	12.6	15.1	18.8	23.8
Lactate (mmol/L)	4.3	5.7	9.4	6.7	3.4	0.8

*Intubated and invasive mechanical ventilation was initiated.
**Extubated.

On the hospital admission, he was comatose with a Glasgow Coma Score (GCS) of 8, a blood pressure (BP) of 77/44 mmHg, and a heart rate (HR) of 48 bpm.

The patient began treatment with intravenous fluid, atropine, glucagon, sodium bicarbonate, and calcium gluconate. Severe bradycardia and hypotension persisted, for which a dopamine infusion was initiated (maximum dose: 7.5 mcg/kg/min).

Laboratory evaluation data are presented in Table 1. Arterial blood gases (FiO$_2$ 0.3) revealed a metabolic acidosis (pH 7.306, PCO$_2$ 34.0 mmHg, PO$_2$ 90.3 mmHg, HCO$_3$ 17.6 mmol/L, and lactate 3.9 mmol/L).

An electrocardiogram was performed and showed a sinus rhythm with 48 bpm; a first-degree atrioventricular block; and the pattern of a complete right bundle branch block.

The condition progressed to refractory shock, and the patient developed an acute renal failure with oliguria. At that time he was admitted in the intensive care unit (ICU).

Aggressive fluid resuscitation and vasopressor support with dopamine, norepinephrine, epinephrine, terlipressin, and dobutamine were initiated with poor hemodynamic response. Progressive worsening of lactic acidosis was observed (Table 2). An intravenous (iv) calcium infusion of 2 g/h was instituted, and renal replacement therapy was initiated (continuous veno-venous hemodiafiltration at

effluent rates of 35 mL/Kg/h) without significant change in his cardiovascular failure.

The patient's level of consciousness deteriorated even further (GCS: 5), and he was subsequently tracheally intubated, and invasive mechanical ventilation was initiated. The patient evolved with a severe bradycardia, needing a temporary pacemaker.

After approximately 9 hours in the ICU, refractory hypotension persisted. At that time, a 20% lipid emulsion infusion was prescribed at 0.5 mL/Kg/h rate, plus (iv) short-acting human insulin at increasing doses reaching a maximum dose of 45 U/h and 30% dextrose in water infusion adjusting infusion rate for the maintenance of euglycaemia.

Approximately 30 min after the initiation of these supportive measures, progressive haemodynamic improvement was observed with the normalisation of lactic acidaemia (Table 2), which allowed a gradual weaning of vasopressor support as well as in the recovery of own cardiac rhythm.

After 48 hours in ICU, the patient was successfully weaned from ventilatory and vasopressor support.

Despite diuresis recovery, the need for renal replacement therapy persisted until haemodynamic stabilisation was observed. Continuous veno-venous haemodiafiltration was stopped and deescalated to intermittent hemodialysis. The patient was discharged from ICU on the 4th day of hospital stay. The patient experienced full recovery of renal function and returned home after 3 days.

The plasma concentration of diltiazem 12 h after ingestion was 4778 ng/mL (therapeutic level: 40–200 ng/mL), that is to say almost 24 times above the upper limit of the therapeutic range.

3. Discussion

In this clinical case, the authors describe a severe CCB poisoning (near 24 × the upper volume of the therapeutic range) that results in a severe refractory shock with multiple organ failure that only recovered with the hyperinsulinaemia-euglycaemia and lipid emulsion treatment.

The cardiovascular effects of CCB poisoning involve the excessive blockage of the L-type calcium channels in the myocardial cell membranes of the cardiac electrical conduction system and the vascular smooth muscle tissue, thereby preventing the entry of calcium into the cells. Therefore, cardiac inotropism, dromotropism, and chronotropism are reduced along with vascular tone. In addition, CCB inhibits the influx of calcium into pancreatic beta cells and peripheral tissue which leads to the decreased excretion of insulin and peripheral resistance to the action of CCB [7, 13, 14]. Conventional therapy for CCB poisoning includes the administration of fluids, calcium salts, glucagon, and vasopressors [5, 6, 15–17].

Extracorporeal elimination by conventional haemofiltration and dialysis is not recommended because these agents bind to plasma proteins and have a large volume of distribution. The molecular adsorbent recirculating system (MARS) was successfully used in one case report of severe diltiazem poisoning [18]. However, this technique is expensive and is not always available in a timely manner.

In our case, there was rapid deterioration of the clinical condition and refractoriness to conventional therapy which was rapidly reversed after the prescription of hyperinsulinaemia-euglycaemia and lipid infusion therapy.

In normal circumstances, myocardial cells use the oxidation of free fatty acids as an energy substrate for aerobic metabolism. In CCB poisoning, the uptake of free fatty acids by the myocardium is decreased, and the myocardium uses glucose as an energy substrate. However, the decrease in tissue perfusion secondary to the excessive blockage of vascular calcium channels complicates the distribution of glucose into the tissue. Simultaneously, hypoinsulinaemia and insulin resistance prevent the uptake of glucose by myocardial cells and vascular smooth muscle, thus limiting the use of glucose as an energy substrate. The lack of energy substrate exacerbates cardiovascular depression which is already compromised by the blocking of the calcium channels.

These mechanisms led to the hypothesis that the administration of high-dose insulin to treat CCB poisoning could compensate for hypoinsulinaemia and insulin resistance and as a result could interrupt the vicious cycle that is responsible for progressive haemodynamic deterioration and, ultimately, patient death. The efficacy and safety of this treatment have been demonstrated in several cases of CCB poisoning [6–8, 10, 12].

Therapeutic hyperinsulinaemia-euglycaemia consists of a continuous infusion of high-dose regular short-acting insulin (0.5–1 UI/kg) with concomitant glucose infusion that is titrated to maintain glycaemia within normal limits, which may necessitate a glucose dosage of 15–30 g/h.

Lipid emulsion has been used to treat poisoning by local anaesthetics. There is insufficient data to support the use of lipid emulsion as a first-line option; however, this therapy has been used as salvage therapy in pharmaceutical poisoning by other lipophilic drugs, particularly CCBs [9, 12]. The exact mechanism of action of this treatment is not known. The most widely accepted theory is that the emulsion acts as a "lipid sink," surrounding a lipophilic drug molecule and rendering it ineffective.

4. Conclusions

The combination of hyperinsulinaemia-euglycaemia and lipid emulsion therapy was effective for the haemodynamic recovery of a patient with refractory cardiogenic shock secondary to severe diltiazem poisoning. The early prescription of these therapies in patients with CCB poisoning may improve their prognosis.

References

[1] I. Kurnatowska, J. Królikowski, K. Jesionowska et al., "Prevalence of arterial hypertension and the number and classes of antihypertensive drugs prescribed for patients late after kidney transplantation," *Annals of Transplantation*, vol. 17, no. 1, pp. 50–57, 2012.

[2] K. A. J. Al Khaja, R. P. Sequeira, and V. S. Mathur, "Rational pharmacotherapy of hypertension in the elderly: analysis of the choice and dosage of drugs," *Journal of Clinical Pharmacy and Therapeutics*, vol. 26, no. 1, pp. 33–42, 2001.

[3] A. C. Bronstein, D. A. Spyker, L. R. Cantilena Jr., B. H. Rumack, and R. C. Dart, "2011 Annual report of the American Association of Poison Control Centers' National Poison Data System (NPDS): 29th annual report," *Clinical Toxicology*, vol. 50, no. 10, pp. 911–1164, 2012.

[4] A. Anusheree, S. W. Yu, Abdul Rehman, and J. Q. Henkle, "Hyperinsulinemia euglycemia therapy for calcium channel blocker overdose," *The Texas Heart Institute Journal*, vol. 39, no. 4, pp. 575–578, 2012.

[5] N. Abeysinghe, J. Aston, and S. Polouse, "Diltiazem overdose: a role for high-dose insulin," *Emergency Medicine Journal*, vol. 27, no. 10, pp. 802–803, 2010.

[6] B. Mégarbane, S. Karyo, and F. J. Baud, "The role of insulin and glucose (hyperinsulinaemia/euglycaemia) therapy in acute calcium channel antagonist and β-blocker poisoning," *Toxicological Reviews*, vol. 23, no. 4, pp. 215–222, 2004.

[7] P. E. R. Lheureux, S. Zahir, M. Gris, A. S. Derrey, and A. Penaloza, "Bench-to-bedside review: hyperinsulinaemia/euglycaemia therapy in the management of overdose of calcium-channel blockers," *Critical Care*, vol. 10, no. 3, article 212, 2006.

[8] S. L. Greene, I. Gawarammana, D. M. Wood, A. L. Jones, and P. I. Dargan, "Relative safety of hyperinsulinaemia/euglycaemia therapy in the management of calcium channel blocker overdose: a prospective observational study," *Intensive Care Medicine*, vol. 33, no. 11, pp. 2019–2024, 2007.

[9] B. J. Wilson, J. S. Cruikshank, K. L. Wiebe, V. C. Dias, and M. C. Yarema, "Intravenous lipid emulsion therapy for sustained release diltiazem poisoning: a case report," *Journal of Population Therapeutics and Clinical Pharmacology*, vol. 19, no. 2, pp. e218–e222, 2012.

[10] L. Min and K. Deshpande, "Diltiazem overdose haemodynamic response to hyperinsulinaemia-euglycaemia therapy: a case report," *Critical Care and Resuscitation*, vol. 6, no. 1, pp. 28–30, 2004.

[11] S. J. Stellpflug, S. J. Fritzlar, J. B. Cole, K. M. Engebretsen, and J. S. Holger, "Cardiotoxic overdose treated with intravenous fat emulsion and high-dose insulin in the setting of hypertrophic cardiomyopathy," *Journal of Medical Toxicology*, vol. 7, no. 2, pp. 151–153, 2011.

[12] V. Montiel, T. Gougnard, and P. Hantson, "Diltiazem poisoning treated with hyperinsulinemic euglycemia therapy and intravenous lipid emulsion," *European Journal of Emergency Medicine*, vol. 18, no. 2, pp. 121–123, 2011.

[13] J. A. Kline, R. M. Raymond, J. D. Schoroeder, and J. A. Watts, "The diabetogeic effects of acute verapamil poisoning," *Toxicology and Applied Pharmacology*, vol. 145, no. 2, pp. 357–362, 1997.

[14] D. F. Blackburn and T. W. Wilson, "Antihypertensive medications and blood sugar: theories and implications," *Canadian Journal of Cardiology*, vol. 22, no. 3, pp. 229–233, 2006.

[15] S. D. Salhanick and M. W. Shannon, "Management of calcium channel antagonist overdose," *Drug Safety*, vol. 26, no. 2, pp. 65–79, 2003.

[16] P. D. Pearigen and N. L. Benowitz, "Poisoning due to calcium antagonists. Experience with verapamil, diltiazem and nifedipine," *Drug Safety*, vol. 6, no. 6, pp. 408–430, 1991.

[17] C. R. DeWitt and J. C. Waksman, "Pharmacology, pathophysiology and management of calcium channel blocker and β-blocker toxicity," *Toxicological Reviews*, vol. 23, no. 4, pp. 223–238, 2004.

[18] M. Belleflamme, P. Hantson, T. Gougnard et al., "Survival despite extremely high plasma diltiazem level in a case of acute poisoning treated by the molecular-adsorbent recirculating system," *European Journal of Emergency Medicine*, vol. 19, no. 1, pp. 59–61, 2012.

15

Guidewire-Related Complications during Central Venous Catheter Placement: A Case Report and Review of the Literature

Faisal A. Khasawneh[1] and Roger D. Smalligan[2]

[1] Division of Critical Care Medicine, Department of Internal Medicine, Texas Tech University Health Sciences Center,
  1400 S. Coulter, Amarillo, TX 79106, USA
[2] Department of Internal Medicine, Texas Tech University Health Sciences Center, 1400 S. Coulter, Amarillo, TX 79106, USA

Correspondence should be addressed to Faisal A. Khasawneh, faisal.khasawneh@ttuhsc.edu

Academic Editors: C. Diez, K. Lenz, and J. Starkopf

Seldinger's technique is widely used to place central venous and arterial catheters and is generally considered safe. The technique does have multiple potential risks. Guidewire-related complications are rare but potentially serious. We describe a case of a lost guidewire during central venous catheter insertion followed by a review of the literature of this topic. Measures which can be taken to prevent such complications are explained in detail as well as recommended steps to remedy errors should they occur.

1. Introduction

In 1953 Seldinger described a simple, over a guidewire, approach for catheter insertion [1]. It offered considerable advantages over the previously used methods, revolutionizing the field of bedside procedures. The Seldinger technique is widely used in the intensive care unit (ICU) to place central venous catheters (CVCs), hemodialysis (HD) catheters, arterial catheters, and chest tubes. Like any other procedure, it has a number of associated potential risks. Guidewire-related complications in particular are rarely reported; nevertheless, when they do occur, they can be accompanied by significant morbidity and mortality. In this paper, a case of a lost guidewire during central venous catheter (CVC) insertion is reported followed by a review of the literature.

2. Case Presentation

A 45-year-old male patient with diabetes mellitus and left-sided nonsmall cell lung cancer was admitted to the ICU with progressive shortness of breath. The patient's acute hypoxemic respiratory failure was attributed to disease progression and possible pneumonia. Failing noninvasive positive pressure ventilation, the patient required intubation and the initiation of mechanical ventilation. A chest X-ray

(Figure 1) was taken shortly afterwards. On the radiograph, he had a well-positioned endotracheal tube, an orogastric tube, a left-sided subclavian CVC, a left-sided chest tube, and multiple superficial leads. There was an additional shadow that could not be easily accounted for. Examining the patient and the bedding offered no explanation for the extra shadow. Sequentially ordered X-rays of the abdomen, pelvis, and right thigh (Figures 2, 3, and 4) revealed a J-shaped guidewire that apparently had been lost but not reported during the left subclavian CVC insertion procedure. With the help of an interventional radiologist, the guidewire was removed successfully without complications.

3. Discussion

Although this case ended without significant harm being caused to the patient, guidewire-related complications with accompanying morbidity and mortality do occur during the insertion of central venous catheters. The high frequency of such CVC placement procedures in emergency rooms, operating rooms, and intensive care units makes the likelihood of seeing an occasional complication quite high. To study this topic in depth, the authors searched PubMed for articles using the search terms "guidewire," "J-wire," "central venous

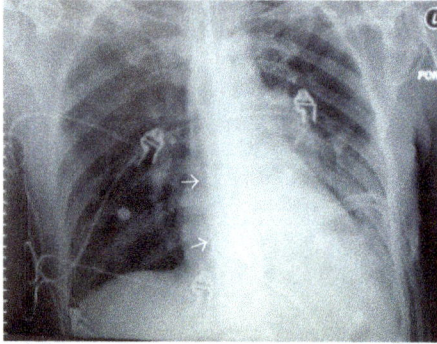

FIGURE 1: Chest X-ray showing an endotracheal tube, an orogastric tube, a left-sided subclavian central venous catheter, a left-sided chest tube, and multiple superficial leads. There is additional shadow (arrow heads) that could not be accounted for.

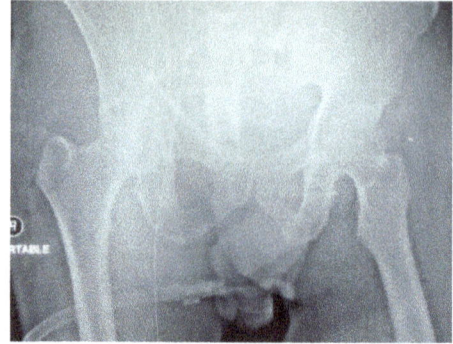

FIGURE 3: Pelvic X-ray showing the guidewire extending into the femoral vein in the right thigh.

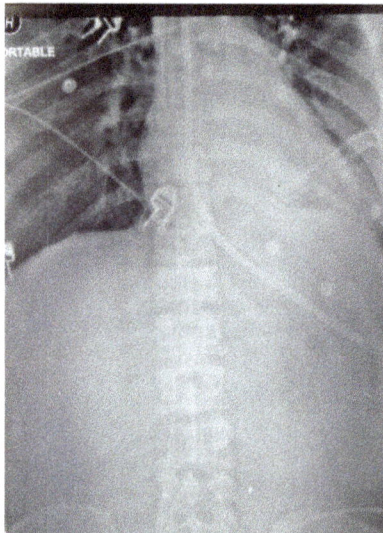

FIGURE 2: Upper abdominal X-ray showing the lost guidewire extending down the inferior vena cava on the right side of the abdomen.

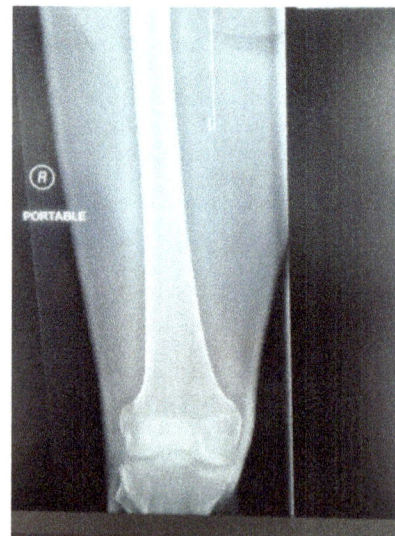

FIGURE 4: Right thigh X-ray showing the J-tip of the lost guidewire medial to the femur.

catheter," and "complications" in various combinations. Studies and case reports written in English as well as their listed references were reviewed for pertinent data.

The most commonly reported guidewire-related complications are listed in Table 1 and will be discussed below.

Cardiac dysrhythmias, most often premature atrial or ventricular contractions, are occasionally reported during subclavian or internal jugular (IJ) CVC insertion [2]. The arrhythmias are typically short lived, resulting from the guidewire touching the endocardium, and resolve when the tip is pulled back a few centimeters [2].

The most common cardiac conduction abnormalities seen during CVC placement are right bundle branch blocks, new left anterior and posterior fascicular blocks, and rarely asystole [3]. The cause of these conduction problems, as described in the case of cardiac dysrhythmias, is also the overzealous advancement of the guidewire. The ease with which a right bundle branch block can be induced is

probably related to the bundle branch's superficial position in the right ventricular endocardium, just inferior to the tricuspid valve [3]. Conduction abnormalities are usually transient and may go unnoticed. However, in a patient with an underlying left bundle branch block, the induction of further conduction defects may lead to a life-threatening complete heart block requiring temporary pacing [3]. The mentioned arrhythmias and conduction problems are essentially avoidable during central venous catheterization since placement should not involve entry into the heart by the guidewire or by the subsequently placed catheter [3].

Perforation of central veins or right-sided cardiac chambers can be catastrophic. In clinical practice, it is often difficult to ascertain what caused the venous perforation; the introducer needle, the guidewire, or the dilator. Nevertheless, the literature reports cases of guidewire-related perforation of the great vessels including the brachiocephalic and subclavian veins [4]. This important complication occurs when excessive force is applied against resistance when introducing the guidewire, especially if the straight or angle

TABLE 1: The most commonly reported guidewire-related complications.

(i) Cardiac dysrhythmias
(ii) Cardiac conduction abnormalities
(iii) Perforation of vessels or cardiac chambers
(iv) Kinking, looping, or knotting of the wire
(v) Entanglement of previously placed intravascular devices
(vi) Breakage of the distal tip of the guidewire with subsequent embolization
(vii) Complete loss of the guidewire within the vascular system

tip wire, rather than J tip style wire, is used. In most instances, bleeding from a small penetrating hole in a vein will stop spontaneously by vasospasm or by external compression of the surrounding tissues [4]. However, serious cases of hemothorax, including fatalities, due to the above complication have been reported [4]. Making a timely diagnosis in such cases requires maintaining a high index of suspicion when there is an unexplained drop in hemoglobin or the development of unilateral pleural effusion ipsilateral to a recently placed or attempted central venous catheterization. Treatment of a serious perforation may necessitate the insertion of a chest tube or an emergent thoracotomy [4].

Perforation of the heart may occur at the time of catheter insertion or any time the catheter tip is placed within the heart chambers [4]. There are at least two reported cases in the literature of heart perforation attributed to the guidewire itself. Both of these complications occurred during the insertion of HD catheters: the first during a subclavian approach leading to a life-threatening cardiac tamponade and the second during an IJ approach leading to a fatal tamponade [5, 6]. Cardiac tamponade usually results from perforation of the right atrium, or less frequently, the right ventricle. Tamponade has also been reported after superior vena cava (SVC) perforation within the pericardium [6]. The possibility of tamponade should be considered when a patient collapses during, or shortly after, placement of a CVC. Other diagnoses to consider in that scenario include tension pneumothorax and air embolism. An emergent chest X-ray or bedside echocardiogram followed by pericardiocentesis can be life saving in such situations.

Another occasional guidewire complication is kinking or looping of the wire itself. Applying force to thread a guidewire through the introducer needle despite significant resistance is likely to cause such a problem [7]. Kinking can also result if the dilator is forced in a direction that diverges from the original path of the wire [7]. If a clinician does not recognize this scenario there is potential for cutting through the vein with possible fatal complications [8]. This type of complication can be avoided by intermittently moving the wire gently in and out as the dilator is being advanced through the subcutaneous tissue. Application of increasing force after looping or kinking sometimes results in knot formation. Both intravascular as well as extravascular knotting have been reported [7]. It is almost exclusively described following the subclavian approach which may be

due to the curved path the vein takes as it loops over the first rib to descend into the SVC [7]. This complication should be suspected when the guidewire cannot be pulled out after successful catheter insertion. In this situation, no force should be used to pull the catheter and wire out, and an immediate X-ray should be ordered. Once the diagnosis is established, interventional radiology should be consulted, and sometimes surgical intervention is necessary.

Entanglement of a guidewire with an existing intravascular apparatus is another reported complication of CVC placement. Special attention is needed in patients with inferior vena cava (IVC) filters since there have been numerous reports of entrapment of guidewires in these filters [9]. It results from over advancement of the guidewire leading to hooking of the J-tip to the filter. Interestingly, IVC filter entrapment with straight guidewires has not been reported [9]. This complication should be suspected when the guidewire cannot be retrieved after catheter placement in a patient with an IVC filter already deployed. In such circumstances, no excessive force should be used to free the wire since this could lead to filter dislodgment and cava perforation [10]. X-ray or examination under fluoroscopy should be ordered promptly followed by interventional radiology consultation once the diagnosis is made.

Tip breakage of a guidewire has been blamed on inherent design flaws [11]. Shearing and breakage of the wire usually results from pulling the wire back through the needle after it has passed the bevel [7]. Hence, if a guidewire fails to pass freely from the introducer needle into the vessel, the careful retraction of the wire through the needle is an option, but it is much safer to withdraw the wire and needle as a single unit.

The inadvertent intravascular insertion of the entire guidewire, as in our case, is a completely avoidable complication [12]. Although the loss of a complete guidewire might cause arrhythmias, vascular damage, and thrombosis, it is usually asymptomatic and is often incidentally found on a routine X-ray done up to several months after the procedure [13]. Holding on to the proximal tip of the wire at all times is fundamental in preventing this mistake. If this complication happens, use of interventional radiology techniques is the preferred method for retrieval and removal [12].

The introduction of an excessive length of guidewire during central venous catheterization explains most of the aforementioned complications. Many reasons stand behind this faulty practice including not knowing its dangerous implications, fear of losing vascular access, absence of marks on the guidewire, use of a circular advancer, and concerns over contamination of the proximal end of the wire. Keeping these possibilities in mind and the fact that the upper limit of safe guidewire insertion in an adult patient is about 18 centimeters might help avoid this risky practice [14].

4. Conclusion

During central venous catheterization, guidewire-related complications are uncommon and essentially preventable. Preventive measures include the following.

(i) Careful selection of catheterization site paying attention to previous attempts and anatomical abnormalities.

(ii) Being aware of the presence of endovascular devices.

(iii) Considering the wire to be a delicate instrument with inherent areas of structural weakness [11]. Thus, on encountering any resistance while advancing or retrieving the wire, force should not be used.

(iv) The wire should not be advanced in the vein more than 18 to 20 centimeters in an adult patient [14].

(v) Using a J-tip style guidewire is a much safer practice.

(vi) The integrity of the guidewire needs to be checked after each attempt of threading the introducer needle and at the end of the procedure.

(vii) The proximal end of the wire should always be held by the operator until the distal tip is completely out of the vessel.

Authors' Contributions

F. A. Khasawneh was the attending physician on the case. F. A. Khasawneh made the diagnosis and took the pictures. F. A. Khasawneh and R. D. Smalligan reviewed the literature and wrote the manuscript.

References

[1] S. I. Seldinger, "Catheter replacement of the needle in percutaneous arteriography; a new technique," *Acta Radiologica*, vol. 39, no. 5, pp. 368–376, 1953.

[2] R. K. Stuart, S. A. Shiroka, P. Akerman et al., "Incidence of arrhythmia with central venous catheter insertion and exchange," *Journal of Parenteral and Enteral Nutrition*, vol. 14, no. 2, pp. 152–155, 1990.

[3] N. T. Eissa and V. Kvetan, "Guide wire as a cause of complete heart block in patients with preexisting left bundle branch block," *Anesthesiology*, vol. 73, no. 4, pp. 772–774, 1990.

[4] Y. Innami, T. Oyaizu, T. Ouchi, N. Umemura, and T. Koitabashi, "Life-threatening hemothorax resulting from right brachiocephalic vein perforation during right internal jugular vein catheterization," *Journal of Anesthesia*, vol. 23, no. 1, pp. 135–138, 2009.

[5] F. Cavatorta, S. Campisi, and F. Fiorini, "Fatal pericardial tamponade by a guide wire during jugular catheter insertion," *Nephron*, vol. 79, no. 3, p. 352, 1998.

[6] P. G. Blake and R. Uldall, "Cardiac perforation by a guide wire during subclavian catheter insertion," *International Journal of Artificial Organs*, vol. 12, no. 2, pp. 111–113, 1989.

[7] K. Z. Khan, D. Graham, A. Ermenyi, and W. R. Pillay, "Case report: managing a knotted Seldinger wire in the subclavian vein during central venous cannulation," *Canadian Journal of Anesthesia*, vol. 54, no. 5, pp. 375–379, 2007.

[8] Z. Jankovic, A. Boon, and R. Prasad, "Fatal haemothorax following large-bore percutaneous cannulation before liver transplantation," *British Journal of Anaesthesia*, vol. 95, no. 4, pp. 472–476, 2005.

[9] F. Y. Vinces, T. V. Robb, K. Alapati et al., "J-tip spring guidewire entrapment by an inferior vena cava filter," *Journal of the American Osteopathic Association*, vol. 104, no. 2, pp. 87–89, 2004.

[10] S. Nanda and L. Strockoz-Scaff, "Images in clinical medicine. A complication of central venous catheterization," *The New England Journal of Medicine*, vol. 356, no. 21, article e22, 2007.

[11] E. Monaca, S. Trojan, J. Lynch, M. Doehn, and F. Wappler, "Broken guide wire—a fault of design?" *Canadian Journal of Anesthesia*, vol. 52, no. 8, pp. 801–804, 2005.

[12] W. Schummer, C. Schummer, E. Gaser, and R. Bartunek, "Loss of the guide wire: mishap or blunder?" *British Journal of Anaesthesia*, vol. 88, no. 1, pp. 144–146, 2002.

[13] M. Auweiler, S. Kampe, M. Zähringer et al., "The human error: delayed diagnosis of intravascular loss of guidewires for central venous catheterization," *Journal of Clinical Anesthesia*, vol. 17, no. 7, pp. 562–564, 2005.

[14] R. T. Andrews, D. A. Bova, and A. C. Venbrux, "How much guidewire is too much? Direct measurement of the distance from subclavian and internal jugular vein access sites to the superior vena cava- atrial junction during central venous catheter placement," *Critical Care Medicine*, vol. 28, no. 1, pp. 138–142, 2000.

16

Early Implementation of THAM for ICP Control: Therapeutic Hypothermia Avoidance and Reduction in Hypertonics/Hyperosmotics

F. A. Zeiler,[1] L. M. Gillman,[2,3] J. Teitelbaum,[4,5] and M. West[1]

[1]Section of Neurosurgery, Department of Surgery, University of Manitoba, Winnipeg, MB, Canada R3A 1R9
[2]Section of Critical Care Medicine, Department of Medicine, University of Manitoba, Winnipeg, MB, Canada R3A 1R9
[3]Section of General Surgery, Department of Surgery, University of Manitoba, Winnipeg, MB, Canada R3A 1R9
[4]Section of Neurocritical Care, Montreal Neurological Institute, McGill University, Montreal, QC, Canada H3A 2B4
[5]Section of Neurology, Montreal Neurological Institute, McGill University, Montreal, QC, Canada H3A 2B4

Correspondence should be addressed to F. A. Zeiler; umzeiler@cc.umanitoba.ca

Academic Editor: Nicolas Nin

Background. Tromethamine (THAM) has been demonstrated to reduce intracranial pressure (ICP). Early consideration for THAM may reduce the need for other measures for ICP control. *Objective.* To describe 4 cases of early THAM therapy for ICP control and highlight the potential to avoid TH and paralytics and achieve reduction in sedation and hypertonic/hyperosmotic agent requirements. *Methods.* We reviewed the charts of 4 patients treated with early THAM for ICP control. *Results.* We identified 2 patients with aneurysmal subarachnoid hemorrhage (SAH) and 2 with traumatic brain injury (TBI) receiving early THAM for ICP control. The mean time to initiation of THAM therapy was 1.8 days, with a mean duration of 5.3 days. In all patients, after 6 to 12 hours of THAM administration, ICP stability was achieved, with reduction in requirements for hypertonic saline and hyperosmotic agents. There was a relative reduction in mean hourly hypertonic saline requirements of 89.1%, 96.1%, 82.4%, and 97.0% for cases 1, 2, 3, and 4, respectively, comparing pre- to post-THAM administration. Mannitol, therapeutic hypothermia, and paralytics were avoided in all patients. *Conclusions.* Early administration of THAM for ICP control could potentially lead to the avoidance of other ICP directed therapies. Prospective studies of early THAM administration are warranted.

1. Introduction

Tromethamine (THAM) is a non-CO_2 generating buffer solution that has been utilized for a variety of clinical applications [1], including the control of intracranial pressure (ICP) [2–4]. Cerebral lactic acidosis after injury has been linked to edema formation and is postulated to be a major contributor to elevated intracranial pressures [5]. Attenuation of such acidosis via non-CO_2 buffer compounds, such as THAM, can allow stability in ICP and an overall reduction in pressure.

Both human and animal studies [6] exist demonstrating the ICP reduction effects of THAM [7]. Recent literature review of the human literature demonstrates an Oxford 2b, GRADE B level of evidence that THAM reduces ICP in traumatic brain injury (TBI) and stroke populations, with minimal adverse effects [8].

Other means of ICP reduction include therapeutic hypothermia (TH), involving external or intravascular cooling of the patient [9, 10]. Though effective in reduction of ICP, this method carries significant morbidity and complications [10]. Thus, if possible, avoidance of TH in ICP control is desired. Early implementation of THAM in patients with ICP issues may provide a treatment that can avoid TH and its inherent complications.

Within we describe 4 cases of patients with elevated ICP in which early administration of THAM led to avoidance of TH and paralytics and a reduction in sedation and hypertonic/hyperosmotic agent usage.

2. Methods

We retrospectively reviewed the charts of 4 patients who received early implementation of THAM therapy for elevated ICP. Data on patient demographics, admission diagnosis, THAM treatment characteristics, pre- and post-THAM hypertonic and hyperosmotic solution requirements, sedation requirements, and patient outcomes were recorded.

3. Results

3.1. THAM Treatment Characteristics. The THAM treatment protocol for all patients was the same. A 0.3 molar solution of THAM was administered, with a 2 mL/kg bolus over 1 hour, followed by a continuous infusion of 1 mL/kg/hr. The mean time to administration of THAM was 1.8 days after injury (range: 1–3 days). The mean duration of THAM therapy was 5.3 days (range: 3–7 days).

3.2. THAM Response

3.2.1. Case 1. A 62-year-old male was admitted after assault with a large right occipital hyperacute epidural hematoma. His initial Glasgow Coma Score (GCS) was 4T. He was emergently taken to the operative room for evacuation of the hematoma. An ICP monitor was placed intraoperatively.

During the first 12 hours postoperatively, his ICP became difficult to control ranging from 15 to 35 mm Hg, with multiple sustained elevations above 20 mm Hg. The total volume of hypertonic saline administered during this time was 840 mL, with the mean hourly 7.3% saline requirements at 44.2 mL/hr. The total amount of mannitol administered was 100 gm. The sedative requirements at this time were as follows: fentanyl 400 mcg/hr, midazolam 20 mg/hr, and propofol 5 mg/kg/hr.

We initiated THAM therapy 19 hours after his operation. Within 6 hours of initiation of THAM treatment, the fluctuations in his ICP above 20 mm Hg reduced dramatically, with 7.3% hypertonic saline administered only once (total volume of 140 mL) during the remainder of his hospital stay. The mean hourly 7.3% saline requirements after THAM were 4.8 mL/hr. No mannitol was required after THAM administration. Therapeutic hypothermia and paralytics were completely avoided. Sedative dosing remained unchanged. No complication related to THAM was identified during the 3 days of therapy.

Unfortunately, given the poor prognosis and magnetic resonance imaging evidence of brainstem and bilateral hemispheric watershed infarcts, it was elected by the family to withdrawal care.

3.2.2. Case 2. A 48-year-old male was admitted after falling down the stairs while intoxicated. His initial GCS on presentation was 5T, and CT of the head demonstrated small right occipital epidural hematoma secondary to a skull fracture over the transverse sinus. Also, there were significant bifrontal lobe contusions. He was admitted to the ICU, and an ICP monitor was placed.

The patient's initial ICP was 24 mm Hg, and prior to THAM therapy it ranged from 15 to 27 mm Hg. On postinjury day number 1, fentanyl was titrated to 150 mcg/hr, midazolam to 15 mg/hr, and propofol to 5 mg/kg/hr. A total of 280 mL of 7.3% hypertonic saline was utilized to control sustained ICP fluctuations above 20. On postinjury day number 2, ICP continued to climb requiring fentanyl at 350 mcg/hr, midazolam at 30 mg/hr, and propofol at 5 mg/kg/hr. The total volume of hypertonic saline utilized in this 24-hour period was 280 mL. On postinjury day number 3, propofol was discontinued due to increasing lactate and was replaced with ketamine at 35 mcg/kg/min. The ICP was increasingly hard to control throughout the day, requiring a total of 560 mL of hypertonic saline to control sustained fluctuations above 20 mm Hg. Over these 72 hours the patient averaged a 15.5 mL/hr of 7.3% hypertonic saline requirement. Thus, THAM therapy was initiated in attempt to avoid hypothermia and paralytics.

Within 12 hours of initiating THAM treatment, ICP fluctuations above 20 mm Hg reduced dramatically. The ICP post-THAM remained between 9 and 20 mm Hg. Over the following 72 hours of THAM therapy, a total of 420 mL of hypertonic saline was utilized (140 mL/day), for a mean 0.6 mL/hr requirement over this period. No mannitol was required post-THAM administration. Therapeutic hypothermia was completely avoided.

The patient was discontinued from THAM therapy after 4 days, was extubated, and eventually transferred to rehabilitation with only minor cognitive deficits. No complication related to THAM was identified.

3.2.3. Case 3. A 56-year-old female was admitted with a Fisher grade 4, Hunt and Hess grade 4 subarachnoid hemorrhage (SAH) secondary to an anterior communicating artery aneurysm. Initial GCS was 5T. After external ventricular drain (EVD) insertion, her GCS improved to 7T, with an opening pressure of 32. The EVD was venting 5–10 mL/hr, open at 20 cm above the tragus, for the duration of her stay in the intensive care unit (ICU). Tranexamic acid was started and continued for the first 72 hours of admission.

Over the first 18 hours of admission her ICP was managed as follows. Aggressive treatment of ICP was conducted utilizing the following sedation: fentanyl titrated to 300 mcg/hr, midazolam titrated to 20 mg/hr, and propofol titrated to 5 mg/kg/hr. Hypertonic saline (7.3%) was administered 3 times for ICP spikes above 20 mmHg, for a total volume of 420 mL. Her mean hourly hypertonic saline requirement was 26.7 mL/hr. Mannitol was given twice for a total of 100 gm, leaving serum osmolarity at 315.

At this point the patient was unable to tolerate lying flat for angiographic management of her ruptured aneurysm. Tromethamine was initiated to avoid hypothermia and paralytics. On postbleed day number 2, her hypertonic saline requirements stayed at 320 mL over the 24-hour period, but a significant reduction in ICP fluctuations above 20 was noted after 12 hours of THAM therapy, allowing a reduction of propofol to 3 mg/kg/hr and complete avoidance of mannitol. On postbleed day number 3, propofol was completely turned off, with ongoing avoidance of mannitol usage. The hypertonic saline requirement over the 24 hours was 140 mL. On postbleed day number 4, mannitol and propofol were avoided, and midazolam was reduced to 20 mg/kg. The total hypertonic requirement was 280 mL over the 24 hours. No further hypertonic saline was needed for postbleed days number 5 to 7. Her mean hourly hypertonic saline requirement after initiation of THAM was 4.7 mL/hr. No complication related to THAM was identified.

On postbleed day number 7, the patient had an acute spike in her ICP to 74, with bilateral blown pupils. Repeat computed tomography (CT) of the brain demonstrated a rebleed from the aneurysm. Sedation and treatment were withdrawn and the patient died. The THAM therapy was administered for a total of 7 days.

3.2.4. Case 4. A 43-year-old male was admitted on postbleed day number 4 with a Fisher grade 4, Hunt and Hess grade 3 SAH secondary to a left posterior communicating artery aneurysm. He presented clinical vasospasm of the left middle cerebral artery territory, with right hemineglect and dysphasia. Emergent microsurgical clipping of his aneurysm was completed with 6 hours of admission, and he was transferred to ICU postoperatively for management of his vasospasm. He had an ICP monitor placed intraoperatively.

He failed hypertensive therapy with mean arterial blood pressure (MABP) of 140 to 150 mm Hg, with no clinical improvement. Continuous intravenous milrinone therapy was initiated with complete resolution of his symptoms and MABP of 90 to 100 mm Hg.

The ICP was fluctuating from 18 to 31 mm Hg during the first 8 hours postoperatively. He received multiple doses of 7.3% hypertonic saline for a total of 700 mL, increasing his serum sodium to 154. The mean hourly hypertonic saline requirement was 87.5 mL/hr during this period prior to THAM. His serum osmolarity at that time was 315. Given the concerns overclouding his clinical exam with sedation during active treatment of symptomatic cerebral vasospasm post-SAH, we elected trial THAM therapy.

Within 6 hours of THAM administration the fluctuations in ICP above 20 were dramatically reduced with ICP ranging from 11 to 23 mm Hg. The requirements for hypertonic saline were reduced to 420 mL over the following 24 hours, after which no hypertonic saline was needed for ICP control during the remaining ICU course. Mannitol usage was avoided completely during THAM treatment. The THAM therapy was continued for a total of 7 days. The patient's mean hourly hypertonic saline requirement after initiation of THAM was 2.6 mL/hr. No complication related to THAM was identified.

At no point was sedation required to control ICP in this patient, thus preserving the neurological examination. On postbleed day number 7, the patient developed worsening focal deficits secondary to vasospasm, requiring angioplasty. These deficits would have likely been missed if on sedatives for ICP control at that time.

The patient eventually recovered from his deficits with mild expressive dysphasia and was transferred to stroke rehabilitation.

4. Discussion

The management of refractory elevated ICP is challenging. Despite maximal management with optimal patient positioning, control of pCO_2 hypertonic/hyperosmotic agents, intravenous sedatives, paralytics, and cerebrospinal fluid (CSF) diversion, ICP control can be difficult.

The use of TH in traumatic brain injury has been extensively investigated as a means of ICP control and neuroprotection [9, 10]. Though data on the impact of TH on patient outcome is unclear, the therapy is quite effective at reduction of increased ICP [9]. The caveat to TH is the complications associated with it implementation. Coagulopathy, hypotension, cardiac dysfunction, and infections complicate TH in all of its applications [10].

Tromethamine provides a non-CO_2 buffering of cerebral lactic acidosis in the setting of brain injury, leading to a reduction in edema formation and ICP reduction [1]. Though not standard front line therapy for elevated ICP, THAM carries the potential to stabilize ICP fluctuations and reduce the need for more aggressive measures, including paralytics and TH.

We reviewed 4 cases of early implementation of THAM for ICP control in 2 TBI and 2 SAH patients. Tromethamine was initiated at a mean of 1.8 days after injury, for a mean duration of 5.3 days. With this small experience we were able to avoid TH in all patients. Similarly, paralytic agents were avoided. After 6 to 12 hours of THAM infusion, significant reductions in the number of sustained ICP fluctuations above 20 mm Hg occurred in all patients. A dramatic reduction in the requirement of hypertonic saline was noted after the initiation of THAM in all patients. The relative reduction in the mean hourly hypertonic saline requirements pre-THAM compared to post-THAM was 89.1%, 96.1%, 82.4%, and 97.0% for cases 1, 2, 3, and 4, respectively. We were able to discontinue propofol usage in case 3, and completely avoid sedation in one patient (case 4) that was suffering from symptomatic cerebral vasospasm. No complications occurred related to THAM therapy. Two patients succumbed to their underlying neuropathology.

We believe this case series displays a few important and interesting findings. First, early implementation of THAM for ICP control is feasible. Second, a dramatic reduction in mean hourly hypertonic saline requirements was displayed in these 4 patients once THAM was initiated. However, this may not necessarily be the response in all patients, and our series only represents a select group. Third, a significant reduction in sustained ICP fluctuations above 20 mm Hg was noted. Fourth, TH and paralytic agents were avoided in all patients. However, given the small patient cohort, this is difficult to interpret. Fifth, sedation reduction was displayed in one SAH patient (case 3). Similarly, sedation avoidance was achieved in case 4, allowing preservation of the neurological examination during symptomatic post-SAH vasospasm. This afforded us the opportunity to determine deterioration of his neurological status leading to angioplasty therapy. Sixth, mannitol usage was avoided in all patients after THAM administration. Finally, no complications related to THAM therapy were identified.

Despite the interesting findings in this series, significant limitations to our study exist. First, the retrospective nature limits our ability to generalize our findings to all patients with elevated ICP. Second, we only have 4 patients in our series; thus our findings are based on a new institutional experience with early THAM for ICP control and may not reflect the experience in a larger series. Third, outcomes related to the underlying neuropathology did not reflect the positive results obtained in the other areas of these patients medical management of their ICP issues. Finally, there exists a significant potential for publication bias with our series given the positive results encountered.

Even though the limitations exist, as outlined, we still believe this study displays the potential that early THAM administration carries in the setting of ICP control. The trend towards reduction in hypertonic/hyperosmotic agent dosing, mannitol, and sedation and avoidance of TH and paralytics warrant further prospective evaluation of early THAM for ICP control in order to determine its effect on these factors. Similarly, the effect of early THAM therapy on patient outcome has yet to be determined.

5. Conclusions

Early THAM administration in the setting of increased ICP carries the potential for avoidance of TH and paralytics and a reduction in the volume of hypertonic/hyperosmotic agents and sedation requirements. Further prospective evaluation of early THAM for ICP control needs to occur.

References

[1] G. G. Nahas, K. M. Sutin, C. Fermon et al., "Guidelines for the treatment of acidemia with THAM," *Drugs*, vol. 55, no. 2, pp. 191–224, 1998.

[2] J. Bardutzky and S. Schwab, "Antiedema therapy in ischemic stroke," *Stroke*, vol. 38, no. 11, pp. 3084–3094, 2007.

[3] J. P. A. H. Jantzen, "Prevention and treatment of intracranial hypertension," *Best Practice & Research Clinical Anaesthesiology*, vol. 21, no. 4, pp. 517–538, 2007.

[4] E. Jüttler, P. D. Schellinger, A. Aschoff, K. Zweckberger, A. Unterberg, and W. Hacke, "Clinical review: therapy for refractory intracranial hypertension in ischaemic stroke," *Critical Care*, vol. 11, no. 5, article 231, 2007.

[5] N. D. Tran, S. Kim, H. K. Vincent et al., "Aquaporin-1-mediated cerebral edema following traumatic brain injury: effects of acidosis and corticosteroid administration," *Journal of Neurosurgery*, vol. 112, no. 5, pp. 1095–1104, 2010.

[6] S. E. Duthie, G. D. Goulin, M. H. Zornow, M. S. Scheller, and B. M. Peterson, "Effects of THAM and sodium bicarbonate on intracranial pressure and mean arterial pressure in an animal model of focal cerebral injury," *Journal of Neurosurgical Anesthesiology*, vol. 6, no. 3, pp. 201–208, 1994.

[7] A. L. Wolf, L. Levi, A. Marmarou et al., "Effect of THAM upon outcome in severe head injury: a randomized prospective clinical trial," *Journal of Neurosurgery*, vol. 78, no. 1, pp. 54–59, 1993.

[8] F. A. Zeiler, J. Teitelbaum, L. M. Gillman, and M. West, "THAM for control of ICP," *Neurocrit Care*, vol. 21, no. 2, pp. 332–344, 2014.

[9] S. Crossley, J. Reid, R. McLatchie et al., "A systematic review of therapeutic hypothermia for adult patients following traumatic brain injury," *Critical Care*, vol. 18, no. 2, article R75, 2014.

[10] N. Badjatia, "Hypothermia in neurocritical care," *Neurosurgery Clinics of North America*, vol. 24, no. 3, pp. 457–467, 2013.

17

Intravenous Lormetazepam during Sedation Weaning in a 26-Year-Old Critically Ill Woman

Alawi Luetz, Bjoern Weiss, and Claudia D. Spies

Department of Anesthesiology and Intensive Care Medicine, Charité-Universitätsmedizin Berlin,
Campus Charité Mitte and Campus Virchow-Klinikum, Augustenburger Platz 1, 13353 Berlin, Germany

Correspondence should be addressed to Alawi Luetz; alawi.luetz@charite.de

Academic Editor: Michael J. Cawley

Recent evidence revealed that sedation is related to adverse outcomes including a higher mortality. Despite this fact, patients sometimes require deep sedation for a limited period of time to control, for example, intracranial hypertension. In particular in these cases, weaning from sedation is often challenging due to emerging agitation, stress, and delirium. The submitted research letter reports a rare case of severe and persisting agitation that was unresponsive to all available treatments. Ultimately, lormetazepam which has recently become available for intravenous use in Germany resolved the problem by stress-reduction and anxiolysis without leading to measurable sedation.

1. Introduction

Sedation in critically ill patients is associated with an increased risk of death within 6 months [1, 2]. Administering drugs with stress-reducing and anxiolytic effects is often necessary to ensure that the patient is calm, alert, and attentive. Despite this fact, patients sometimes require deep sedation for a limited period of time to control, for example, intracranial hypertension or tolerate prone positioning. In particular in these cases, weaning from sedation is often challenging due to agitation, stress, and additional symptoms that may be associated with delirium.

2. Case Presentation

The 26-year-old, female, patient was admitted to our intensive care unit (ICU) from an external hospital, suffering from severe acute respiratory distress syndrome due to community-acquired pneumonia. At the time of admission, she was mechanically ventilated and deeply sedated (Richmond Agitation Sedation Scale (RASS) −5) with continuous infusion of midazolam and propofol. Analgesia was performed with continuous infusion of sufentanil. Beside starting an empiric antimicrobial therapy, we used prone positioning to stabilise oxygenation. After clinical situation

regarding respiration had improved, we initiated daily spontaneous awakening trials (SATs). However, during SATs, the patient was severely agitated (RASS +3) and delirious (confusion assessment method for the ICU (CAM-ICU) positive) and required immediate deep sedation due to respiratory deterioration.

During the SATs the Behavioural Pain Scale was always <6. We initiated a symptom-oriented therapy for delirium with haloperidol and clonidine without remarkable success.

A computerised tomography scan (day 5) showed an infarction of the right cerebellar hemisphere and signs of increased intracranial pressure which made a constant deep sedation necessary. Furthermore, the patient suffered from a pulmonary reinfection with a consecutive CO_2-retention. Therefore, an extracorporeal lung-assist (pECLA) was necessary to optain normocapnia and control intracranial pressure consecutively. After improvement of the clinical situation, we restarted daily SATs. Following, we faced the same problem of severe agitation. Symptom-oriented treatment of delirium was continued with haloperidol and alpha-2-agonists (clonidine followed by dexmedetomidine).

A cranial magnetic resonance imaging showed residues of very small cortical and subcortical bleedings which were classified to be of septic-embolic pathogenesis. However, in accordance with our neurosurgeons and neurologists,

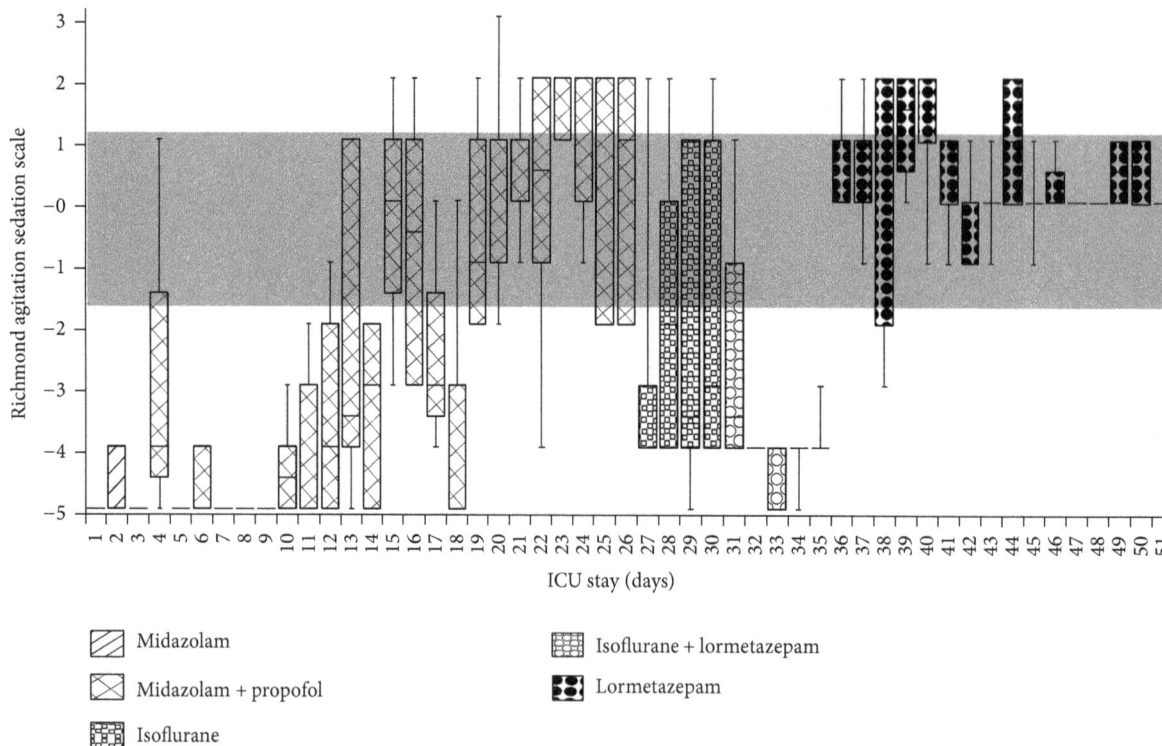

FIGURE 1: Levels of sedation and agitation. Measurement with the Richmond Agitation Sedation Scale (RASS) during intensive care unit treatment. The shadow indicates RASS −1 to 0 (no sedation). Analgesia was performed with continious infusion of sufentanil until discharge from our intensive care unit.

these findings could not explain agitated delirium during the SATs. A lumbar puncture revealed no pathological findings.

In order to stop propofol infusion and to reduce admnistration of midazolam, we perfomed inhalative sedation with isoflurane (day 27). Although we were able to stop propofol and midazolam infusion, we were not able to achieve a RASS between −2 and +1.

On day 31 after ICU admission, we started intravenous administration of lormetazepam which is newly available for iv use in Germany. The initial infusion rate was 0.36 μg/kg/hr. Even though the patient was less agitated during SATs, we still measured RASS peaks of >1. Consequently, we increased the amount of continuously administered lormetazepam which lead to a constant improvement. On day 36, the patient had a RASS of 0 for several hours (Figure 1). At this time, the patient received continuous lormetazepam infusion with an unexpected high dose of 33 mg/day (Figure 2), dexmedetomidine infusion of 1.4 μh/kg/hr, and 3 × 2 mg haloperidol intravenously. Even though the patient was still CAM-ICU positive but not agitated, we started weaning the patient from the ventilator. Furthermore, we reduced administration of dexmedetomidine and sufentanil about 10% per day. In order to maintain a RASS of 0 to −1, lormetazepam infusion had to be increased to a maximum dose of 39 mg/day (Figure 2). Because of the persistent positive CAM-ICU, we decided to use quetiapine instead of haloperidol for antipsychotic therapy. Within the next 2 weeks, the patient was successfully weaned from the respirator. With ICU discharge (day 51), sufentanil and dexmedetomidine infusion were stopped.

After 3 consecutive days without delirium, antipsychotic therapy was stopped as well. Two milligrams of lormetazepam was administered orally every 8 hours.

No obvious relationship between an increase of liver enzymes and the administration of lormetazepam was determined. In fact, blood concentrations of the alanine transaminase (ALT) and the gamma-glutamyl transpeptidase (GGT) tended to decrease with the start of lormetazepam infusion (Figure 3). Blood concentrations of the aspartate transaminase (AST), creatinine, and urea were normal during all times of lormetazepam infusion.

3. Discussion

Since 2009, intravenous lormetazepam is approved for anxiolysis and sedation in critically ill patients in Germany. Unlike many other hypnotics, the distribution of lormetazepam is associated with less alteration of rapid eye movement sleep [3]. Furthermore, lormetazepam showed superior anxiolytic properties compared to other benzodiazepines when used for premedication [4]. Lormetazepam is metabolised independently from cytochrome-P450 enzymes and inactivated by glucoronidation. The resulting inactive metabolites are renally excreted afterwards. The elimination half-life of lormetazepam after intravenous administration is therefore constantly 8–12 hours and shorter than the half-life of lorazepam.

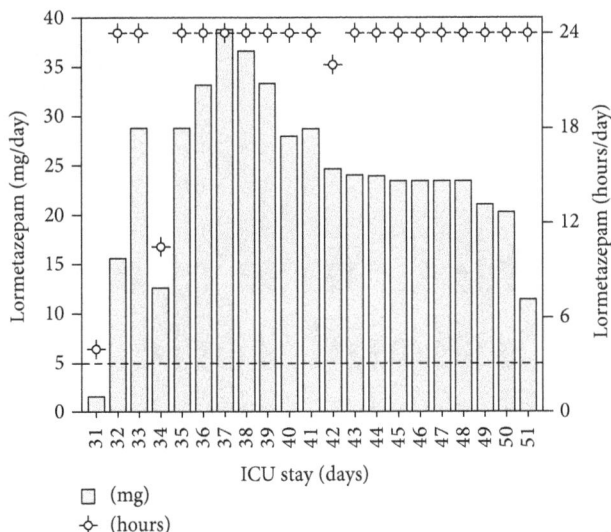

FIGURE 2: Duration and amount of intravenous administered lormetazepam per day. mg = milligram.

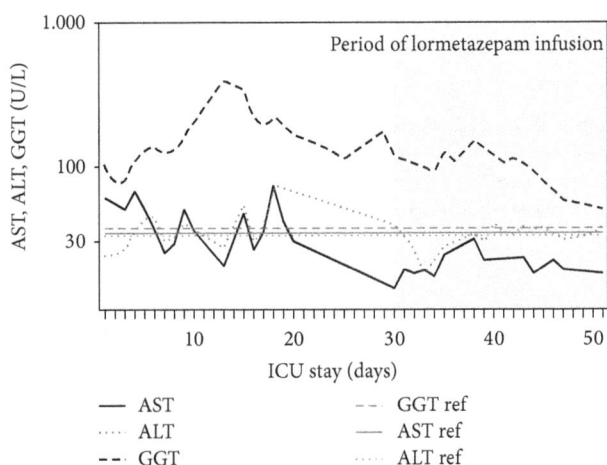

FIGURE 3: Blood concentrations of different liver enzymes during ICU treatment. (AST, aspartate transaminase; ALT, alanine transaminase; GGT, gamma-glutamyl transpeptidase). The grey lines (GGT ref, AST ref, and ALT ref) indicate the upper threshold levels for the corresponding enzymes; ref = reference.

In our case, lormetazepam was able to sufficiently treat agitation without sedating the patient (RASS > −2). Clinically, it seemed that lormetazepam caused predominantly anxiolytic effects accompanied by an improved navigability of the drug.

From the pharmacodynamic point of view, benzodiazepines act by indirect activation of the $GABA_A$ receptor that either enhance or reduce the inhibitory effects of GABA [5]. The majority of brain $GABA_A$ receptors contain α-, β-, and γ-subunits. Studies could show that variations in the α-subunit are the main determinants of benzodiazepines pharmacology. Löw and colleagues could show that the anxiolytic effect of benzodiazepines is mediated by α_2-$GABA_A$ receptors but not by α_3-$GABA_A$ receptors [6]. Because nonselective benzodiazepines, exemplified by diazepam, act by enhancing

the inhibitory effects of GABA at (A) receptors containing either an α_1, α_2, α_3, or α_5 subunit, such compounds possess a relatively narrow window between doses that produce anxiolysis and those that cause sedation. That is probably why, in the clinical setting, the proven anxiolytic efficacy of benzodiazepines is often superimposed by their sedative effect. A hypothesis for the different clinical effect of lormetazepam compared to lorazepam and midazolam might be that lormetazepam exerts its effect by α_2-$GABA_A$-receptor-agonistic activity, which is likely to be responsible for the antianxiety-like effects of benzodiazepines.

Although we needed remarkable higher daily doses as recommended by the manufacturer, continuous, intravenous administration of lormetazepam was safe, without any observed side effects, related to the drug.

Randomized controlled trials are needed to investigate whether administration of lormetazepam compared to othere benzodiazepines can be benificial for the ICU patient.

Authors' Contribution

All listed authors made substantial contributions to conception and design, acquisition of data, analysis and interpretation of data, drafting the paper, revising it critically for important intellectual content, and final approval of the version to be published.

Acknowledgments

Alawi Luetz is participant in the Charité Clinical Scientist Program funded by the Charité-Universitätsmedizin Berlin and the Berlin Institute of Health.

References

[1] Y. Shehabi, R. Bellomo, M. C. Reade et al., "Early intensive care sedation predicts long-term mortality in ventilated critically ill patients," *The American Journal of Respiratory and Critical Care Medicine*, vol. 186, no. 8, pp. 724–731, 2012.

[2] P. L. Watson, A. K. Shintani, R. Tyson, P. P. Pandharipande, B. T. Pun, and E. W. Ely, "Presence of electroencephalogram burst suppression in sedated, critically ill patients is associated with increased mortality," *Critical Care Medicine*, vol. 36, no. 12, pp. 3171–3177, 2008.

[3] W. M. Hermann, L. Holler, and C. Haag, "On the distribution of REM and NREM sleep under two benzodiazepines with comparable receptor affinity but different kinetics properties," *Pharmacopsychiatry*, vol. 20, no. 6, pp. 270–277, 1987.

[4] C.-J. Jakobsen, J.-J. Jensen, W. Hansen, and N. Grabe, "Oral lormetazepam in premedication: a comparison with diazepam," *Anaesthesia*, vol. 41, no. 8, pp. 870–873, 1986.

[5] W. Sieghart and G. Sperk, "Subunit composition, distribution and function of GABA(A) receptor subtypes," *Current Topics in Medicinal Chemistry*, vol. 2, no. 8, pp. 795–816, 2002.

[6] K. Löw, F. Crestani, R. Keist et al., "Molecular and neuronal substrate for the selective attenuation of anxiety," *Science*, vol. 290, no. 5489, pp. 131–134, 2000.

18

Spinal Cord Infarction in the Course of a Septic Shock: About One Case and Review of the Literature

P. Henin, A. Molderez, V. Huberlant, and H. Trine

Groupe Jolimont, Centre Hospitalier de Jolimont, 159 rue Ferrer, 7100 Haine Saint Paul, Belgium

Correspondence should be addressed to V. Huberlant; vhuberlant@hotmail.com

Academic Editor: Kurt Lenz

We report the case of a patient admitted to our intensive care unit in the course of a septic shock, secondary to cholangitis. After rapid hemodynamic stabilization, antibiotherapy, and endoscopic extraction of bile ducts stones, she appeared to have developed flaccid paraplegia. The suspected diagnosis of medullar ischemia was confirmed by typical MRI findings. This case stresses the potential pathogenic role of hypotension in medullar ischemia and the place of magnetic resonance imaging (MRI) as a reliable diagnostic tool.

1. Introduction

Medullar ischemia is a rare and severe condition [1] that can lead to death or persistent paraplegia [2–4].

Its most usual etiologies are thoracoabdominal aortic surgery, trauma, or cardiovascular diseases. It can also be due to deep hypotension and global ischemia [4–6].

We report a seldom case of medullar ischemia occurring in the course of a septic shock. We also describe the typical magnetic resonance imaging (MRI) findings, most accurate tool for diagnosis confirmation [1, 3, 4, 7–10].

2. Case Report

A 55-year-old Caucasian woman was admitted through the Emergency Room with severe abdominal pain and dehydration. Her main past medical history included diabetes, active alcoholism, smoking, chronic pancreatitis, and hypercholesterolemia. She had a recent episode of acute on chronic alcoholic pancreatitis, with transient acute renal failure. She was transferred to our intensive care unit in septic shock with severe hypotension (MAP < 40 mmHg at the time of admission) and transient sinus bradycardia.

She also had fever, clinical jaundice, and peripheral signs of hypoperfusion. The neurological exam showed impaired consciousness but no motor or sensitive deficit.

Laboratory data showed lactic metabolic acidosis, acute renal failure, and cholestasis. There was no coagulation disorder.

An abdominal CT scan showed hepatic steatosis, pancreatic calcifications, gallbladder hydrops and lithiasis, and enlargement of the extrahepatic bile ducts. Ultrasonography confirmed the suspected diagnosis of cholangitis: enlargement of the choledochus (12 mm), occluded in its distal part by a 9 mm lithiasis.

Within the first hour, the MAP was restored to normal range (>65 mmHg). She received empirical antibiotherapy (Amoxicillin-Clavulanate) and an urgent ERCP was performed, with successful extraction of the common bile duct stone.

On the next day, her clinical exam confirmed the recovery of stable hemodynamic parameters, with normal urine output. Lactic acidosis was corrected, and renal function and liver enzymes were improving.

Unfortunately, the patient appeared to have developed complete flaccid paraplegia. A thorough neurological exam showed a sensory (pain and temperature) and motor deficit at T10 level and loss of sphincter control. We suspected spinal cord ischemia.

Somatosensory evoked potentials were compatible with that diagnosis.

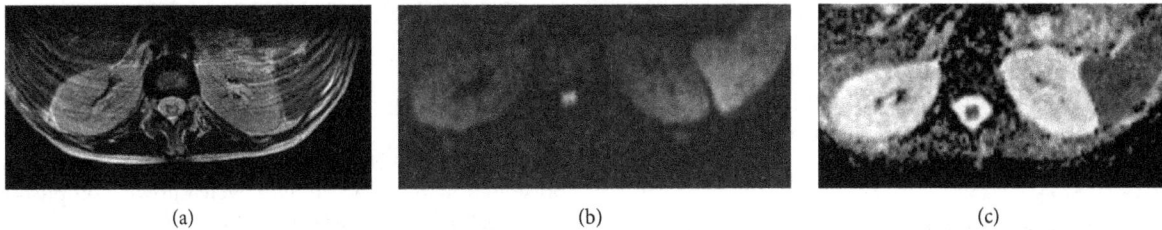

FIGURE 1: (a) The sagittal T2-weighted image shows a hyperintense lesion of the conus medullaris. (b) High signal is observed at the corresponding level on axial DWI. (c) Low ADC value on the ADC map confirmed the hypothesis of spinal cord infarction.

MRI demonstrated on the sagittal T2-weighted image a hyperintense lesion of the conus medullaris and high signal was observed at the corresponding level on axial DWI (Diffusion Weighted Imaging); low ADC (Apparent Diffusion Coefficient) value on the ADC map confirmed the hypothesis of spinal cord infarction (Figure 1).

The patient remained stable and further recovered from all her biological disorders. Bacteriology remained negative and antibiotics were discontinued on day 5.

Unfortunately, apart from discrete contraction of the proximal muscles of the right leg, the patient did not recover from her neurologic disorder and had persistent flaccid paraplegia, abolition of temperature and pain sensitivity, and sphincter dysfunction, despite thorough multidisciplinary rehabilitation.

She died a few months later in the rehabilitation center, in the course of an acute myocardial infarct.

3. Discussion

Acute onset of paraplegia is rarely seen in the ICU setting. The differential diagnosis will mainly be orientated by clinical context: recent history of trauma, lumbar or epidural puncture, recent aortic surgery, recent history of hemodynamic instability (shock or global hypoperfusion), cardiovascular comorbidities, especially with thromboembolic events, anticoagulant therapies, systemic inflammatory diseases, or cancers.

We can distinguish extramedullar and medullar etiologies.

Extramedullar etiologies include polyradiculitis (Guillain-Barre syndrome) [11] or can be part of the clinical manifestations of ion disorders [12] like hyperkaliemia or hypercalcemia. Their onset will usually be more subacute. Psychogenic disorders can also mimic paraplegia [13].

Medullar etiologies are more relevant to our discussion. They can be traumatic: vertebral trauma with cord lesion [14], through mechanisms of transection, compression, contusion, or vascular compromise, and spinal epidural bleeding after puncture [15].

Medullar etiologies can also be nontraumatic: medullar ischemia or thromboembolism, as discussed in this case report, spinal bleeding, spontaneous [16] or under anticoagulant therapy [17], tumor, or abscess compression [18, 19].

Other nontraumatic medullar etiologies of paraplegia can be seen, but their course is usually more subacute, not as sudden as in our case, and will often be part of a more complex clinical situation: hepatic myelopathy in liver cirrhosis [20], paraneoplastic necrotizing myelopathy [21], systemic inflammatory diseases like multiple sclerosis or sarcoidosis [22–24], or infectious diseases like viral or bacterial myelitis (e.g., Lyme's disease or CMV). Some (around 15%) cases of transverse myelitis remain unclear and are referred to as idiopathic [25].

Medullar ischemia is a rare diagnosis [1]. Its incidence is difficult to evaluate and few series are published [1–7, 9, 10, 26–28]. Anterior spinal artery syndrome (ASAS) is the most usual clinical presentation [1]. This syndrome results from an infarction of the anterior two-thirds of the spinal cord. The midthoracic level is usually seen as the watershed zone for ischemic vulnerability, but some authors argue that lower (lumbar or lumbosacral) levels seem most vulnerable to global ischemic events [4, 29].

The common symptoms are sudden weakness under the level of ischemia, flaccid paraplegia, areflexia, urinary bladder and anal sphincter dysfunction, and loss of pain and temperature perception without proprioceptive disorder (no involvement of the posterior third of the spinal cord) [4]. The onset is usually sudden, with maximal impairment often reached within the first hour [10]. Severity of impairment can be defined using the American Spinal Injury Association (ASIA) scoring [8] as follows:

(1) Complete: no motor or sensory function is found in the lowest sacral segment (S4-S5).

(2) Incomplete: sensory function is found below neurologic level and in S4-S5; no motor function is found below neurologic level.

(3) Incomplete: motor function is preserved below neurologic level and more than half of the key muscle groups below neurologic level have a muscle grade less than 3.

(4) Incomplete: motor function is preserved below neurologic level and at least half of the key muscle groups below neurologic level have a muscle grade greater than 3.

(5) Normal: sensory and motor function is normal.

Initial impairment can be mild (ASIA scoring C or D), in about 40 to 50% of all cases, moderate (ASIA B), or severe (ASIA A), each around 25% [5, 10].

Etiologies of ASAS are multiple. The most common causes are surgery of the thoracoabdominal aorta, trauma, all vascular disorders like thromboembolism and inflammatory diseases, and global hypoxic-ischemic events such as cardiac arrest or severe hypotension [4, 9, 10]. Cardiovascular risk factors such as hypertension are common among patients with ASAS [2, 5, 7].

The best diagnostic tool for ASAS is neuroimaging with MRI. The typical findings are focal cord swelling with increased T2 signal in the central part of the spinal cord and in DWI (Diffusion Weighted Imaging), an increased medullar signal associated with a low ADC (Apparent Diffusion Coefficient) value [6, 10–12, 30].

The prognosis of ASAS is variable and can range from full recovery to long term persistence of complete paraplegia, loss of sensitivity, sphincter dysfunction, and chronic pain. The percentage of different outcomes is difficult to evaluate, depending on the author and because of the relatively small size of published series [1–7, 9, 10, 26–28, 31]. Death occurs in less than 10% [1, 5, 6] to more than 20% [9] of cases. Complete or satisfactory (ambulatory) recovery seems to occur in 25% of the survivors according to the pessimistic [9] and up to more than 50% according to the optimistic authors [1, 2]. Complete persistent impairment (wheelchair dependence, bladder catheter, loss of sensitivity, and chronic pain) also ranges from 20 [5] to more than 50% [9], depending on authors. The remaining patients will have partial recovery and a mix of motor, sensory, and autonomic sequelae.

Recovery occurs mainly in the first 2 to 4 weeks [4], but meaningful improvement can occur after several months in a significant minority of cases [10].

All authors agree that severity of the initial impairment is associated with a poor outcome [2, 4, 6, 9, 10]. The correlation between age at onset and outcome is disputed. Some authors find a better prognosis in younger patients [10], while others describe a poorer prognosis below age of 55 years [2].

Severe hypotension is a recognized etiological factor of spinal cord ischemia [29, 32], and our case shows the potential deleterious consequences of sepsis related shock on medullar perfusion. It stresses the importance of quickly restoring a MAP above 65 mmHg according to the surviving sepsis campaign guidelines [33], especially in patients with cardiovascular risk factors, in order to prevent, among other complications, medullar ischemia.

There is no specific therapy for ASAS. Treatment in the acute phase is thus mainly supportive. Selective injection of Dexamethasone and Urokinase in the Adamkiewicz artery (arteria radicularis magna) has been proposed in a small group of 3 patients [28].

During thoracoabdominal aortic surgery, lumbar CSF drainage can be used to protect medullar perfusion. The rationale is to maintain a spinal perfusion pressure (MAP − intrathecal pressure) above 70 to 80 mmHg, by supporting hemodynamics and draining CSF to maintain intrathecal pressure below 10 mmHg [34].

Other techniques are proposed in order to reduce the incidence of perioperative medullar ischemia, such as perioperative somatosensory evoked potentials [35], induced hypothermia [36], intrathecal papaverine [37], or epidural cooling [38].

4. Conclusion

Spinal ischemia is a severe condition. Its most common presentation is ASAS. It is a well known complication of thoracoabdominal surgery but can also result from traumatic, cardiovascular, or systemic disorders and from severe hypotension and global ischemia.

Its onset is sudden, and its prognosis is variable, from recovery to persistent paraplegia or death.

A severe initial impairment is related to a poorer prognosis, but recovery can occur even in severe cases, and delayed recoveries are not exceptional.

This case report shows the potential consequences of septic shock on medullar perfusion and stresses the importance of rapidly restoring MAP, according to the surviving sepsis campaign.

It also shows the key diagnostic role of MRI and its typical findings in cases of ASAS.

Competing Interests

The authors declare no conflict of interests.

References

[1] T. A. Sandson and J. H. Friedman, "Spinal cord infarction. Report of 8 cases and review of the literature," *Medicine (Baltimore)*, vol. 68, no. 5, pp. 282–292, 1989.

[2] K. Nedeltchev, T. J. Loher, F. Stepper et al., "Long-term outcome of acute spinal cord ischemia syndrome," *Stroke*, vol. 35, no. 2, pp. 560–565, 2004.

[3] C. Masson, J. P. Pruvo, J. F. Meder et al., "Spinal cord infarction: clinical and magnetic resonance imaging findings and short term outcome," *Journal of Neurology, Neurosurgery and Psychiatry*, vol. 75, no. 10, pp. 1431–1435, 2004.

[4] S. Salvador de la Barrera, A. Barca-Buyo, A. Montoto-Marqués, M. E. Ferreiro-Velasco, M. Cidoncha-Dans, and A. Rodriguez-Sotillo, "Spinal cord infarction: prognosis and recovery in a series of 36 patients," *Spinal Cord*, vol. 39, no. 10, pp. 520–525, 2001.

[5] W. P. Cheshire, C. C. Santos, E. W. Massey, and J. F. Howard Jr., "Spinal cord infarction: etiology and outcome," *Neurology*, vol. 47, no. 2, pp. 321–330, 1996.

[6] C. E. Robertson, R. D. Brown Jr., E. F. M. Wijdicks, and A. A. Rabinstein, "Recovery after spinal cord infarcts: long-term outcome in 115 patients," *Neurology*, vol. 78, no. 2, pp. 114–121, 2012.

[7] S. Weidauer, M. Nichtweiss, H. Lanfermann, and F. E. Zanella, "Spinal cord infarction: MR imaging and clinical features in 16 cases," *Neuroradiology*, vol. 44, no. 10, pp. 851–857, 2002.

[8] American Spinal Injury Association, *International Standards for Neurological Classification of Spinal Cord Injury*, American Spinal Injury Association, Chicago, Ill, USA, 2002.

[9] M.-Y. Cheng, R.-K. Lyu, Y.-J. Chang et al., "Spinal cord infarction in Chinese patients: clinical features, risk factors, imaging and prognosis," *Cerebrovascular Diseases*, vol. 26, no. 5, pp. 502–508, 2008.

[10] J. Novy, A. Carruzzo, P. Maeder, and J. Bogousslavsky, "Spinal cord ischemia: clinical and imaging patterns, pathogenesis, and outcomes in 27 patients," *Archives of Neurology*, vol. 63, no. 8, pp. 1113–1120, 2006.

[11] T. Solomon and H. Willison, "Infectious causes of acute flaccid paralysis," *Current Opinion in Infectious Diseases*, vol. 16, no. 5, pp. 375–381, 2003.

[12] S. Evers, A. Engelien, V. Karsch, and M. Hund, "Secondary hyperkalaemic paralysis," *Journal of Neurology Neurosurgery and Psychiatry*, vol. 64, no. 2, pp. 249–252, 1998.

[13] J. Stone, C. Warlow, and M. Sharpe, "The symptom of functional weakness: a controlled study of 107 patients," *Brain*, vol. 133, no. 5, pp. 1537–1551, 2010.

[14] J. R. Chapman and P. A. Anderson, "Thoracolumbar spine fractures with neurologic deficit," *Orthopedic Clinics of North America*, vol. 25, no. 4, pp. 595–612, 1994.

[15] M. T. Pitkänen, U. Aromaa, D. A. Cozanitis, and J. G. Förster, "Serious complications associated with spinal and epidural anaesthesia in Finland from 2000 to 2009," *Acta Anaesthesiologica Scandinavica*, vol. 57, no. 5, pp. 553–564, 2013.

[16] R. H. Thiele, Z. A. Hage, D. L. Surdell, S. L. Ondra, H. H. Batjer, and B. R. Bendok, "Spontaneous spinal epidural hematoma of unknown etiology: case report and literature review," *Neurocritical Care*, vol. 9, no. 2, pp. 242–246, 2008.

[17] J. Furlan, G. W. Hawryluk, J. Austin, and M. G. Fehlings, "Spinal haemorrhage during anticoagulant regimen for thromboprophylaxis: a unique form of central nervous system haemorrhage," *Journal of Neurology, Neurosurgery and Psychiatry*, vol. 83, no. 7, pp. 746–752, 2012.

[18] R. J. Sevick and C. J. Wallace, "MR imaging of neoplasms of the lumbar spine," *Magnetic Resonance Imaging Clinics of North America*, vol. 7, no. 3, pp. 539–553, 1999.

[19] R. O. Darouiche, "Spinal epidural abscess," *New England Journal of Medicine*, vol. 355, no. 19, pp. 2012–2020, 2006.

[20] R. Nardone, T. Buratti, A. Oliviero, A. Lochmann, and F. Tezzon, "Corticospinal involvement in patients with a portosystemic shunt due to liver cirrhosis: A MEP Study," *Journal of Neurology*, vol. 253, no. 1, pp. 81–85, 2006.

[21] V. J. Ojeda, "Necrotizing myelopathy associated with malignancy. A clinicopathologic study of two cases and literature review," *Cancer*, vol. 53, no. 5, pp. 1115–1123, 1984.

[22] R. Bakshi, P. R. Kinkel, L. L. Mechtler et al., "Magnetic resonance imaging findings in 22 cases of myelitis: comparison between patients with and without multiple sclerosis," *European Journal of Neurology*, vol. 5, no. 1, pp. 35–48, 1998.

[23] M. Harzheim, U. Schlegel, H. Urbach, T. Klockgether, and S. Schmidt, "Discriminatory features of acute transverse myelitis: a retrospective analysis of 45 patients," *Journal of the Neurological Sciences*, vol. 217, no. 2, pp. 217–223, 2004.

[24] S. Saleh, C. Saw, K. Marzouk, and O. Sharma, "Sarcoidosis of the spinal cord: literature review and report of eight cases," *Journal of the National Medical Association*, vol. 98, no. 6, pp. 965–974, 2006.

[25] J. De Seze, C. Lanctin, C. Lebrun et al., "Idiopathic acute transverse myelitis: application of the recent diagnostic criteria," *Neurology*, vol. 65, no. 12, pp. 1950–1953, 2005.

[26] M. Shinoyama, T. Takahashi, H. Shimizu, T. Tominaga, and M. Suzuki, "Spinal cord infarction demonstrated by diffusion-weighted magnetic resonance imaging," *Journal of Clinical Neuroscience*, vol. 12, no. 4, pp. 466–468, 2005.

[27] R. G. Nogueira, R. Ferreira, P. E. Grant et al., "Restricted diffusion in spinal cord infarction demonstrated by magnetic resonance line scan diffusion imaging," *Stroke*, vol. 43, no. 2, pp. 532–535, 2012.

[28] H. Baba, K. Tomita, T. Kawagishi, and S. Imura, "Anterior spinal artery syndrome," *International Orthopaedics*, vol. 17, no. 6, pp. 353–356, 1993.

[29] N. Duggal and B. Lach, "Selective vulnerability of the lumbosacral spinal cord after cardiac arrest and hypotension," *Stroke*, vol. 33, no. 1, pp. 116–121, 2002.

[30] M. M. Thurnher and R. Bammer, "Diffusion-weighted MR imaging (DWI) in spinal cord ischemia," *Neuroradiology*, vol. 48, no. 11, pp. 795–801, 2006.

[31] E. Iseli, A. Cavigelli, V. Dietz, and A. Curt, "Prognosis and recovery in ischaemic and traumatic spinal cord injury: clinical and electrophysiological evaluation," *Journal of Neurology Neurosurgery and Psychiatry*, vol. 67, no. 5, pp. 567–571, 1999.

[32] C.-C. Lin, S.-Y. Chen, C. Lan, T. Ting-Fang Shih, M.-C. Lin, and J.-S. Lai, "Spinal cord infarction caused by cardiac tamponade," *American Journal of Physical Medicine and Rehabilitation*, vol. 81, no. 1, pp. 68–71, 2002.

[33] R. P. Dellinger, M. M. Levy, A. Rhodes et al., "Surviving sepsis campaign: international guidelines for management of severe sepsis and septic shock: 2012," *Critical Care Medicine*, vol. 41, no. 2, pp. 580–637, 2013.

[34] H. Takayama and M. A. Borger, "Preventing spinal cord injury during thoracic aortic surgery: simpler than we thought?" *Journal of Thoracic and Cardiovascular Surgery*, vol. 149, no. 1, pp. 366–368, 2015.

[35] J. D. Galla, M. A. Ergin, S. L. Lansman et al., "Use of somatosensory evoked potentials for thoracic and thoracoabdominal aortic resections," *Annals of Thoracic Surgery*, vol. 67, no. 6, pp. 1947–1952, 1999.

[36] G. Di Luozzo, "Visceral and spinal cord protection during thoracoabdominal aortic aneurysm repair: clinical and laboratory update," *Journal of Thoracic and Cardiovascular Surgery*, vol. 145, no. 3S, pp. S135–S138, 2013.

[37] B. Lima, E. R. Nowicki, E. H. Blackstone et al., "Spinal cord protective strategies during descending and thoracoabdominal aortic aneurysm repair in the modern era: the role of intrathecal papaverine," *Journal of Thoracic and Cardiovascular Surgery*, vol. 143, no. 4, pp. 945–952.e1, 2012.

[38] R. P. Cambria, J. K. Davison, C. Carter et al., "Epidural cooling for spinal cord protection during thoracoabdominal aneurysm repair: a five-year experience," *Journal of Vascular Surgery*, vol. 31, no. 6, pp. 1093–1102, 2000.

19

Management of Calcium Channel Antagonist Overdose with Hyperinsulinemia-Euglycemia Therapy: Case Series and Review of the Literature

Shiwan K. Shah,[1] Sanjeev Kumar Goswami,[2] Rajesh V. Babu,[2] Gulshan Sharma,[2] and Alexander G. Duarte[2]

[1] *Department of Internal Medicine and Pediatrics, University of Texas Medical Branch, 301 University Boulevard, Route 0354, Gaveston, TX 77555, USA*
[2] *Department of Pulmonary, Allergy, and Critical Care, University of Texas Medical Branch, Gaveston, TX 77555, USA*

Correspondence should be addressed to Shiwan K. Shah, skshah@utmb.edu

Academic Editors: P. Kopterides and K. Lenz

Calcium channel antagonists (CCAs) are commonly involved in drug overdoses. Standard approaches to the management of CCA overdoses, including fluid resuscitation, gut decontamination, administration of calcium, glucagon, and atropine, as well as supportive care, are often ineffective. We report on two patients who improved after addition of hyperinsulinemia-euglycemia (HIE) therapy. We conclude with a literature review on hyperinsulinemia-euglycemia therapy with an exploration of the physiology behind its potential use.

1. Introduction

Calcium channel antagonists (CCAs) are widely prescribed for the treatment of cardiovascular diseases and have been demonstrated to be efficacious in the management of hypertension, cardiac arrhythmias, and angina. However, toxicity associated with overdose may produce serious, life-threatening complications, including bradycardia, hypotension, metabolic acidosis, and shock. In 2004, 10,513 cases of CCA toxicity were reported in the United States, resulting in 62 deaths [1]. Standard approach to the management of CCA overdose consists of intravenous fluid resuscitation, gut decontamination, administration of calcium, glucagon, and atropine, and supportive care. In severe cases, the development of bradycardia and hypotension may require placement of a temporary pacemaker and administration of vasopressors and inotropes. In many cases, however, the shock is refractory to inotropes and vasopressors, leading to cardiovascular collapse and death. Interestingly, recent case reports have described novel, successful management of CCA toxicity with euglycemic insulin therapy. We present our

experience and review of the management of CCA toxicity with high-dose hyperinsulinemia-euglycemia (HIE therapy).

Case 1. A 40-year-old male with HIV, hepatitis C, and hypertension was admitted for hypotension, six hours after ingestion of approximately fifty extended release diltiazem pills in a suicide attempt (180 mg pills, 9 grams total). On arrival to the emergency department, vital signs were blood pressure of 70/40 mmHg; pulse of 87 min^{-1}; respiratory rate of 35 min^{-1}; temperature of 37°C and SpO$_2$ 80% (FiO$_2$ 0.50). The patient was intubated secondary to respiratory distress and was initially given 4 liters of intravenous normal saline followed by intravenous calcium and glucagon. Gut decontamination with activated charcoal administration via nasogastric tube was undertaken. Over the next several hours, additional fluids, glucagon, and calcium were given, with minimal improvement in the blood pressure or pulse: 75/42, pulse 82 min^{-1}, respectively. Despite initiation of dopamine, norepinephrine, and epinephrine infusions, blood pressures did not improve, and he developed acute renal failure noted by a decrease in urine output and rise in creatinine from 1.1 to 2.7 mg/dL. Seventeen hours after the initial overdose, the patient was started on intravenous insulin, with no bolus and an initial rate of 10 units (0.11 units/kg). A 10% dextrose infusion was started and titrated to maintain an appropriate glucose concentration. The insulin infusion was increased over the next four hours to a max of 35 IU (0.4 units/kg) per hour. Within three hours after starting the insulin infusion, his blood pressure increased to 142/43 mmHg, and vasopressor requirements decreased. He was weaned off the epinephrine within 10 hours after starting the insulin infusion, weaned off the dopamine within 11 hours after starting the insulin infusion, and weaned off the norepinephrine within 21 hours after starting the insulin infusion. He was extubated 72 hours after initial presentation. The insulin drip was discontinued on the third hospital day following resolution of shock. No significant adverse effects were noted from the insulin therapy, and renal replacement therapy was not required.

Case 2. A 51-year-old African-American male with hypertension and bipolar disorder presented to our hospital after an intentional overdose of amlodipine, hydrochlorothiazide, bupropion, and quetiapine. Of note, he ingested approximately thirty amlodipine 10 mg tablets (total 300 mg). Initial physical exam revealed a lethargic, afebrile male with blood pressure 84/56 mmHg, pulse 92 min^{-1}, respiratory rate 28 min^{-1}, and SpO$_2$ of 97% (FiO$_2$ 0.21). Examination was notable for regular rate and rhythm and bilateral crackles on chest auscultation. Initial laboratory findings included a creatinine 3.2 mg/dL, glucose of 452 mg/dL, and serum lactic acid 6.9 mmol/L. Subsequently, an arterial blood gas obtained on a nonrebreather mask revealed a metabolic acidosis: pH 7.25, PaCO$_2$ 33 mmHg, PaO$_2$ 78 mmHg, bicarbonate 15 mEq/L. Chest radiographs showed bilateral interstitial infiltrates. He was given a total of 5 liters of normal saline, activated charcoal, and calcium chloride, but remained hypotensive with blood pressure 70/40 mmHg. He required intubation and mechanical ventilation. Despite administration of a norepinephrine infusion, and subsequently, phenylephrine infusion, he remained hypotensive. Continuous venovenous hemodiafiltration was initiated for renal failure. Thirty-six hours after presentation, intravenous insulin (no bolus, initial rate of 10 U/hr, 0.12 U/kg) and infusion of 10% dextrose (titrated to maintain an appropriate glucose concentration) were initiated. Insulin was titrated to 40 IU/hour (approximately 0.5 U/kg) and one day after insulin initiation, improvements in hemodynamics were noted. Over the following five days, the vasopressor and insulin infusion were gradually weaned off. He was extubated on hospital day 11 and transferred to the general medical floor where he continued to improve. After discharge, a serum amlodipine level obtained at time of admission was discovered to be 60 ng/mL (therapeutic levels 3–11 ng/mL). The only complication that developed as a result of therapy was hypophosphatemia, nadir of 0.9 mg/dL, which rapidly improved with phosphate replacement.

2. Discussion

Since being introduced almost fifty years ago, CCAs have become one of the most frequently prescribed class of medications. This significant usage has led to increasing reports of toxicity and in 2004, a national survey of poison control centers found 10,513 cases of CCA toxicity with 62 subsequent deaths [1].

2.1. Review of CCA Pharmacology. CCAs can be divided into two major categories: dihydropyridines and nondihydropyridines [2, 3]. Dihydropyridines (amlodipine, felodipine, nicardipine, and nifedipine) block L-type calcium channels, preferentially in the vascular smooth muscle, resulting in smooth muscle relaxation. These drugs have little myocardial depressant activity at therapeutic levels and in fact may increase cardiac output due to the reflex tachycardia. Nondihydropyridines (diltiazem and verapamil) block myocardial and smooth muscle L-type calcium channels, leading to myocardial depression and inhibition of electrical activity. However, two important points need to be noted. First, dihydropyridines are smooth muscle selective, not smooth muscle-specific, and in toxic concentrations may lead to myocardial depression and impaired cardiac conduction. Secondly, CCA, especially at high doses, can block sodium channels and can cause QRS prolongation, similar to tricyclic antidepressants.

In addition to actions on the heart and vascular smooth muscle, CCAs often have an effect on the pancreas. Calcium entry into the pancreatic beta cells via L-type calcium channels is essential for insulin release. Thus, CCA toxicity frequently results in hyperglycemia with relative hypoinsulinemia.

2.2. Clinical Findings of CCA Toxicity. Patients who overdose on CCAs often present with hypotension and bradycardia. The hypotension results from vasodilation and decreased cardiac output (due to the bradycardia and myocardial depression). The bradycardia is often secondary to sinus arrest, and patients often have an AV or ventricular escape rhythm. Due to the myocardial depression, patients may present with pulmonary edema. These patients often have an altered mental status, and they are often hyperglycemic due to insulin resistance, as mentioned earlier.

2.3. Management of CCA Toxicity. Management of CCA toxicity focuses on restoring cardiac function and systemic blood pressure (Table 2). Supportive care and gastrointestinal decontamination are the standard approaches. In addition, specific pharmacologic therapies available for CCA overdose include calcium, glucagon, adrenergic agents, and sodium bicarbonate. When pharmacological measures prove ineffective, cardiac pacing, intra-aortic balloon counterpulsation, and extracorporeal bypass may play important roles.

Initial therapy consists of securing the airway as many patients with CCA toxicity have an altered mental status. In addition, some of the therapies, such as glucagon, are associated with a significant risk of vomiting; thus, the importance of a secure airway cannot be overstated. In a hypotensive patient, an intravenous fluid bolus of 1-2 liters is warranted, especially in the absence of overt pulmonary edema. If hypotension persists, intravenous inotropes and vasopressors are warranted. Detoxification may include gastric lavage especially when a patient presents within 1-2 hours of ingestion. Other useful detoxification measures include the use of activated charcoal in patients within the first two hours of ingestion. However, especially with sustained release formulations, the use of activated charcoal up to 4 hours after ingestion has been documented to be effective. Lastly, whole-gut lavage with polyethylene glycol solution may be useful in selected cases of ingestion of sustained release tablets, although adverse outcomes have been reported with this treatment modality, especially in patients who are already hemodynamically unstable or who have ileus [4].

Intravenous calcium is a frequently used agent for calcium channel overdose. The goal is to competitively overcome the antagonism of the CCAs. However, not all patients respond to intravenous calcium administration, and the benefit may be temporary [5]. Calcium may be given either as calcium gluconate or calcium chloride. While calcium chloride contains three times more calcium for the same volume, calcium gluconate is less irritating to the veins and is preferred in most instances. Calcium salts can be given in bolus doses or administered as a continuous infusion [5]. A typical dosing would start with a 0.6 mL/kg bolus of calcium gluconate (0.2 mL/kg bolus of calcium chloride), followed by a continuous infusion of 0.6–1.5 mL/kg/hr of calcium gluconate (0.2–0.5 mL/kg/hr of calcium chloride), and the infusion rate titrated to hemodynamic response. Importantly, ionized calcium levels should be monitored, with the goal being two times the normal. While calcium salt administration is recommended for treatment of CCA toxicity, significant overdose with cardiovascular instability rarely responds to calcium as a single agent, and other measures are instituted.

Glucagon is another frequently recommended antidote for CCA overdose. Glucagon stimulates adenyl cyclase via G proteins, resulting in increased intracellular cyclic AMP which in turn leads to stimulation of muscle contraction. The clinical effect of glucagon resides in its positive inotropic and chronotropic effects as confirmed in multiple animal studies [6]. However, many of the results from animal studies have not been confirmed in human clinical trials [6]. The initial glucagon dose is 50–150 microgram/kg given as intravenous bolus or 3 to 10 mg in a 70 kg patient. The bolus may be repeated every 3–5 minutes to clinical effect, followed by infusions of the effective dose every hour. Main side effects of this therapy are nausea, vomiting, hyperglycemia, and ileus. The significant incidence of vomiting mandates ensuring a protected airway prior to glucagon administration.

Sodium bicarbonate is another potentially useful therapy in treatment of CCA overdose. In an acidemic environment, CCA binding to the L-type calcium channel is increased. Thus, treatment of the acidemia may improve the hemodynamic status. In addition, CCAs, especially in high doses, may also inhibit fast sodium channels, leading to QRS prolongation, similar to tricyclic antidepressants [6]. If the QRS duration is longer than 120 milliseconds, a 1-2 mEq/kg bolus of sodium bicarbonate may be warranted.

Yet, in spite of the supportive care previously mentioned above, many patients often continue to experience clinical deterioration. In the past several years, hyperinsulinemia-euglycemia (HIE) therapy has gained wider acceptance as part of the treatment for CCA toxicity as described in multiple case reports and animal studies [7–21]. CCA toxicity often results in hyperglycemia from decreased insulin production due to the blockage of the L-type calcium channels in the pancreas. Another consequence of hypoinsulinemia is impairment of the myocardial energy supply. In most instances, the myocardium uses free fatty acids for energy. However, in a shock state, the myocardium switches to glucose use, dependent on insulin. With hypoinsulinemia and acquired insulin resistance, myocardial cells are unable to use glucose as an energy source, leading to decreased myocardial contractility and hypotension. HIE therapy may lead to reversal of cardiovascular collapse in CCA toxicity by improving myocardial utilization of carbohydrates as well as by clearing the cytosol of lactic acid and other glycolytic byproducts. In addition, insulin has direct positive inotropic activity that may contribute to its clinical effects [6, 22, 23].

Animal studies have indicated the role of insulin as an inotropic agent as well as the beneficial effects of insulin therapy in CCA poisoning. In a prospective randomized controlled trial, verapamil toxicity was induced in thirty mongrel dogs. The dogs were randomized to one of the following groups: control, calcium chloride, hyperinsulinemia-euglycemia, epinephrine, or glucagon. HIE treatment was reported to lead to larger increases in both myocardial glucose and lactate uptake thereby associated with improved cardiac performance. Importantly, all animals in the HIE group survived compared to 80% survival rate in the epinephrine group and a 60% survival rate in the glucagon group; a 50% survival in the calcium chloride groups and 0% in the control group [8].

However, no randomized controlled trials have yet been performed to evaluate the role of high-dose insulin therapy in human subjects with CCA overdose. Yet, hyperinsulinemia-euglycemia therapy appears to offer clinical benefit in management of acute myocardial infarction (AMI) and after coronary artery bypass grafting (CABG) surgery, although it goes by another name: glucose-insulin-potassium (GIK) therapy. A meta-analysis by Fath-Ordoubadi reported GIK therapy reduced inhospital mortality after acute myocardial infarction [24]. Another meta-analysis exploring the use of GIK in cardiac surgery, reported that GIK therapy may improve postoperative recovery of contractile function and reduce the incidence of atrial arrhythmias after CABG or heart valve replacement [25].

Most of the human data for HIE therapy in CCA toxicity is limited to published case reports [9–20, 26–29]. Table 1 summarizes the case reports and series in the literature that have used hyperinsulinemia therapy for CCA overdose in adults. These cases have involved the treatment of overdoses of diltiazem (9 cases), verapamil (10 cases), and amlodipine CCAs (9 cases). The dosing of the insulin bolus ranged from

TABLE 1: Case reports of calcium channel antagonist overdose using hyperinsulinemia therapy with clinical outcomes.

CCA ingested	Dose range (mg)	Number of patients (%)	Insulin bolus (IU/kg)	Insulin infusion (IU/kg/hr)	Duration of treatment	Survival N (%)
Verapamil	2000–5800	10 (40)	0–1000 units (no IU/kg reported)	0–1	8–33 hours	9 (90)
Diltiazem	900–10080	9 (24)	0-1	0.2–1.5	6–8 hours	6 (67)
Amlodipine	30–1000	9 (36)	0-1	0–2.64	6–49 hours	8 (88)

TABLE 2: Typical treatment modalities.

(1) Decontamination/supportive therapy:

　(a) activated charcoal: single dose of 50 g for adults;

　(b) polyethylene glycol whole bowel irrigation: 2L/hr in adults until rectal effluent is clear;

　(c) intravenous fluids;

　(d) atropine: 1 mg IV (can be repeated up to 3 mg total).

(2) Antidotes:

　(a) calcium salts:

　　(i) calcium chloride: 10–20 mL of a 10% solution administered over 10 min (can repeat dose if no effect);

　　(ii) calcium gluconate: 30–60 mL of a 10% solution (dose can be repeated if no effect);

　　(iii) continuous infusion with either salt: 0.5 meq of Ca/kg/hr;

　(b) glucagon: 5 mg IV bolus, can be repeated twice at 10 min intervals.

(3) PDI (e.g., amrinone and milrinone).

(4) Adrenergic agents (e.g., norepinephrine and dopamine, etc.).

(5) HIE:

　(a) regular insulin bolus of 0.1 U/kg IV and then continuous infusion of 0.2–0.5 U/kg/hr;

　(b) dextrose 25 to 50 g bolus followed by a continuous infusion of 0.5 g glucose/kg/hr that can be titrated to appropriate blood glucose.

(6) Invasive therapy:

　(a) transvenous pacing;

　(b) intraaortic balloon pump;

　(c) cardiopulmonary bypass;

　(d) extracorporeal membrane oxygenation.

0 to 1000 IU though only about half of the patients received a bolus, and the maintenance insulin infusion ranged from 0–2.64 IU/kg/hr. Current recommendations for the use of insulin therapy in CCA overdose consist of intravenous bolus administration of 1 IU/kg followed by an infusion of 0.5 IU/kg/hr. The duration of therapy ranged from 6 to 96 hours. In these reports and as well as our case series, hyperinsulinemia therapy resulted in hemodynamic improvement in the majority of treated patients, and 23 (82%) of the patients receiving therapy survived. Some authors have suggested that late onset of hyperinsulinemia-euglycemia is associated with lack of survival; however, in our patients, improvement was demonstrated up to 36 hours post presentation [6, 29].

Notably, hypoglycemia and hypokalemia are the main adverse effects of HIE therapy; therefore, serum glucose and electrolytes should be closely monitored. As suggested by Boyer, it is reasonable to administer 25 grams of glucose (1 ampule of D50) prior to initiation of HIE therapy if the blood glucose is less than 200 mg/dL, and similarly, to administer 40 mEq of potassium chloride intravenously if the potassium level is less than 2.5 meq/L.

Although no definitive guidelines regarding HIE therapy in human CCA overdose have been published, there is enough empirical evidence to warrant strong consideration of this therapy for treatment of CCA overdose. More research is warranted to answer questions such as which patient populations would benefit most from this treatment, at what point in the treatment timeline should this therapy be instituted, and what are the optimal doses.

3. Conclusion

CCA poisoning is on the rise due to increased use for a number of cardiovascular indications. CCA overdose, whether intentional or accidental, can be lethal. HIE therapy has been shown to be beneficial in multiple animal studies as well as the majority of case series. HIE therapy should be considered early in the presentation of CCA toxicity in order to improve cardiac contractility and hemodynamics. Close monitoring of serum glucose and electrolytes is advised to prevent potential adverse effects.

References

[1] W. A. Watson, T. L. Litovitz, G. C. Rodgers Jr. et al., "2004 Annual report of the American Association of Poison Control Centers Toxic Exposure Surveillance System," *American Journal of Emergency Medicine*, vol. 23, no. 5, pp. 589–666, 2005.

[2] M. Spedding and R. Paoletti, "Classification of calcium channels and the sites of action of drugs modifying channel function," *Pharmacological Reviews*, vol. 44, no. 3, pp. 363–876, 1992.

[3] D. R. Abernethy and J. B. Schwartz, "Calcium-antagonist drugs," *The New England Journal of Medicine*, vol. 341, no. 19, pp. 1447–1457, 1999.

[4] K. L. Cumpston, S. E. Aks, T. Sigg, and E. Pallasch, "Whole bowel irrigation and the hemodynamically unstable calcium channel blocker overdose: primum non nocere," *Journal of Emergency Medicine*, vol. 38, no. 2, pp. 171–174, 2010.

[5] S. D. Salhanick and M. W. Shannon, "Management of calcium channel antagonist overdose," *Drug Safety*, vol. 26, no. 2, pp. 65–79, 2003.

[6] W. Kerns II, "Management of beta-adrenergic blocker and calcium channel antagonist toxicity," *Emergency Medicine Clinics of North America*, vol. 25, no. 2, pp. 309–331, 2007.

[7] M. T. Meyer, E. Stremski, and M. C. Scanlon, "Successful resuscitation of a verapamil intoxicated child with a dextrose-insulin infusion," *Clinical Intensive Care*, vol. 14, no. 3-4, pp. 109–113, 2003.

[8] J. A. Kline, E. Leonova, and R. M. Raymond, "Beneficial myocardial metabolic effects of insulin during verapamil toxicity in the anesthetized canine," *Critical Care Medicine*, vol. 23, no. 7, pp. 1251–1263, 1995.

[9] E. W. Boyer and M. Shannon, "Treatment of calcium-channel-blocker intoxication with insulin infusion," *The New England Journal of Medicine*, vol. 344, no. 22, pp. 1721–1722, 2001.

[10] T. H. Yuan, W. P. Kerns II, C. A. Tomaszewski, M. D. Ford, and J. A. Kline, "Insulin-glucose as adjunctive therapy for severe calcium channel antagonist poisoning," *Journal of Toxicology. Clinical Toxicology*, vol. 37, no. 4, pp. 463–474, 1999.

[11] M. Marques, E. Gomes, and J. de Oliveira, "Treatment of calcium channel blocker intoxication with insulin infusion: case report and literature review," *Resuscitation*, vol. 57, no. 2, pp. 211–213, 2003.

[12] L. Rasmussen, S. E. Husted, and S. P. Johnsen, "Severe intoxication after an intentional overdose of amlodipine," *Acta Anaesthesiologica Scandinavica*, vol. 47, no. 8, pp. 1038–1040, 2003.

[13] L. B. Verbrugge and H. B. van Wezel, "Pathophysiology of verapamil overdose: new insights in the role of insulin," *Journal of Cardiothoracic and Vascular Anesthesia*, vol. 21, no. 3, pp. 406–409, 2007.

[14] L. Min and K. Deshpande, "Diltiazem overdose haemodynamic response to hyperinsulinaemia-euglycaemia therapy: a case report," *Critical Care and Resuscitation*, vol. 6, no. 1, pp. 28–30, 2004.

[15] N. S. Harris, "Case records of the Massachusetts General Hospital. Case 24-2006. A 40-year-old woman with hypotension after an overdose of amlodipine," *The New England Journal of Medicine*, vol. 355, no. 6, pp. 602–611, 2006.

[16] N. P. Patel, M. E. Pugh, S. Goldberg, and G. Eiger, "Hyperinsulinemic euglycemia therapy for verapamil poisoning: case report," *American Journal of Critical Care*, vol. 16, no. 5, pp. 518–520, 2007.

[17] S. L. Greene, I. Gawarammana, D. M. Wood, A. L. Jones, and P. I. Dargan, "Relative safety of hyperinsulinaemia/euglycaemia therapy in the management of calcium channel blocker overdose: a prospective observational study," *Intensive Care Medicine*, vol. 33, no. 11, pp. 2019–2024, 2007.

[18] H. Azendour, L. Belyamani, M. Atmani, H. Balkhi, and C. Haimeur, "Severe amlodipine intoxication treated by hyperinsulinemia euglycemia therapy," *Journal of Emergency Medicine*, vol. 38, no. 1, pp. 33–35, 2010.

[19] E. W. Boyer, P. A. Duic, and A. Evans, "Hyperinsulinemia/euglycemia therapy for calcium channel blocker poisoning," *Pediatric Emergency Care*, vol. 18, no. 1, pp. 36–37, 2002.

[20] S. W. Smith, K. L. Ferguson, R. S. Hoffman, L. S. Nelson, and H. A. Greller, "Prolonged severe hypotension following combined amlodipine and valsartan ingestion," *Clinical Toxicology*, vol. 46, no. 5, pp. 470–474, 2008.

[21] C. L. Morris-Kukoski, A. K. Biswas, M. Parra, and C. Smith, "Insulin euglycemia therapy for accidental nifedipine overdose [abstract]," *Journal of Toxicology. Clinical Toxicology*, vol. 38, article 577, 2000.

[22] U. N. Das, "Insulin: an endogenous cardioprotector," *Current Opinion in Critical Care*, vol. 9, no. 5, pp. 375–383, 2003.

[23] L. Proano, W. K. Chiang, and R. Y. Wang, "Calcium channel blocker overdose," *American Journal of Emergency Medicine*, vol. 13, no. 4, pp. 444–450, 1995.

[24] F. Fath-Ordoubadi and K. J. Beatt, "Glucose-insulin-potassium therapy for treatment of acute myocardial infarction: an overview of randomized placebo-controlled trials," *Circulation*, vol. 96, no. 4, pp. 1152–1156, 1997.

[25] W. Bothe, M. Olschewski, F. Beyersdorf, and T. Doenst, "Glucose-insulin-potassium in cardiac surgery: a meta-analysis," *Annals of Thoracic Surgery*, vol. 78, no. 5, pp. 1650–1657, 2004.

[26] T. Hasin, D. Leibowitz, M. Antopolsky, and T. Chajek-Shaul, "The use of low-dose insulin in cardiogenic shock due to combined overdose of verapamil, enalapril and metoprolol," *Cardiology*, vol. 106, no. 4, pp. 233–236, 2006.

[27] J. Herbert, C. O'Malley, J. Tracey, R. Dwyer, and M. Power, "Verapamil overdosage unresponsive to dextrose/insulin therapy [abstract]," *Journal of Toxicology. Clinical Toxicology*, vol. 39, pp. 293–294, 2001.

[28] R. Place, A. Carlson, J. Leiken, and P. Hanashiro, "Hyperinsulin therapy in the treatment of verapamil overdose [abstract]," *Journal of Toxicology. Clinical Toxicology*, vol. 38, pp. 576–577, 2000.

[29] K. Cumpston, M. Mycyk, E. Pallash et al., "Failure of hyperinsulinemia/euglycemia therapy in severe diltiazem overdose [abstract]," *Journal of Toxicology. Clinical Toxicology*, vol. 40, article 618, 2002.

20

Disseminated Necrotizing Leukoencephalopathy Complicating Septic Shock in an Immunocompetent Patient

Pedro Gaspar-da-Costa,[1] **Sofia Reimão,**[2,3] **Sandra Braz,**[1,3]
João Meneses Santos,[1,3] **and Rui M. M. Victorino**[1,3]

[1]*Department of Internal Medicine, Hospital de Santa Maria and Faculty of Medicine of Lisbon, Lisbon, Portugal*
[2]*Department of Neurologic Imaging, Hospital de Santa Maria and Faculty of Medicine of Lisbon, Lisbon, Portugal*
[3]*Faculty of Medicine of Lisbon, Lisbon, Portugal*

Correspondence should be addressed to Pedro Gaspar-da-Costa; pgasparcosta@gmail.com

Academic Editor: Gerhard Pichler

Disseminated necrotizing leukoencephalopathy (DNL) is characterized by multiple microscopic foci of white matter necrosis. DNL was initially thought to be exclusively associated with immunosuppression conditions but it has been recently described in immunocompetent patients in septic shock. A 90-year-old immunocompetent woman with no previous neurological impairment presented with septic shock and drowsiness that responded well to therapy with clinical improvement and a full neurological recovery. Unexpectedly deterioration with progression to coma occurred. Investigation excluded other causes and Magnetic Resonance Imaging (MRI) was consistent with the diagnosis of DNL showing bilateral multifocal white matter lesions with a nonvascular pattern with restricted diffusion. Neurological impairment persisted with progression to death. DNL is an unexpected diagnosis in an immunocompetent patient. We compared the present case to those found in the literature of DNL complicating septic shock and discuss the antemortem diagnosis based on MRI findings.

1. Introduction

Disseminated necrotizing leukoencephalopathy (DNL), also known as multiple necrotizing leukoencephalopathy (MNL), is a clinical entity with a poorly understood pathobiology [1]. It was first described in 1975 [2] by Rubinstein et al. in four children with leukemia and one child with Burkitt's lymphoma with central nervous system involvement that were under treatment with high dose systemic and intrathecal chemotherapy. Since then DNL has been identified in all age groups and in other immunosuppression states, such as Acquired Immunodeficiency Syndrome (AIDS) [1–6].

DNL has also been named pontine leukoencephalopathy due to reports of preferential involvement of this central nervous system area [6, 7], although there is consistent evidence that most patients have disseminated and multifocal white matter lesions [4, 6]. It was initially described as a rare complication of these specific immunocompromised patients but recent studies identified a possible link with the state of immune deregulation in septic shock [1, 8]. Typical histopathologic findings are microscopic multifocal white matter foci of necrosis, oedema, axonal swelling, and demyelinization [6] with diverse clinical manifestations such as a pyramidal syndrome, cerebellar dysfunction, behaviour alterations, and coma [1–12]. No specific clinical signs or symptoms are associated with the disease and the brain involvement of leukemia or lymphoma and the frequent use of intravenous sedation in septic patients further confound the clinical manifestations of DNL [1, 8]. Although definite confirmation relies on histology, Magnetic Resonance Imaging (MRI) is fundamental for the diagnosis of DNL in view of the characteristic features of bilateral multifocal supra and infratentorial white matter lesions with a nonvascular distribution with restricted diffusion [3, 13].

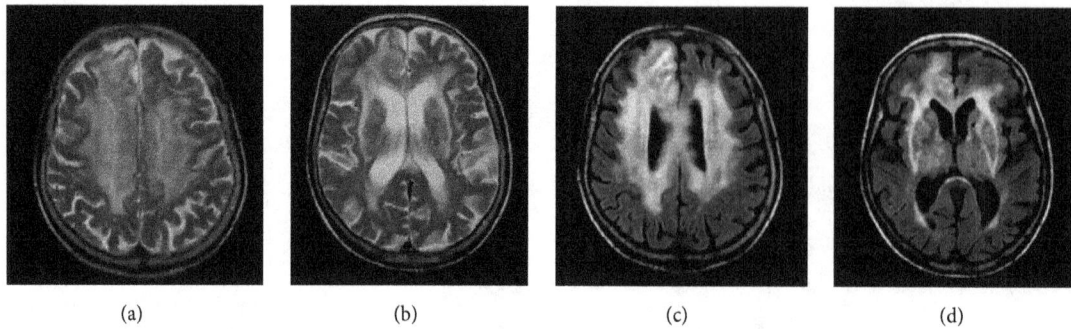

(a)   (b)   (c)   (d)

FIGURE 1: Axial T2 weighted (a, b) and FLAIR (c, d) MR imaging showing extensive white matter hyperintensity signal changes with a confluent pattern in periventricular and deep white matter of the cerebral hemispheres, without vascular distribution, more extensive on the right frontal region and involving all segments of the corpus callosum.

The present case illustrates the rarely reported unexpected association between septic shock and DNL and the importance of the MRI in the diagnosis of this clinical entity with poor prognosis.

2. Case Report

A 90-year-old women with known diagnosis of hypertension and otherwise healthy presented with drowsiness, abdominal pain, nausea, vomiting, fever, tachycardia, and hypotension with a blood pressure of 88/62 mmHg. Heart, lung, and abdominal observation were unremarkable. Neurological examination showed no focal or meningeal signs. Laboratory tests revealed thrombocytopenia (85000/uL) and a significant increase in leukocytes (16860/uL), neutrophils (15800/uL), C-reactive protein (18.1 mg/dL), blood urea nitrogen (93 mg/dL), and creatinine (2.8 mg/dL). Urinalysis had significant leukocyturia (>500 leukocytes/uL) and arterial blood gas analysis showed hyperlactacidemia (38 mg/dL) and metabolic acidosis (HCO_3^-: 19.8 mmol/L). Her chest roentgenography and electrocardiogram had no significant changes and the renal ultrasound found pathologic alterations in the right kidney with slight pyelocaliceal dilation and perirenal fluid. A diagnosis of acute pyelonephritis was made and the laboratory and hemodynamic parameters were consistent with septic shock and multiple organ failure.

Blood and urine cultures were obtained and prompt broad spectrum antibiotic therapy was initiated. Concurrent fluid resuscitation and hemodynamic support were provided and after a transient 24-hour worsening period, a steady progressive improvement was noted. *Escherichia coli* was isolated from both blood and urine samples and antibiotic adequacy was confirmed. Over the following days, clinical improvement was evident with full neurological recovery to previous cognition status, absence of fever, nausea, and abdominal pain. Laboratory tests also had a favourable evolution with a recovery of kidney failure and haematological dysfunction. Significant decrease in the inflammatory markers was also noted.

The patient had no previously neurocognitive impairment and the initial drowsiness resolved alongside with the global improvement. Despite this initial response, on the 5th day of hospitalization, there was sudden neurological deterioration to coma. No meningeal or focal signs were apparent and there was no evidence of tonic or clonic movements. Examination also excluded neurologic or hemodynamic signs of intracranial hypertension. Laboratory reevaluation was unremarkable and metabolic causes were excluded, namely, hypoglycemia, dysnatremia, uraemia, and hyperammonemia. Iatrogenic pharmacological causes were also absent.

This sudden neurological deterioration was unexpected and thus a diagnostic approach for other possible causes such as vascular, epileptic, and septic encephalopathy was done. Brain Computerized Tomography (CT) scan revealed a possible ischemic cortical and subcortical right frontal lesion with attenuation of the adjacent sulci. There were no haemorrhages, hydrocephalus, or midline shifts. As this possible ischemic lesion did not explain the neurological status, an electroencephalography was performed and showed slow bilateral frontal and temporal activity with periodical 1 to 2 Hz discharges. This was not diagnostic of status epilepticus and was suggestive of a low epileptic threshold. Neurologic and neurophysiologic specialist consultation was obtained and valproic acid was initiated, without neurologic benefit. A brain Magnetic Resonance Imaging (MRI) was then performed and showed bilateral supra and infratentorial multifocal white matter lesions, with a pattern that did not follow vascular territorial distribution (Figures 1, 2, 3, and 4), involvement of the corpus callosum with restricted diffusion (Figures 1 and 3), and areas of necrosis (Figure 2). These MRI findings led to the diagnosis of DNL and that was further supported by the exhaustive investigation of other alternative causes. Lumbar puncture was not obtained; however meningitis and encephalitis were not relevant differential diagnosis in the absence of meningeal signs and fever and with a progressive reduction of inflammatory biomarkers.

In the following days the state of coma persisted and the patient eventually died as a consequence of persistent neurological dysfunction. Pathological necropsy studies were

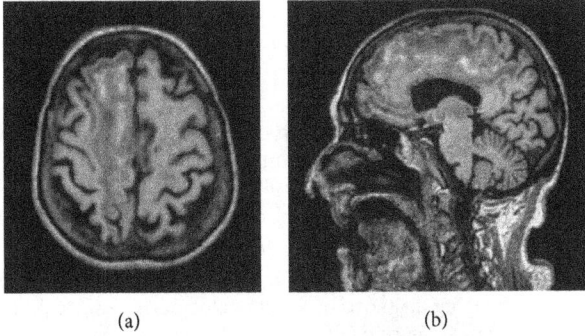

FIGURE 2: Axial (a) and sagittal (b) T1 weighted MR images. Linear spontaneous hyperintensity of the cortex in the frontoparietal convexity, compatible with laminar necrosis.

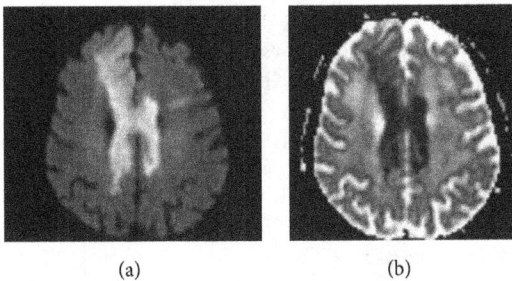

FIGURE 3: MR diffusion weighted images. DWI (a) and ADC map (b) with significant restricted diffusion of the corpus callosum bilaterally in all the segments and in the right anterior frontal and parietal region.

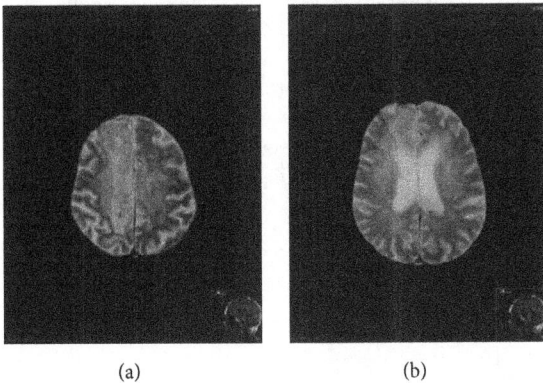

FIGURE 4: Axial T2*. Punctate hypointensity foci of magnetic susceptibility diffusely in the central and subcortical cerebral white matter, without vascular distribution, corresponding to hemosiderin deposition.

considered unnecessary by the combined consideration of MRI findings typical of DNL and thorough exclusion of an alternative diagnosis.

3. Discussion

DNL in immunocompetent patients has increasingly been recognized and the diagnosis is challenging not only because of its rarity but also as a result of the nonspecificity of the clinical manifestations. Moreover, both the immuno-compromised and the septic shock patients usually have parallel confounding factors which contribute do decreased level of consciousness, particularly intravenous sedatives, and analgesics [8]. The identification of the typical MRI pattern was determinant in our case, in view of the importance and specificity of these findings documented in the medical literature [3, 13]. Still, in many cases, particularly in critically ill patients, the diagnosis is established postmortem after necropsy [1, 2, 6, 8].

The pathobiology of DNL remains unclear [1]. In regard to the association between DNL and septic shock, Sharshar et al. found evidence of higher levels of systemic TNF-α, IL-1β, IL-6, IL-8, and IL-10, at days one, three, four, and eight of hospitalization in one case, in comparison to two septic shock controls [1]. Despite their small study population, they postulated a possible correlation between those values and DNL [1]. Interestingly, IL-1β and TNF-α have been proposed to have a role in axonal damage, mediation of neurotoxic factors, regulation of nitric oxide synthase, and apoptotic neuronal death. IL-1β can also augment vascular permeability causing brain oedema in other clinical settings [1, 14–20].

There are two reported cases in patients with septic shock with no evidence of previous immunodeficiency [1, 8] which were diagnosed postmortem in contrast to our case where the MRI findings together with an exhaustive exclusion of other causes allowed an antemortem diagnosis.

The relationship between DNL and septic shock raises additional questions, namely, in the interpretation and classification of the septic encephalopathy (SE) syndrome. SE is a common finding with a variable range of clinical manifestations that can be present in about one-third of the patients with septic shock [8]. It is considered a brain or autonomic dysfunction complicating septic shock and the pathogenic mechanism can involve septic embolism in central nervous system, endotoxinemia, immunologic deregulation, vascular ischemic or hemorrhagic complications, metabolic disturbances, and leukoencephalopathy such as posterior reversible leukoencephalopathy [8]. Thus, it is possible to look at DNL as one of the possible causes of SE, rather than an alternative diagnosis, and increased awareness about this relationship will probably identify additional cases where DNL is the primary brain change in patients who would otherwise be diagnosed as having unclassified SE.

In conclusion, we present a case of a patient with septic shock without previous immunodeficiency with severe and fatal neurologic dysfunction, in which a DNL diagnosis was established antemortem on the basis of the typical MRI findings, and after the thorough exclusion of an alternative diagnosis.

References

[1] T. Sharshar, F. Gray, F. Poron, J. C. Raphael, P. Gajdos, and D. Annane, "Multifocal necrotizing leukoencephalopathy in septic shock," *Critical Care Medicine*, vol. 30, no. 10, pp. 2371–2375, 2002.

[2] L. J. Rubinstein, M. M. Herman, T. F. Long, and J. R. Wilbur, "Disseminated necrotizing leukoencephalopathy: a complication of treated central nervous system leukemia and lymphoma," *Cancer*, vol. 35, no. 2, pp. 291–305, 1975.

[3] J. Matsubayashi, K. Tsuchiya, T. Matsunaga, and K. Mukai, "Methotrexate-related leukoencephalopathy without radiation therapy: distribution of brain lesions and pathological heterogeneity on two autopsy cases," *Neuropathology*, vol. 29, no. 2, pp. 105–115, 2009.

[4] J. Robb, L. Chalmers, A. Rojiani, and M. Chamberlain, "Multifocal necrotizing leukoencephalopathy: an unusual complication of acute leukemia," *Archives of Neurology*, vol. 63, no. 7, pp. 1028–1029, 2006.

[5] J. Y. Kim, S. T. Kim, D. Nam, J. Lee, K. Park, and D. Kong, "Leukoencephalopathy and disseminated necrotizing leukoencephalopathy following intrathecal methotrexate chemotherapy and radiation therapy for central nerve system lymphoma or leukemia," *Journal of Korean Neurosurgical Society*, vol. 50, no. 4, pp. 304–310, 2011.

[6] K. H. Anders, P. Scott Becker, J. K. Holden et al., "Multifocal necrotizing leukoencephalopathy with pontine predilection in immunosuppressed patients: a clinicopathologic review of 16 cases," *Human Pathology*, vol. 24, no. 8, pp. 897–904, 1993.

[7] Vinters H. V., Anders K. H., and Barach P., "Focal pontine leukoencephalopathy in immunosuppressed patients," *Arch Pathol Lab Med*, vol. 2, no. 111, pp. 192–196, 1987.

[8] T. Sharshar, D. Annane, G. L. De La Grandmaison, J. P. Brouland, N. S. Hopkinson, and F. Gray, "The neuropathology of septic shock," *Brain Pathology*, vol. 14, no. 1, pp. 21–33, 2004.

[9] Y. Nakazato, Y. Ishida, and M. Morimatsu, "Disseminated necrotizing leukoencephalopathy," *Acta Pathologica Japonica*, vol. 30, no. 4, pp. 659–670, 1980.

[10] T. Mizutani, Y. Morimatsu, and K. Hayakawa, "Necrotizing leukoencephalopathy and treated multiple myeloma. an autopsy case without intrathecal chemotherapy or irradiation of the brain," *Pathology International*, vol. 34, no. 3, pp. 655–662, 1984.

[11] S. Raghavendra, M. D. Nair, T. Chemmanam, T. Krishnamoorthy, V. V. Radhakrishnan, and A. Kuruvilla, "Disseminated necrotizing leukoencephalopathy following low-dose oral methotrexate," *European Journal of Neurology*, vol. 14, no. 3, pp. 309–314, 2007.

[12] T. Shimura, S. Nakazawa, Y. Akutsu, M. Matsumoto, M. Kazuhara, and D. Yoshida, "Disseminated necrotizing leukoencephalopathy accompanied with multiple calcium deposits following antineoplastic and radiation therapy in a case with intracranial germ cell tumor: computerized tomographical study," *No Shinkei Geka*, vol. 17, no. 6, pp. 573–577, 1989.

[13] S. W. Atlas, R. I. Grossman, R. J. Packer et al., "Magnetic resonance imaging diagnosis of disseminated necrotizing leukoencephalopathy," *Journal of Computed Tomography*, vol. 11, no. 1, pp. 39–43, 1987.

[14] A. Burke-Gaffeyy and A. K. Keenan, "Modulation of human endothelial cell permeability by combinations of the cytokines interleukin-1 α/β, tumor necrosis factor-α and interferon-γ," *Immunopharmacology*, vol. 25, no. 1, pp. 1–9, 1993.

[15] K. Jellinger, "Neuroaxonal dystrophy: its natural history and related disorders," in *Progress in Neuropathology*, H. M. Zimmerman, Ed., pp. 129–180, Grune and Stratton, New York, NY, USA, 1973.

[16] H. G. Jenkins and H. Ikeda, "Tumour necrosis factor causes an increase in axonal transport of protein and demyelination in the mouse optic nerve," *Journal of the Neurological Sciences*, vol. 108, no. 1, pp. 99–104, 1992.

[17] T. Kita, T. Tanaka, N. Tanaka, and Y. Kinoshita, "The role of tumor necrosis, factor-α in diffuse axonal injury following fluid-percussive brain injury in rats," *International Journal of Legal Medicine*, vol. 113, no. 4, pp. 221–228, 2000.

[18] U. Gimsa, S. V. A. Peter, K. Lehmann, I. Bechmann, and R. Nitsch, "Axonal damage induced by invading T cells in organotypic central nervous system tissue in vitro: involvement of microglial cells," *Brain Pathology*, vol. 10, no. 3, pp. 365–377, 2000.

[19] K. M. Boje and P. K. Arora, "Microglial-produced nitric oxide and reactive nitrogen oxides mediate neuronal cell death," *Brain Research*, vol. 587, no. 2, pp. 250–256, 1992.

[20] E. Änggård, "Nitric oxide: mediator, murderer, and medicine," *The Lancet*, vol. 343, no. 8907, pp. 1199–1205, 1994.

21

Early Recognition of Foreign Body Aspiration as the Cause of Cardiac Arrest

Muhammad Kashif, Hafiz Rizwan Talib Hashmi, and Misbahuddin Khaja

Division of Pulmonary and Critical Care Medicine, Department of Medicine, Bronx Lebanon Hospital Center, Bronx, NY 10457, USA

Correspondence should be addressed to Muhammad Kashif; mkashif@bronxleb.org

Academic Editor: Ricardo Oliveira

Foreign body aspiration (FBA) is uncommon in the adult population but can be a life-threatening condition. Clinical manifestations vary according to the degree of airway obstruction, and, in some cases, making the correct diagnosis requires a high level of clinical suspicion combined with a detailed history and exam. Sudden cardiac arrest after FBA may occur secondary to asphyxiation. We present a 48-year-old male with no history of cardiac disease brought to the emergency department after an out-of-hospital cardiac arrest (OHCA). The patient was resuscitated after 15 minutes of cardiac arrest. He was initially managed with therapeutic hypothermia (TH). Subsequent history suggested FBA as a possible etiology of the cardiac arrest, and fiberoptic bronchoscopy demonstrated a piece of meat and bone lodged in the left main stem bronchus. The foreign body was removed with the bronchoscope and the patient clinically improved with full neurological recovery. Therapeutic hypothermia following cardiac arrest due to asphyxia has been reported to have high mortality and poor neurological outcomes. This case highlights the importance of early identification of FBA causing cardiac arrest, and we report a positive neurological outcome for postresuscitation therapeutic hypothermia following cardiac arrest due to asphyxia.

1. Introduction

Foreign body aspiration is uncommon in the adult population but can be associated with life-threatening airway obstruction. Symptoms can range from cough, dyspnea, choking, and acute asphyxiation leading to cardiorespiratory arrest [1]. Cardiac arrest due to foreign body aspiration is relatively less common in adults likely due to larger airway diameters [2]. Poor neurologic status, irrespective of the primary cardiac arrest arrhythmia, is the predominant cause of death among survivors of OHCA [3]. TH is indicated in survivors of OHCA from several causes with favorable outcome. However, studies specifically focusing on the outcome of TH after asphyxial cardiac arrest showed good neurologic outcomes in a very small number of patients [4, 5]. The TH maintenance times were not uniform in some of those patients. Here, we present an unusual case of asphyxial cardiac arrest secondary to foreign body aspiration with complete neurological recovery after early bronchoscopy removal and TH.

2. Case Presentation

A 48-year-old male was brought to the emergency department in cardiac arrest after collapsing at a grocery store. Bystanders called emergency medical services (EMS). The patient was found to have pulseless electrical activity (PEA), and EMS initiated cardiopulmonary resuscitation. During the resuscitation, the patient was bag-ventilated and intubated. Following administration of three doses of intravenous epinephrine (1 mg in 10 mL), the cardiac rhythm converted to ventricular tachycardia, and, after two shocks of 360 J, the patient reverted to sinus rhythm with good cardiac output. The total duration of cardiopulmonary resuscitation was 15 minutes.

The patient's past medical history was significant only for controlled hypertension. There was no history of smoking, illegal drug use, or other behaviors that might increase his risk of cardiac disorders. He had no family history of sudden cardiac arrest and no reported allergies. His medications

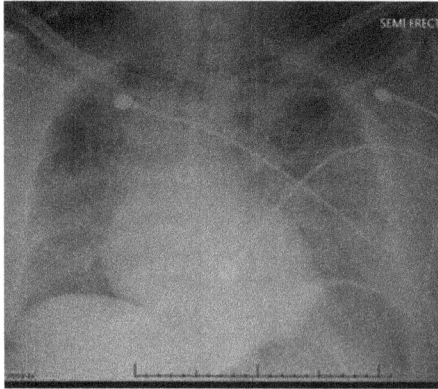

FIGURE 1: Chest radiograph shows endotracheal tube in position.

3. Discussion

Foreign body aspiration (FBA) is a dangerous and potentially life-threatening event. In the United States, death from FBA is the fourth leading cause of accidental home and community deaths, but the occurrence of FBA is less common in the adult population compared to children and the elderly [6].

Vegetable matter and inorganic objects such as toy parts are also commonly aspirated objects in children, whereas adults aspirate food particles, medication tablets, dental pieces, and a variety of other inorganic substances. Choking while eating, leading to severe dyspnea followed by respiratory and cardiac arrest, may be initially misdiagnosed as myocardial ischemia. Tracheobronchial foreign body aspiration has a range of possible outcomes, including immediate resolution, recurrent pulmonary disease, recurrent pneumonia and a right lower lobe lung abscess, asphyxia, and death [7].

Aspiration of dietary or nondietary foreign bodies may occur as a result of choking while eating, in patients under anesthesia, during seizures, while a person is intoxicated, or as an accidental event while an object is held in the mouth. The risk of FBA is increased in the presence of oropharyngeal dysfunction, which may occur due to a neurologic disorder or as the result of certain sedating medications.

Aspiration events can vary widely in presentation due to factors such as patient age, degree of airway obstruction, and baseline neurologic status. These events can range from unobserved, asymptomatic episodes to complete airway obstructions with acute asphyxia and cardiorespiratory collapse. In the case of an acute airway obstruction, a conscious patient may have symptoms of aphonia, dysphagia, odynophagia, the hand-to-the-throat choking sign, stridor, facial swelling, and/or prominence of the neck veins. Clinical exam in these patients may identify absent air entry on chest auscultation, marked respiratory distress, and tachycardia [8]. In complete airway obstruction, however, asphyxiation quickly leads to hypoxia and collapse. In unconscious or sedated patients, the presentation of FBA is often less apparent, and the first sign of airway obstruction may be the inability to ventilate with a bag-valve mask. Untreated, complete airway obstruction quickly leads to cyanosis, respiratory distress, and death [9].

Making the correct diagnosis requires an awareness of the circumstances in which the aspiration event occurred, as well as consideration of subtle clues in the clinical presentation. Imaging modalities may be useful in certain cases. In addition to asphyxia and respiratory failure, other potential causes of cardiac arrest include cardiac disorders, drowning, drug use, exsanguination, and chest trauma. Lethal FBA can be avoided by immediate removal of the obstructing piece of foreign material [10], but prompt, life-saving treatment requires the diagnosis of FBA as the cause of asphyxia.

During resuscitation following an acute event, establishing a secure and patent airway is the most important goal. Available medical and surgical approaches include oropharyngeal airways, endotracheal intubation (transnasal or oral), tracheotomy, cricothyroidotomy, fiberoptic intubation, and the administration of racemic epinephrine, corticosteroids, and helium-oxygen mixtures. The addition of laser therapy,

included daily losartan (100 mg) and hydrochlorothiazide (25 mg).

Physical exam on arrival to the emergency department revealed a middle-aged, intubated patient with a temperature of 98.6 F, pulse rate of 98 beats per minute, respiratory rate of 18 breaths per minute, and blood pressure of 98/65 mm Hg. His oxygen saturation was 100% while on a ventilator receiving 40% FiO_2. He had no conjunctival pallor. Auscultation of the lungs demonstrated bilateral air entry with no adventitious sounds. Precordial exam revealed normal heart sounds with no murmur, rub, or gallop. Abdominal exam revealed no hepatosplenomegaly. Glasgow Coma Scale (GCS) score was three on initial assessment. Electrocardiogram showed normal sinus rhythm with T wave inversions in I, AVL, and V3–V6. Portable chest radiograph revealed an appropriately placed endotracheal tube (ETT) (Figure 1). Computed Tomography (CT) of the brain did not reveal any significant pathology. No arrhythmias were identified during cardiac monitoring. Cardiac enzymes and an initial echocardiogram did not show any ischemia.

The patient was deemed a candidate for postresuscitation hypothermia and was managed according to the current hypothermia guidelines. Cardiac catheterization was performed and demonstrated patent coronary vessels. Further history was then provided by family members, who reported that the patient was choking on food prior to his collapse. In the absence of another clear etiology for cardiac arrest and with no significant arrhythmias or ischemia identified, foreign body aspiration was considered as the most plausible explanation for the patient's arrest. The patient underwent bronchoscopy, revealing a piece of meat and bone lodged in the left main stem bronchus (Figures 2(a) and 2(c)). During the retrieval process, pieces of foreign body were dislodged in the right mainstem (Figure 2(b)). Biopsy forceps were used to remove the foreign body (Figure 2(d)). Follow-up flexible bronchoscopy performed 48 hours later revealed complete removal of the foreign body and diffuse tracheobronchial mucosal edema. The patient went on to have an excellent clinical recovery and was discharged after 15 days in the hospital, with no cardiac, respiratory, or neurological sequelae.

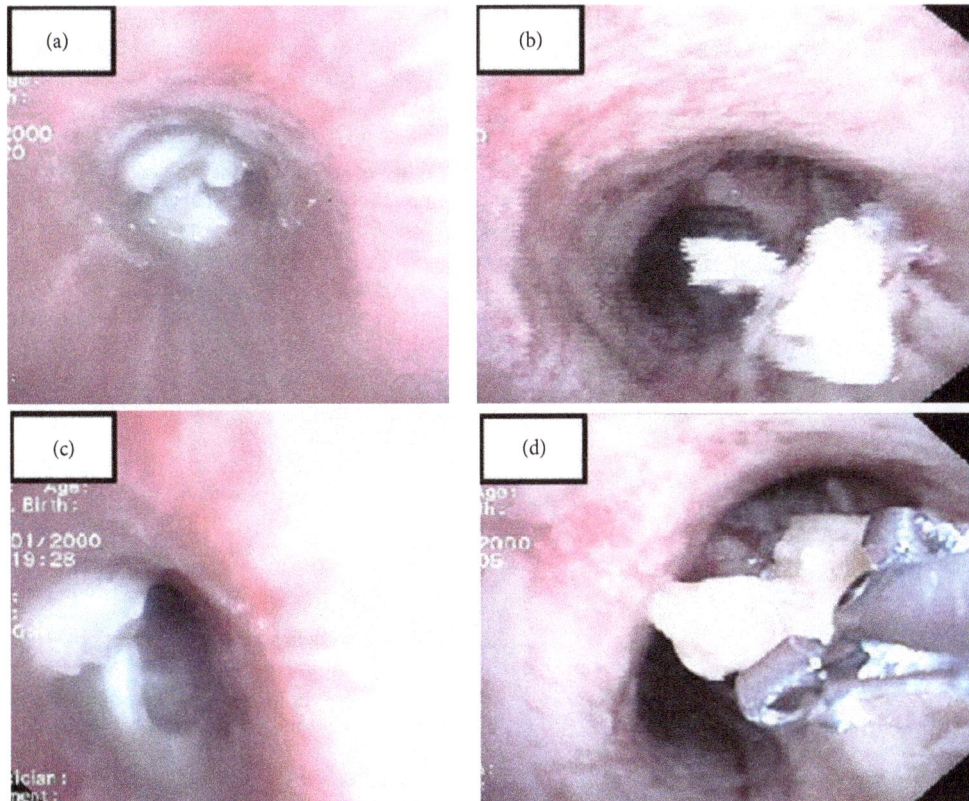

FIGURE 2: (a, c) Foreign body in the left main stem bronchus; (b) foreign body in the right main stem; (d) forceps retrieving the foreign body.

bronchoscopic dilation, and airway stenting may also be helpful [11]. Fiberoptic bronchoscopy is the diagnostic test of choice for the initial diagnosis of FBA in adults [12, 13].

Reports from the Mayo Clinic have demonstrated that the flexible bronchoscope was successful in the extraction of 100% of airway FBs in 26 children and 89% of FBs in 61 adults [14].

Rigid bronchoscopy is recommended if fiberoptic bronchoscopy fails; for foreign bodies that are centrally located or embedded in scar tissue; and for the removal of sharp objects that might cause mucosal trauma during manipulation [15].

In this case, the patient was found on bronchoscopy to have a foreign body located in the left main stem bronchus. This location contrasts with the finding in children that aspirated foreign bodies are more often lodged in the right main stem bronchus, likely due to the anatomy of the right main stem bronchus, which is shorter, larger in diameter, and at a less acute angle to the trachea than the left. The patient appeared to have initially had a complete airway obstruction, resulting in asphyxia and cardiac arrest. It is plausible that the foreign body obstructing the airway was pushed by the endotracheal tube into the left main stem bronchus, allowing for ventilation and resuscitation from the arrest.

For patients who experience out-of-hospital cardiac arrest, neurologic injury is the most common cause of death. In addition, for patients who regain spontaneous circulation, neurologic injury contributes to high inpatient mortality and morbidity rates [3]. Therapeutic hypothermia is indicated after out-of-hospital cardiac arrest for comatose, hemodynamically stable patients who experienced nonperfusing ventricular tachycardia, and ventricular fibrillation prior to resuscitation [5]. A study of therapeutic hypothermia following resuscitation from asphyxial cardiac arrest reported a 46.8% survival rate, but, in this cohort, good neurologic outcomes were reported in only a small percentage of patients (5.4%) [16].

For survivors of cardiac arrest, neuroprotection from therapeutic hypothermia has been attributed to a reduction in cerebral metabolism at reduced temperatures, estimated as a 6–10% reduction in cerebral metabolism for each reduction of one degree Celsius. Reduced brain metabolic activity prevents the progression of a cytotoxic cascade caused by free oxygen radicals, resulting in decreased cellular apoptosis between 48 and 72 hours after the arrest; decreased cerebral inflammatory responses; and improved blood-brain barrier integrity [17]. Some level 4 evidence suggests that survivors of out-of-hospital cardiac arrests from several causes may benefit from therapeutic hypothermia [18]. The target temperature for TH varies widely due to the variability in the updated recommended goal temperatures (ranging from 32°C to 36°C) in the 2015 AHA Guidelines. It is reasonable that the target temperature be maintained for at least 24 hours after achieving target temperature [19]. In this case, the patient went on to an excellent clinical outcome after receiving therapeutic hypothermia following out-of-hospital cardiac arrest with an initially nonshockable rhythm (PEA) and 15 minutes of resuscitation.

4. Conclusion

Tracheobronchial foreign body aspiration is a serious medical problem with clinical manifestations ranging from acute asphyxiation to insidious lung damage. This case highlights the importance of early identification and management of acute airway obstruction caused by foreign body aspiration, as well as the value of postresuscitation hypothermia for improving postcardiac arrest neurological outcomes.

Abbreviations

FBA: Foreign body aspiration
PEA: Pulseless electrical activity
ETT: Endotracheal tube
GCS: Glasgow Coma Scale
OHCA: Out-of-hospital cardiac arrest.

Authors' Contribution

Muhammad Kashif searched the literature and wrote the paper. Hafiz Hashmi conceived and edited the paper. Misbahuddin Khaja supervised the patient treatment and critically revised and edited the paper. All authors have made significant contributions to the paper and have reviewed it before submission. All authors have read and approved the final paper.

References

[1] S. V. Dhadke, A. L. Chaudhari, N. S. Deshpande, V. N. Dhadke, and S. A. Sangle, "Foreign body in left main bronchus," *Journal of the Association of Physicians of India*, vol. 63, no. 7, pp. 70–71, 2015.

[2] S. C. Wong and S. M. Tariq, "Cardiac arrest following foreign-body aspiration," *Respiratory Care*, vol. 56, no. 4, pp. 527–529, 2011.

[3] S. Laver, C. Farrow, D. Turner, and J. Nolan, "Mode of death after admission to an intensive care unit following cardiac arrest," *Intensive Care Medicine*, vol. 30, no. 11, pp. 2126–2128, 2004.

[4] B. K. Lee, K. W. Jeung, H. Y. Lee, and J. H. Lim, "Outcomes of therapeutic hypothermia in unconscious patients after near-hanging," *Emergency Medicine Journal*, vol. 29, no. 9, pp. 748–752, 2012.

[5] M. Holzer, "Targeted temperature management for comatose survivors of cardiac arrest," *The New England Journal of Medicine*, vol. 363, no. 13, pp. 1256–1264, 2010.

[6] F. Baharloo, F. Veyckemans, C. Francis, M.-P. Biettlot, and D. O. Rodenstein, "Tracheobronchial foreign bodies: presentation and management in children and adults," *Chest*, vol. 115, no. 5, pp. 1357–1362, 1999.

[7] B. Pritt, M. Harmon, M. Schwartz, and K. Cooper, "A tale of three aspirations: foreign bodies in the airway," *Journal of Clinical Pathology*, vol. 56, no. 10, pp. 791–794, 2003.

[8] S. Jacobson, "Upper airway obstruction," *Emergency Medicine Clinics of North America*, vol. 7, no. 2, pp. 205–217, 1989.

[9] S. I. Sersar, W. H. Rizk, M. Bilal et al., "Inhaled foreign bodies: presentation, management and value of history and plain chest radiography in delayed presentation," *Otolaryngology—Head and Neck Surgery*, vol. 134, no. 1, pp. 92–99, 2006.

[10] A. M. Berzlanovich, M. Muhm, E. Sim, and G. Bauer, "Foreign body asphyxiation—an autopsy study," *The American Journal of Medicine*, vol. 107, no. 4, pp. 351–355, 1999.

[11] L. S. Aboussouan and J. K. Stoller, "Diagnosis and management of upper airway obstruction," *Clinics in Chest Medicine*, vol. 15, no. 1, pp. 35–53, 1994.

[12] C. A. Righini, N. Morel, A. Karkas et al., "What is the diagnostic value of flexible bronchoscopy in the initial investigation of children with suspected foreign body aspiration?" *International Journal of Pediatric Otorhinolaryngology*, vol. 71, no. 9, pp. 1383–1390, 2007.

[13] N. Jamshed, K. Madan, M. Ekka, and R. Guleria, "Successful flexible bronchoscopic management of a large-sized aspirated partial denture," *BMJ Case Reports*, 2014.

[14] K. L. Swanson, "Airway foreign bodies: what's new?" *Seminars in Respiratory and Critical Care Medicine*, vol. 25, no. 4, pp. 405–411, 2004.

[15] V. Oke, R. Vadde, P. Munigikar et al., "Use of flexible bronchoscopy in an adult for removal of an aspirated foreign body at a community hospital," *Journal of Community Hospital Internal Medicine Perspectives*, vol. 5, no. 5, Article ID 28589, 2015.

[16] J. H. Wee, Y. H. You, H. Lim et al., "Outcomes of asphyxial cardiac arrest patients who were treated with therapeutic hypothermia: a multicentre retrospective cohort study," *Resuscitation*, vol. 89, pp. 81–85, 2015.

[17] R. G. Geocadin, M. A. Koenig, X. Jia, R. D. Stevens, and M. A. Peberdy, "Management of brain injury after resuscitation from cardiac arrest," *Neurologic Clinics*, vol. 26, no. 2, pp. 487–506, 2008.

[18] M. W. Donnino, L. W. Andersen, K. M. Berg et al., "ILCOR ALS Task Force. Temperature management after cardiac arrest: an advisory statement by the advanced life support task force of the international liaison committee on resuscitation and the american heart association emergency cardiovascular care committee and the council on cardiopulmonary, critical care, perioperative and resuscitation," *Circulation*, vol. 132, no. 25, pp. 2448–2456, 2015.

[19] M. Leary, A. L. Blewer, G. Delfin, and B. S. Abella, "Variability in postarrest targeted temperature management practice: implications of the 2015 guidelines," *Therapeutic Hypothermia and Temperature Management*, vol. 5, no. 4, pp. 184–187, 2015.

22

Tension Pneumothorax and Subcutaneous Emphysema Complicating Insertion of Nasogastric Tube

Narjis AL Saif, Adel Hammodi, M. Ali Al-Azem, and Rasheed Al-Hubail

Critical Care Department, King Fahad Specialist Hospital, P.O. Box 15215, Dammam 31444, Saudi Arabia

Correspondence should be addressed to Adel Hammodi; adelali34@gmail.com

Academic Editor: Moritoki Egi

Nasogastric tube has a key role in the management of substantial number of hospitalized patients particularly the critically ill. In spite of the apparent simple insertion technique, nasogastric tube placement has its serious perhaps fatal complications which need to be carefully assessed. Pulmonary misplacement and associated complications are commonplace during nasogastric tube procedure. We present a case of tension pneumothorax and massive surgical emphysema in critically ill ventilated patient due to inadvertent nasogastric tube insertion and also discussed the risk factors, complication list, and arrays of techniques for safer tube placement.

1. Introduction

Nasogastric tube insertion is a common procedure in hospitalized, particularly critically ill patients. Simple yet serious, this procedure may carry severe complications, increasing the odds of morbidity and mortality. The interactions between patient and procedure risk factors probably aggravate the range of drawbacks. Training, observation, and confirmation techniques would help to prevent or at least minimize the complication and maximize safe practice.

2. Case Report

2.1. History. Sixty-year-old male patient was known to have type II diabetes mellitus, hypertension, 4-year postrenal transplant, and hepatitis C cirrhosis. The patient was admitted to the hospital complaining of watery diarrhea that proved to be due to cytomegalovirus (CMV) colitis. During hospital stay, he developed respiratory distress and hypoxia, so he was transferred to the intensive care unit (ICU).

2.2. Assessment and ICU Course. The patient was intubated with no airway difficulty, connected to mechanical ventilation with SIMV/pressure support mode, FiO_2 0.4, and PEEP of $12 \, cmH_2O$ to maintain oxygen saturation of 95%. His chest X-ray showed bilateral airspace disease that was suggestive

of CMV pneumonitis. The patient was in a shock status requiring norepinephrine infusion of 18 micrograms/min. The patient was sedated with fentanyl and propofol targeting Richmond Agitation Sedation Scale (RASS) of −2.

In order to establish enteral feeding, attempts of insertion of nasogastric tube had failed. By the third attempt, a 16-French size, stylet-stiffened polyurethane nasogastric tube was inserted without difficulty.

The aspiration via the inserted NG tube revealed a 300 mL of clear yellow fluid. However, insufflations with 50 mL of air and auscultation at epigastric area were equivocal.

After NG tube insertion, chest X-ray showed misplaced NG tube at the right main bronchus down to the right pleural space and development of new 7.8 mm right sided pneumothorax (Figure 1, chest X-ray). The NG tube had been immediately removed and PEEP was decreased to $5 \, cmH_2O$. Over few minutes, the patient became progressively hypotensive and hypoxic, requiring higher doses of norepinephrine infusion and FiO_2 of 60% to maintain 95% saturation. Right sided chest tube was inserted and the repeated X-ray revealed new subcutaneous emphysema (Figure 2). Using direct laryngoscopy technique, nasogastric tube was inserted under vision.

Over the following seven days, the patient condition had improved and the patient was successfully extubated and noninvasive ventilation was applied electively for few hours.

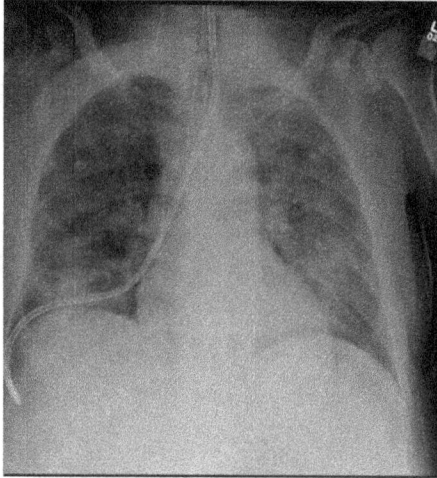

FIGURE 1

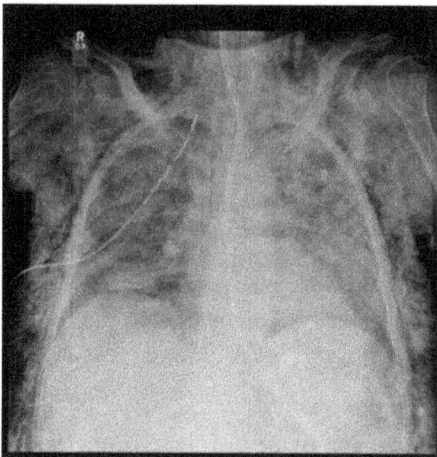

FIGURE 2

3. Discussion

Nasogastric tube (NGT) placement is a frequently performed procedure for hospitalized, particularly critically ill patients. Though it seems a simple procedure, it may carry potential life-threatening complications due to misplacement. These complications may be exacerbated by the delay in recognition or removal of misplaced tube.

In one prospective series of 740 NGT insertions in ICU patients, there was a 2% incidence of tracheopulmonary complications with a mortality of 0.3%, with pneumothoraces being the most frequent complication [1]. Other thoracic complications include erroneous bronchial placement, leading to atelectasis, pneumonia, and lung abscess (Table 1).

While the enteral nutrition is devoid of risk of complications associated with central venous catheter insertion for parental nutrition, the hazard of pulmonary complications with feeding tube insertion is comparable to that of central line [2].

Arrays of risk factors which individually or synergistically lead to NGT malposition are summarized in Table 2.

Our patient had developed an iatrogenic tension pneumothorax secondary to misplaced NG tube as a result of intricately involved potential risk factors, namely, impairment of conscious level, being critically ill, and the presence of endotracheal tube. All those factors compromise the airway reflexes, swallowing mechanism, and patient's ability to report shortness of breath or chest discomfort associated with displaced NGT. In addition, the blind insertion of NGT, stylet-stiffened feeding tube, and multiple attempts of insertion are well recognized predisposing factors of NGT complications [3, 4].

In the presented case, bedside tests were done in order to confirm appropriate positioning, starting with aspiration of gastric fluid which was falsely positive due to extraction of the yellowish pleural effusion. Then, air insufflation test was performed revealing worrisome auscultation sounds for possible tracheopulmonary insertion; for that reason, the tube was not used for feeding and a chest X-ray was requested, though it is not our routine institutional protocol, done, and confirmed a malposition NGT into the right pleural space. Criticizing the lack of the institutional protocol was addressed clearly by Weinberg and Skewes who concluded that the adoption of rigid protocols that include a mandatory radiograph immediately after the insertion of feeding tubes shows an alarming rate of 1–3% risk of feeding tubes lodging at any site in the airway down to the lung [5].

The traditional bedside techniques of gastric aspiration and insufflation test lack specificity and sensitivity and often give false reassurance that the NGT is properly positioned [6, 7].

Several suggested confirmatory tests are depicted elaborately in the literature including clinical, radiological, and laboratory investigations (Table 3).

Nevertheless, chest X-ray after insertion of feeding tube is considered a gold standard confirmatory test [6], which prevents additional complications.

In an endeavor to prevent rather than reduce the NGT insertion drawbacks, many trials and techniques had been described. In 1989, Roubenoff and Ravich proposed a two-step protocol for nasogastric tube insertion. In this procedure, the feeding tube is initially advanced blindly to 30 cm and then its position is verified by chest radiograph. After radiographic confirmation of the tube position in the esophagus, the tube is further inserted into its adequate length and a second radiograph is taken to check the final location [7].

Marderstein et al. applied that protocol at their institution and found that the rate of nasogastric tube induced pneumothorax decreased from 0.38% to 0.09%. While improving patient safety, it is a time-consuming protocol, exposing the patient to two X-rays and questioning its cost-effectiveness [3].

Additionally, the observation of the aspirate character to predict proper placement is subjective and has limited value which could be deceiving as what had occurred with our case [8].

Having inadequate conventional confirmatory methods, several new techniques are developed to overcome the misplacement and related complications. In addition to fluoroscopic and endoscopic based approaches, another device that

TABLE 1: Complications of nasogastric tubes insertion.

Organ/system	Complication	
Nasopharyngeal	Hemorrhage	
	Ulceration	
	Oropharyngeal coiling	
	Eustachian tube misplacement	
Larynx	Trauma	
	Ulceration	
	Vocal cord dysfunction	
	Vocal cord paralysis	
Gastrointestinal	Coiling	Knotted tube
	Hemorrhage	Reflex esophagitis
	Ulceration	Pneumoperitoneum
	Perforation	Esophageal feeding
	Tracheoesophageal fistula	Sepsis
Pleuropulmonary (2%)	Aspiration of gastric content/enteral feed: pneumonitis, pneumonia, empyema, abscess, and sepsis Bronchial misplacement: atelectasis, collapse, pulmonary hemorrhage, and perforation	Intrapleural placement: pneumothorax (60%), haemothorax, hydrothorax, and bronchopleural fistula Airway obstruction: early or late; respiratory distress and ventilator failure
Mediastinal	Mediastinal misplacement	
	Mediastinitis	
	Pneumomediastinum	
Others	Nasogastric tube syndrome (upper airway obstruction secondary to ulceration of postcricoid region causing vocal cord abduction paralysis)	
	Intracranial misplacement	
	Erosion to large vessels	

TABLE 2: Factors increasing the risk of nasogastric tube misplacement.

NGT factors	Technique factors	Patient factors
(i) Fine bore	(i) Inexperienced operator	(i) Altered mental status
(ii) Stiff monofilament core	(ii) Incorrect patient position	(ii) Critically ill patients
(iii) Stiffening wire	(iii) Blind insertion	(iii) Endotracheal intubation
(iv) Absent radiopaque marker	(iv) Incorrect NGT length	(iv) Tracheostomy
(v) Flexible polymer constriction	(v) Repeated attempts	(v) Use of sedation
		(vi) Use of neuromuscular blocker agents
		(vii) Anatomical facial abnormalities
		(viii) Facial trauma/inhalation injury
	(vi) Insufficient lubricant	(ix) Anticoagulation/thrombophilia
		(x) Upper airway/esophageal injury
		(xi) Nasopharyngeal pathology
		(xii) Following lung transplant

allows for real time localization of the feeding tube tip was assessed by Young et al. with promising success rates [9]. This technology uses a signaling device at the end of the NGT which is traced by an external sensor with feedback signals as it passes through stomach, pylorus, and duodenum.

4. Conclusion

Airway and other significant complications rates pertinent to NGT insertion are considerable. Institutional protocol is required to reduce the substantial risk of tube misplacement of NGT.

Considering the potential life-threatening complications that may occur in case of displaced nasogastric tube, especially in critically ill patient, alternative essential confirmatory methods need to be discovered.

Capnometry method has the highest specificity and sensitivity among the other known bedside methodologies. Carbon dioxide detection monitoring may detect the respiratory displacement of the feeding tube and consequently

TABLE 3: Techniques used to confirm NG position.

The technique	Comment
Insufflation test	(i) Unreliable in small tubes or those with guide wire because of reduced airflow (ii) 20% false positive results [10, 11]
Gastric aspiration	(i) Normal gastric aspirate is clear to slightly yellow (ii) Altered in gastrointestinal bleeding and bowel obstruction
Aspirated fluid pH and bilirubin	(i) A pH less than 5 and bilirubin less than 5 mg/dL identified 98% of gastric sites (ii) A pH greater than 5 and bilirubin less than 5 mg/dL identified 100% of the respiratory sites [12]
Capnometry	Reported high specificity and sensitivity rate [13, 14]
Capnography	Capnography was as accurate as colorimetric device for detecting CO_2 during placement of NG tubes [15]
Magnetic guidance	(i) Relatively new technique (ii) Rule out the presence of the NGT in stomach and lung

contribute to the prevention of pulmonary complications. Nevertheless, the other techniques still aimed at early detection of anticipated adverse events rather than prevention.

Experienced operator, periprocedural risk assessment, proper technique of placement, and postprocedure confirmations are the fundamental recommendations for safe NGT insertions.

References

[1] A. J. Rassias, P. A. Ball, and H. L. Corwin, "A prospective study of tracheopulmonary complications associated with the placement of narrow-bore enteral feeding tubes," *Critical Care*, vol. 2, no. 1, pp. 25–28, 1998.

[2] H. Al-Jahdali, K. L. Irion, C. Allen, D. M. de Godoy, and A. N. Khan, "Imaging review of procedural and periprocedural complications of central venous lines, percutaneous intrathoracic drains, and nasogastric tubes," *Pulmonary Medicine*, vol. 2012, Article ID 842138, 18 pages, 2012.

[3] E. L. Marderstein, R. L. Simmons, and J. B. Ochoa, "Patient safety: effect of institutional protocols on adverse events related to feeding tube placement in the critically ill," *Journal of the American College of Surgeons*, vol. 199, no. 1, pp. 39–50, 2004.

[4] P.-C. Wang, G.-Y. Tseng, H.-B. Yang, K.-C. Chou, and C.-H. Chen, "Inadvertent tracheobronchial placement of feeding tube in a mechanically ventilated patient," *Journal of the Chinese Medical Association*, vol. 71, no. 7, pp. 365–367, 2008.

[5] L. Weinberg and D. Skewes, "Pneumothorax from intrapleural placement of a nasogastric tube," *Anaesthesia and Intensive Care*, vol. 34, no. 2, pp. 276–279, 2006.

[6] J. B. Pillai, A. Vegas, and S. Brister, "Thoracic complications of nasogastric tube: review of safe practice," *Interactive Cardiovascular and Thoracic Surgery*, vol. 4, no. 5, pp. 429–433, 2005.

[7] R. Roubenoff and W. J. Ravich, "Pneumothorax due to nasogastric feeding tubes: report of four cases, review of the literature, and recommendations for prevention," *Archives of Internal Medicine*, vol. 149, no. 1, pp. 184–188, 1989.

[8] N. A. Metheny, R. Schnelker, J. McGinnis et al., "Indicators of tube site during feeding," *Journal of Neuroscience Nursing*, vol. 37, no. 6, pp. 320–325, 2005.

[9] R. J. Young, M. J. Chapman, R. Fraser, R. Vozzo, D. P. Chorley, and S. Creed, "A novel technique for post-pyloric feeding tube placement in critically ill patients: a pilot study," *Anaesthesia & Intensive Care*, vol. 33, no. 2, pp. 229–234, 2005.

[10] R. Benya, S. Langer, and S. Mobarhan, "Flexible nasogastric feeding tube tip malposition immediately after placement," *Journal of Parenteral and Enteral Nutrition*, vol. 14, no. 1, pp. 108–109, 1990.

[11] N. A. Metheny, L. Smith, and B. J. Stewart, "Development of a reliable and valid bedside test for bilirubin and its utility for improving prediction of feeding tube location," *Nursing Research*, vol. 49, no. 6, pp. 302–309, 2000.

[12] C. E. Araujo-Preza, M. E. Melhado, F. J. Gutierrez, T. Maniatis, and M. A. Castellano, "Use of capnometry to verify feeding tube placement," *Critical Care Medicine*, vol. 30, no. 10, pp. 2255–2259, 2002.

[13] Joanna Briggs Institute, "Methods for determining the correct nasogastric tube placement after insertion in adults," *Best Practice*, vol. 14, no. 1, 2010.

[14] S. M. Burns, R. Carpenter, and J. D. Truwit, "Report on the development of a procedure to prevent placement of feeding tubes into the lungs using end-tidal CO_2 measurements," *Critical Care Medicine*, vol. 29, no. 5, pp. 936–939, 2001.

[15] S. M. Burns, R. Carpenter, C. Blevins et al., "Detection of inadvertent airway intubation during gastric tube insertion: capnography versus a colorimetric carbon dioxide detector," *American Journal of Critical Care*, vol. 15, no. 2, pp. 188–195, 2006.

23

Malignant Catatonia Warrants Early Psychiatric-Critical Care Collaborative Management: Two Cases and Literature Review

Julia Park,[1] **Josh Tan,**[1] **Sylvia Krzeminski,**[1] **Maryam Hazeghazam,**[2] **Meghana Bandlamuri,**[1] **and Richard W. Carlson**[1,3,4]

[1]*Department of Medicine, Maricopa Medical Center, Phoenix, AZ, USA*
[2]*Department of Psychiatry, Maricopa Medical Center, Phoenix, AZ, USA*
[3]*College of Medicine, University of Arizona, Phoenix, AZ, USA*
[4]*College of Medicine, Mayo Clinic, Scottsdale, AZ, USA*

Correspondence should be addressed to Julia Park; tojuliapark@gmail.com

Academic Editor: Gil Klinger

Malignant catatonia (MC) is a life-threatening manifestation which can occur in the setting of an underlying neuropsychiatric syndrome or general medical illness and shares clinical and pathophysiological features and medical comorbidities with the Neuroleptic Malignant Syndrome (NMS). The subsequent diagnosis and definitive therapy of MC are typically delayed, which increases morbidity and mortality. We present two cases of MC and review recent literature of MC and NMS, illustrating factors which delay diagnosis and management. When clinical features suggest MC or NMS, we propose early critical care consultation and stabilization with collaborative psychiatric management.

1. Introduction

MC, previously termed "lethal catatonia," is the most severe manifestation within the spectrum of catatonic syndromes. Catatonia is defined as immobility, rigidity, mutism, posturing, excessive motor activity, stupor, negativism, staring, and echolalia. MC represents a life-threatening manifestation that can develop in the context of a neuropsychiatric syndrome or general medical illness and includes behavioral changes, movement disturbances, and autonomic dysregulation [1–5].

Schizophrenia is the most commonly cited inciting condition, although major depression and various toxic-metabolic etiologies have also been implicated. Typical symptoms of MC include catalepsy, stupor, mutism, waxy flexibility, negativism, posturing, autonomic dysfunction, rigidity, fever, and muscle injury [4, 6–10].

Although the potential lethal consequences of MC are well known, diagnosis is often difficult and typically delayed. Due to the fact that both MC and NMS have similar biochemical and neuropharmacologic disturbances, similar clinical features can be seen in both disorders. Current concepts suggest that NMS and malignant catatonia represent a spectrum with biochemical and neuropharmacologic disturbances that involve disturbances of dopamine and GABAergic receptors [11, 12].

The predominant pathophysiology of NMS is central dopamine receptor blockade in the hypothalamus that results in autonomic dysregulation [13]. However, as many patients with either MC or NMS respond to benzodiazepines, it is thought that both share a single biochemical pathway of reduced $GABA_A$ inhibition of the frontal corticostriatal tracts [6, 12].

Standard treatment of MC includes initiation of benzodiazepines and electroconvulsive therapy (ECT). Prior to this approach, the mortality of MC typically exceeded 50%. Recent management strategies which include combined ECT and benzodiazepines result in decreases in morbidity and mortality [14]. Dąbrowski et al. reported full recovery to baseline in up to 80% of patients with this approach [14, 15]. However delay of treatment continues to remain a concerning issue, as recent studies reveal treatment delays are on average 60 days prior to initiation of treatment with benzodiazepines or ECT [16].

We describe two patients with MC that illustrate the problems of misdiagnosis, delayed identifications, and management of critical cardiopulmonary and metabolic disturbances which lead to further delays of definitive therapy. We review clinical features and current management of MC and NMS and propose guidelines for prompt and ongoing collaborative management between psychiatry and critical care services when MC is suspected.

1.1. Case 1. A 55-year-old male with a history of schizophrenia who was noncompliant of medications presented to the hospital with catatonic symptoms and autonomic instability. During the hospital stay, the patient exhibited worsening catatonia, mutism, anorexia, leukocytosis, and autonomic instability. He was treated with rehydration, electrolyte replacement, antibiotics for aspiration pneumonia, and nasoenteral tube feeding. The clinical picture was initially thought to be most consistent with catatonic schizophrenia and the patient was transferred to a psychiatric facility for ECT after fourteen days of medical therapy. During ECT without protection of airway, the patient developed a cardiac arrest with pulseless ventricular tachycardia that was related to dehydration, pneumonia, and sepsis. He was resuscitated, intubated, and admitted to the ICU. The patient had additional complications which included Methicillin Sensitive *Staphylococcus aureus* (MSSA) pneumonia, ischemic colitis, and Vancomycin Resistant Enterococcus (VRE) Urinary Tract Infection (UTI). From the initial presentation to the facility after the cardiac arrest, the diagnosis was delayed by 15 days. Benzodiazepines were initiated at the time of diagnosis and ECT was initiated after medical stabilization that required a total of 26 days from initial presentation. The patient slowly showed signs of clinical improvement in mental status. He was discharged to an extended care inpatient psychiatric facility after nearly 16 months of inpatient psychiatric care.

1.2. Case 2. A 20-year-old male was admitted to inpatient psychiatric care due to acute psychosis. He developed autonomic instability, catatonia, mutism, waxy flexibility, and agitation. He was transferred to a medicine service for treatment of suspected MC. After a poor response to benzodiazepines, institution of ECT was delayed from the time of diagnosis by seventeen days. The delay in treatment was primarily related to exclusion of alternative diagnoses. Critical care was consulted 7 days after admission for MC. The patient was ultimately given a total of 12 sessions of ECT, which resulted in gradual improvement after each dose. During the hospital stay, the patient developed multiple complications including dehydration, urinary tract infection due to *Escherichia coli*, and aspiration pneumonia. The patient's mental status improved. He was discharged home after 4 months of inpatient psychiatric care.

2. Review and Discussion

The cases presented herein illustrate that MC is an emergent and life-threatening illness that is accompanied by multiorgan dysfunction, including cardiopulmonary and metabolic defects requiring concurrent ICU and psychiatric care [1]. Both patients presented in this article suffered severe complications, including cardiopulmonary crisis, infections, dehydration, and prolonged hospital stay. We propose that suspicion of MC should prompt collaborative psychiatric and critical care management with early use of ECT if there is inadequate response to benzodiazepines therapy [7, 17].

We agree with Tuerlings et al. that the high mortality associated with MC is related in part to the failure of rapid and efficient exclusion of alternative diagnoses [18, 19]. The authors reported that delay to first and second treatment was 15 and 60 days, respectively [18]. A decrease in this delay should be a major goal as treatment delay and longer duration of symptoms without treatment have been associated with poorer clinical response [20]. We propose that organic causes be promptly narrowed by psychiatric history, medications changes, overdoses, metabolic derangements, and central nervous system infections. Any suspicion of MC should prompt admission to a critical care unit and stabilization as the diagnostic process proceeds. Currently, no biomarkers exist for MC to assist in diagnosis, although there appears to be an association of elevated d-dimer in the disease [21]. Use of this marker may be helpful in expediting detection of this disease. We further postulate that favorable outcomes may be achieved by collaborative management between critical care and psychiatry, with earlier detection and exclusion of alternative diagnoses, and prompt management of complications associated with MC.

Similarities exist between NMS and MC, thus confounding the picture of a potentially life-threatening disease. Therefore, a comparison of the differences and similarities between the two syndromes is warranted [7, 22–26]. Typically, MC is predominantly manifested by bizarre behavior and mutism, posturing, and catalepsy and with psychiatric disturbances. In contrast, NMS is classically linked to exposure of a neuroleptic agent or atypical antipsychotic, with prominent features of rigidity, autonomic dysfunction, fever, and stupor [4, 11, 26]. Both MC and NMS may lead to muscle injury, aspiration, and metabolic disturbance due to hyperthermia and altered mental status. However, prodromes of MC have psychiatric undertones of psychosis, agitation, stupor, mutism, or anxiety while NMS would present with acute onset of autonomic instability and extrapyramidal side effects after antipsychotic exposure [4, 11, 26]. Therefore, if history excludes exposure to an antipsychotic, the diagnosis of MC would be apparent [3, 4, 22].

Unfortunately, this defining characteristic may be blurred for providers, as the majority of patients with MC have a psychiatric history and therefore have been treated with antipsychotics.

In many instances, the deduction to the diagnosis of NMS or MC requires several days, during which time patients may

TABLE 1: Complications associated with patient's clinical features.

Clinical features	Potential complications
Autonomic instability	Hypotension, hypertension, arrhythmias, myocardial ischemia, rhabdomyolysis, hemodynamic instability
Decreased movement	Thromboembolic disease, pressure ulcers, rhabdomyolysis
Decreased oral intake	Dehydration, hypovolemia, electrolyte derangements, inability to take oral medications
Catalepsy	Decreased airway clearance, aspiration pneumonia, hypoxemia, pneumonia

already develop medical comorbidities. One of the largest series that reviewed the clinical course of MC was reported by Tuerlings et al. (2010). The mean lag time from first catatonic symptoms to first treatment with benzodiazepines or ECT was 15 days on average. The time lag between the first and second treatment was approximately 27 days. Reported overall improvement with treatment was 76% and complete remission was 58%. Mortality was 9%. Virtually, it is impossible to differentiate NMS from MC on clinical presentation and course. Importantly, both conditions require the same treatment consisting of withdrawal of antipsychotics and initiation of benzodiazepines and ECT as first-line treatments [18].

Whether the diagnosis is MC or NMS, both of the conditions have life-threatening consequences and therefore need ICU and psychiatric collaboration. Alternative diagnoses must be swiftly excluded and benzodiazepines must be utilized within 24 hours as first-line treatment for MC and NMS [18]. Additionally, ECT has been theorized as effective second- if not first-line treatment. ECT should be supplemented after or additionally with benzodiazepines [27–29]. Benzodiazepines are theorized to improve MC and NMS by increasing GABA$_A$ activity. Likewise, the use of ECT may involve GABA activity by inducing a neural storm with increased GABA transmission and clinical improvement [7, 27].

MC typically has a complicated course that involves multiple medical comorbid conditions such as dehydration, aspiration pneumonia, electrolyte disturbances, cardiopulmonary instability, and thromboembolic phenomena. Table 1 lists symptoms and clinical features and associated complications. Psychiatric care including the use of benzodiazepines and ECT is important, but identifying the appropriate level of medical support is crucial [5, 6, 19]. The psychiatric management includes sedative care and ECT treatment for up to 7 days. We suggest that critical care consultation and protection of airway may facilitate safer ECT by close monitoring and prompt care for life-threatening arrhythmias, airway protection, aspiration, hemodynamic instability, ischemia, and fluid and electrolyte balance [17, 30, 31].

3. Conclusion

The previous cases and review describe MC from diagnosis to management and complications. Delays or subtherapeutic treatment with ineffective and less aggressive methods increase morbidity and mortality [16].

No standardized treatment protocols exist for complications of MC, thus causing a delay and hindrance to proper treatment. Prompt identification and institution of life-saving treatments of ECT and pharmacologic therapy with benzodiazepines can be achieved by early critical care consultation for appropriate level of care that is equipped for attention to fluid-electrolyte balance, cardiopulmonary stabilization, and thermoregulation.

Competing Interests

The authors declare that they have no competing interests.

References

[1] M. A. Oldham and H. B. Lee, "Catatonia vis-à-vis delirium: the significance of recognizing catatonia in altered mental status," General Hospital Psychiatry, vol. 37, no. 6, pp. 554–559, 2015.

[2] P. M. Sadr, M. Hazeghazam, M. Bailon et al., "Management of a severe form of malignant catatonia: useful lessons in diagnosis and management," in Proceedings of the American Psychiatric Association Annual Meeting, San Francisco, Calif, USA, March 2013.

[3] V. R. Velamoor, "Neuroleptic malignant syndrome," Drug Safety, vol. 19, no. 1, pp. 73–82, 1998.

[4] E. Castillo, R. T. Rubin, and E. Holsboer-Trachsler, "Clinical differentiation between lethal catatonia and neuroleptic malignant syndrome," The American Journal of Psychiatry, vol. 146, no. 3, pp. 324–328, 1989.

[5] A. F. Gross, F. A. Smith, and T. A. Stern, "Dread complications of catatonia: a case discussion and review of the literature," Primary Care Companion to the Journal of Clinical Psychiatry, vol. 10, no. 2, pp. 153–155, 2008.

[6] G. L. Fricchione, A. F. Gross, J. C. Huffman, G. Bush, and T. A. Stern, "Catatonia, neuroleptic malignant syndrome, and serotonin syndrome," in Massachusetts General Hospital Handbook of General Hospital Psychiatry, Elsevier, 2016, https://www.clinicalkey.com/#!/content/book/3-s2.0-B9781437719277000212.

[7] M. Fink, "Catatonia: a syndrome appears, disappears, and is rediscovered," Canadian Journal of Psychiatry, vol. 54, no. 7, pp. 437–445, 2009.

[8] M. M. Woodbury and M. A. Woodbury, "Neuroleptic-induced catatonia as a stage in the progression toward neuroleptic malignant syndrome," Journal of the American Academy of Child and Adolescent Psychiatry, vol. 31, no. 6, pp. 1161–1164, 1992.

[9] W. W. Fleischhacker, B. Unterweger, J. M. Kane, and H. Hinterhuber, "The neuroleptic malignant syndrome and its differentiation from lethal catatonia," Acta Psychiatrica Scandinavica, vol. 81, no. 1, pp. 3–5, 1990.

[10] A. Francis, "Catatonia: diagnosis, classification, and treatment," Current Psychiatry Reports, vol. 12, no. 3, pp. 180–185, 2010.

[11] F. U. Lang, S. Lang, T. Becker, and M. Jäger, "Neuroleptic malignant syndrome or catatonia? Trying to solve the catatonic dilemma," Psychopharmacology, vol. 232, no. 1, pp. 1–5, 2015.

[12] B. T. Carroll, "The universal field hypothesis of catatonia and neuroleptic malignant syndrome," *CNS Spectrums*, vol. 5, no. 7, pp. 26–33, 2000.

[13] G. Northoff, "Catatonia and neuroleptic malignant syndrome: psychopathology and pathophysiology," *Journal of Neural Transmission*, vol. 109, no. 12, pp. 1453–1467, 2002.

[14] M. Dąbrowski and T. Parnowski, "Clinical analysis of safety and effectiveness of electroconvulsive therapy," *Psychiatria Polska*, vol. 46, no. 3, pp. 345–360, 2012.

[15] O. Freudenreich, S. H. Nejad, A. Francis, and G. L. Fricchione, "Psychosis, mania, and catatonia," in *Textbook of Psychosomatic Medicine: Psychiatric Care of the Medically Ill*, J. L. Levenson, Ed., American Psychiatric, Washington, DC, USA, 2011.

[16] J. A. Van Waarde, J. H. A. M. Tuerlings, B. Verwey, and R. C. Van Der Mast, "Electroconvulsive therapy for catatonia: treatment characteristics and outcomes in 27 patients," *The Journal of ECT*, vol. 26, no. 4, pp. 248–252, 2010.

[17] F. Luchini, P. Medda, M. Mariani, M. Mauri, C. Toni, and G. Perugi, "Electroconvulsive therapy in catatonic patients: efficacy and predictors of response," *World Journal of Psychiatry*, vol. 5, no. 2, pp. 182–192, 2015.

[18] J. H. A. M. Tuerlings, J. A. van Waarde, and B. Verwey, "A retrospective study of 34 catatonic patients: analysis of clinical care and treatment," *General Hospital Psychiatry*, vol. 32, no. 6, pp. 631–635, 2010.

[19] B. K. Boyarsky, M. Fuller, and T. Early, "Malignant catatonia-induced respiratory failure with response to ECT," *The Journal of ECT*, vol. 15, no. 3, pp. 232–236, 1999.

[20] J. C. Narayanaswamy, P. Tibrewal, A. Zutshi, R. Srinivasaraju, and S. B. Math, "Clinical predictors of response to treatment in catatonia," *General Hospital Psychiatry*, vol. 34, no. 3, pp. 312–316, 2012.

[21] S. Haouzir, X. Lemoine, M. Petit et al., "The role of coagulation marker fibrin D-dimer in early diagnosis of catatonia," *Psychiatry Research*, vol. 168, no. 1, pp. 78–85, 2009.

[22] J. W. Y. Lee, "Neuroleptic-induced catatonia: clinical presentation, response to benzodiazepines, and relationship to neuroleptic malignant syndrome," *Journal of Clinical Psychopharmacology*, vol. 30, no. 1, pp. 3–10, 2010.

[23] D. A. C. White, "Catatonia and the neuroleptic malignant syndrome—a single entity?" *The British Journal of Psychiatry*, vol. 161, pp. 558–560, 1992.

[24] V. R. Velamoor, "Neuroleptic malignant syndrome," *Drug Safety*, vol. 19, no. 1, pp. 73–82, 1998.

[25] M. Koch, S. Chandragiri, S. Rizvi, G. Petrides, and A. Francis, "Catatonic signs in neuroleptic malignant syndrome," *Comprehensive Psychiatry*, vol. 41, no. 1, pp. 73–75, 2000.

[26] S. Caroff, S. Mann, and P. Keck, "Specific treatment of the neuroleptic malignant syndrome," *Biological Psychiatry*, vol. 44, no. 6, pp. 378–381, 1998.

[27] S. C. Mann, S. N. Caroff, H. R. Bleier, R. E. Antelo, and H. Un, "Electroconvulsive therapy of the lethal catatonia syndrome," *Convulsive Therapy*, vol. 6, no. 3, pp. 239–247, 1990.

[28] J. M. Hawkins, K. J. Archer, S. M. Strakowski, and P. E. Keck Jr., "Somatic treatment of catatonia," *International Journal of Psychiatry in Medicine*, vol. 25, no. 4, pp. 345–369, 1995.

[29] J. M. Davis, P. G. Janicak, P. Sakkas, C. Gilmore, and Z. Wang, "Electroconvulsive therapy in the treatment of the neuroleptic malignant syndrome," *Convulsive Therapy*, vol. 7, no. 2, pp. 111–120, 1991.

[30] W. V. McCall, S. C. Mann, F. E. Shelp, and S. N. Caroff, "Fatal pulmonary embolism in the catatonic syndrome: two case reports and a literature review," *The Journal of Clinical Psychiatry*, vol. 56, no. 1, pp. 21–25, 1995.

[31] W. M. McDonald, T. W. Meeks, W. V. McCall, and C. F. Zorumski, "Electroconvulsive therapy," in *The American Psychiatric Publishing Textbook of Psychopharmacology*, 2009, http://psychiatryonline.org/doi/full/10.1176/appi.books.9781585623860.as44.

24

Early Diagnosis of Nonconvulsive Status Epilepticus Recurrence with Raw EEG of a Bispectral Index Monitor

Aristide Ntahe (iD)

Département d'Anesthésie-Réanimation, Hôpital Saint-Louis, Assistance Publique-Hôpitaux de Paris, 1 Avenue Claude Vellefaux, 75010 Paris, France

Correspondence should be addressed to Aristide Ntahe; aristide.ntahe@yahoo.fr

Academic Editor: Chiara Lazzeri

Background. Seizures are frequent in ICU and their diagnosis is challenging, often delayed or missed. Their diagnosis requires a conventional EEG recording. When cEEG is not available, there is no consensus on how patients should be monitored when there is high risk of seizure. This case illustrates how a bispectral index monitor allowed an early diagnosis of an NCSE recurrence. *Case Presentation.* A NCSE was diagnosed at the admission. cEEG was not available and then a bispectral index (BIS) monitor was placed and processed parameters were monitored as usual. During the first and second day, both conventional and BIS's EEG showed patterns of burst suppression and the BIS value varied between 25 and 35 while the suppression ratio (SR) varied between 20 and 35. On the third day, while hypnotic drugs were withdrawn progressively, raw EEG of the BIS monitor showed spikes, spikes waves, and polyspikes without significant variation of BIS and SR values. Even if processed parameters stayed between their usual ranges, the typical aspect of the real time EEG raised concern for NCSE recurrence. An unplanned conventional EEG recording was urgently requested, and the diagnosis was confirmed and treated. *Conclusion.* Primitive and secondary brain injuries can lead to seizures which are often purely electrical. Even though BIS monitors cannot substitute the conventional EEG, processed parameters and raw EEG should be always analysed jointly. In the present case, seizure was suspected only on the aspect of real time EEG which showed spikes, spikes waves, and polyspikes.

1. Background

Hypoxic-ischaemic brain injury is one of the most feared complications following cardiac arrest. If present, the incidence of seizures and status epilepticus is high and associated with poor outcome [1]. Managing status epilepticus without continuous EEG (cEEG) is very challenging especially if it is a nonconvulsive status epilepticus (NCSE). Bispectral index (BIS) is one among other technologies used to monitor hypnotic drug's effect in operating room and in intensive care units (ICU). BIS monitors display 2 numbers named BIS and suppression ratio (SR) which are derived from analysis of frontal EEG signal by a single sensor (with multiples electrodes) placed on the forehead. This case showed how the raw EEG signal of BIS monitor allowed a rapid diagnosis of a NCSE recurrence.

2. Case Presentation

A 75-year-old woman was admitted in ICU after a cardiac arrest with return of spontaneous circulation, caused by tension pneumothorax. Now-flow and low-flow were 1 minute and 17 minutes, respectively. She was admitted 1 hour after the event, without sedation. Lungs were mechanically ventilated, the pleural drain was in place, pulse oximetry was 100% /FiO2 0.5, arterial pressure and heart rate were 160/70 mmHg and 110bpm, respectively, with norepinephrine at an infusion rate of 1mg/h, and temperature and glycaemia were 36.5°C and 8 mmol/L, respectively. There was no any sign of pneumothorax. Fever was actively treated without inducing hypothermia.

She was unconscious (Glasgow Coma Scale: 3/15), with a conserved bilateral photomotor reflexes. She had intermittent

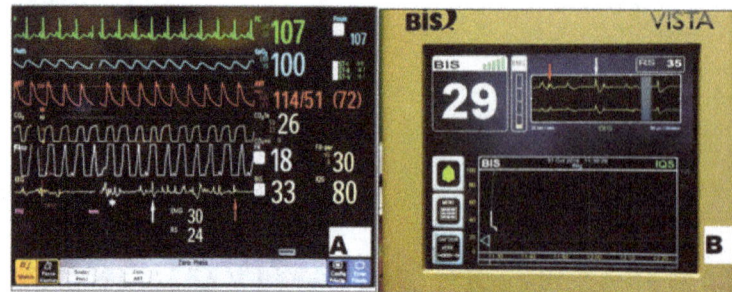

FIGURE 1: PANEL A: 2 channels sensors (BIS Quatro) connected to a Philips module: real time EEG shows polyspikes (white star), spikes (white arrow), and spike-wave (red arrow). IQS = signal quality index. RS= suppression ratio. PANEL B: 2-channel sensor (BIS Quatro) connected to a BIS VISTA module: real time EEG shows spike-wave (red arrow) and spike (white arrow). IQS = signal quality index. RS= suppression ratio.

bilateral ocular revulsion and bilateral shoulders tremor. Propofol was initiated by a bolus followed by a continuous infusion and the movements of the eyes and shoulders ceased immediately. One hour later a 13 channels EEG (Figure S1 in supplementary figures) diagnosed a NCSE as a pattern of generalized periodic spike-waves evolving in generalized rhythmic spike-waves at 1 Hz with high amplitude (> 200 μV), without response to stimulation. Midazolam was initiated by a bolus followed by a continuous infusion which permitted to achieve a burst suppression pattern (Figure S2 in supplementary figures). A 4-channel sensor connected to BIS VISTA[5] monitor was placed, in order to monitor the two processed parameters and showed an isoelectric signal (Figure S3 in supplementary figures).

On day 2 Clobazam and levetiracetam were added to ensure a bridging between IV and oral antiepileptic drugs. Conventional EEG recording showed a pattern of burst suppression and raw EEG from BIS monitor showed an isoelectric signal.

On day 3, the 4-channel sensor was replaced by a 2-channel sensor which was connected to patient's bedside monitoring. Propofol and midazolam were both decreased progressively. Few hours later (Figure 1, video 1, and figure S4), while there were no any abnormal movements, raw EEG of BIS monitor connected to a Philips BIS module [panel A] and secondarily to a BIS VISTA module [panel B] showed a pattern of high voltage with irregular morphology, alternating with isoelectric signal, evoking spikes (white arrows), spike-waves (red arrows), and polyspikes (white star). BIS and SR values did not show significant variations.

Although it was not planned at that moment to request a conventional EEG recording, given the high suspicion of NCSE recurrence, the neurophysiology team was urgently contacted and the NCSE recurrence was confirmed and treated. The conventional EEG showed continuous generalized rhythmic spikes and spike-waves, sharply countered, of medium amplitude at 1-1.5 Hz (Figure S5 in supplementary figures). Unfortunately the patient died on the fifth day.

3. Discussion

The context of sudden brain aggression, the bilateral stereotyped movements, the EEG pattern, the clinical and EEG

responses following propofol, and midazolam injections and withdrawal are all in favour of a NCSE, according to recent definitions [2].

Seizures are frequent in ICU, independently of the presence of primitive brain lesion, and are subclinical in the majority of cases [3–5]; this put the ICU's patients at high risk for secondary brain injury, poor neurologic outcome, and increase mortality [6–8]. Diagnosis of nonconvulsive seizures or status epilepticus can be very challenging and is often delayed or simply missed. One reason is that there are multiple causes of altered mental status in ICU; the second major reason is availability of EEG equipment and interpreting staff. In 2015 the American clinical neurophysiology society issued recommendations on the use of critical care cEEG, focusing on the importance of each care centre to have a program development and improvement and indicating the contexts in which patients should be monitored with a cEEG [9]. According to those recommendations, patients suffering from hypoxic-ischaemic brain injury should be monitored with cEEG.

When cEEG is not available, there is no consensus on how patients should be monitored when there is high risk of seizure. Simplified bedside EEG monitors are more available and offer a real time analysis of brain function. Most of them display one or more channels continuous EEG and their diagnostics performance is directly correlated with the numbers of electrodes used. Average sensitivity is 68% with 4 channels montage [10] and can reach 92.5% with seven electrodes montage [11]. Users should keep in mind that all brain areas are not covered and that brief seizures can be easily missed.

Other bedside monitors can provide quantitative EEG(qEEG) which facilitates interpretation of prolonged EEG recording. Among them, those which provide amplitude-integrated EEG (aEEG) are widely used in clinical practice especially in pediatric ICUs but studies are scarce in adult ICUs. In one study, using a 1-channel montage, authors found a sensitivity of 40% for the identification of seizure by nonexperts ICUs physicians [12]. Another type of quantitative EEG frequently used is compressed spectral array, which can identify seizure patterns with a very good accuracy [13, 14]. However qEEG do not allow instantaneous diagnosis of seizure.

In the case presented here, NCSE was diagnosed at the admission with a conventional EEG. Because a cEEG is not available in our centre, a BIS monitor was placed. BIS monitoring is based on EEG analysis and monitors usually display at the same time a simplified frontal EEG signal and a BIS value between 0 and 100. The BIS value is derived from correlation of the phases between frequency components of the EEG. These monitors also display a SR value which corresponds of the percentage of time in which the EEG is isoelectric over a 63 seconds period.

In ICU, BIS monitors are used in different contexts when patients have intracranial hypertension BIS and SR values are used to titrate barbiturate treatment [10, 11]; when patients have refractory status epilepticus, BIS and SR values are used to guide the depth of sedation if cEEG is not available because there is a strong correlation between BIS and SR values and the burst rate monitored with conventional EEG [12, 13].

The reliability of BIS and SR values depends entirely on a good EEG signal quality, but in routine clinical practice, physicians tend to focus essentially on this two processed parameters. In the present case neither BIS nor SR values changed markedly at the moment the real time EEG started to show seizure patterns, which means that the NCSE recurrence could have been missed or diagnosed with delay. The diagnostic value of the real time EEG of BIS monitor is high because it diagnoses well a recruiting rhythm, spikes, and spikes waves during generalized tonic-clonic seizures [15].

Even though BIS monitors are easy to handle, learning how to interpret EEG signal is a lengthy process, but the benefits for patients are important, because the neurological outcome depends on rapid diagnosis and treatment.

It is important to remember that BIS monitors cannot substitute the conventional EEG, but when a BIS monitor is used, processed parameters and raw EEG should be analysed jointly, and when a rhythm and/or amplitude variations appear on the real time EEG, seizure should be sought.

4. Conclusion

In ICU, primitive and secondary brain injuries can lead to seizures which are often purely electrical. When a bispectral index monitor is used, real time EEG should be monitored and interpreted according to the context to detect signs of seizure, even if processed parameters values are unremarkable.

List of Abbreviations

aEEG: Amplitude-integrated EEG
BIS: Bispectral index
cEEG: Continuous electroencephalogram
EEG: Electroencephalogram
ICU: Intensive care unit
NCSE: Nonconvulsive status epilepticus
qEEG: Quantitative EEG
SR: Suppression ratio.

Supplementary Materials

I expect the case report to have a high pedagogical value, so there are one principal figure (Figure 1) and one principal video (video 1). There are 5 supplementary figures (figure S1-figure S2-figure S3-figure S4-figure S5): each one is supposed to help the editorial board to confirm the accuracy and the relevance of the case report. Also they will help readers if necessary. (i) **Figure S1** is a conventional electroencephalogram recorded at the admission of the patient which confirmed the nonconvulsive status epilepticus. (ii) **Figure S2** is as the figure S2, a conventional electroencephalogram recorded few hours later, which confirmed that the nonconvulsive status epilepticus was well treated. (iii) **Figure S3** is an electroencephalogram, recorded on day 2, which is displayed by a BISvista monitor connected to a bilateral sensor. (iv) **Figure S4**, as figure S3, is an electroencephalogram, recorded on day 3, which is displayed by a BISvista monitor connected to unilateral sensor. (v) **Figure S5**, as figures S1 and S2, is a conventional electroencephalogram recorded on day 3, which confirmed the nonconvulsive status epilepticus recurrence. The complete files (30 minutes EEG recording for each supplementary figure) are available if they are needed. **Figure S1**: Day 1: 10-20 system EEG: diagnosis of NCSE. **Figure S2**: Day 1: 10-20 system EEG: burst suppression. **Figure S3**: Day 2: PDF format generated by BIS VISTA module: burst suppression 4 channels sensor EEG. **Figure S4**: Day 3: PDF format generated by BIS VISTA module: spikes, spikes waves, and 2-channel sensor. **Figure S5**: Day 3: 10-20 system EEG: diagnosis of NCSE recurrence. *(Supplementary Materials)*

References

[1] F. Sadaka, D. Doerr, J. Hindia, K. P. Lee, and W. Logan, "Continuous electroencephalogram in comatose postcardiac arrest syndrome patients treated with therapeutic hypothermia: outcome prediction study," *Journal of Intensive Care Medicine*, vol. 30, no. 5, pp. 292–296, 2015.

[2] S. Beniczky, L. J. Hirsch, P. W. Kaplan et al., "Unified EEG terminology and criteria for nonconvulsive status epilepticus," *Epilepsia*, vol. 54, no. 6, pp. 28-29, 2013.

[3] J. Claassen, S. A. Mayer, R. G. Kowalski, R. G. Emerson, and L. J. Hirsch, "Detection of electrographic seizures with continuous EEG monitoring in critically ill patients," *Neurology*, vol. 62, no. 10, pp. 1743–1748, 2004.

[4] M. Oddo, E. Carrera, J. Claassen, S. A. Mayer, and L. J. Hirsch, "Continuous electroencephalography in the medical intensive care unit," *Critical Care Medicine*, vol. 37, no. 6, pp. 2051–2056, 2009.

[5] E. J. Gilmore, N. Gaspard, H. A. Choi et al., "Acute brain failure in severe sepsis: a prospective study in the medical intensive care unit utilizing continuous EEG monitoring," *Intensive Care Medicine*, vol. 41, no. 4, pp. 686–694, 2015.

[6] N. S. Abend, D. H. Arndt, J. L. Carpenter et al., "Electrographic seizures in pediatric ICU patients: Cohort study of risk factors and mortality," *Neurology*, vol. 81, no. 4, pp. 383–391, 2013.

[7] K. L. Wagenman, T. P. Blake, S. M. Sanchez et al., "Electrographic status epilepticus and long-term outcome in critically ill children," *Neurology*, vol. 82, no. 5, pp. 396–404, 2014.

[8] P. Kurtz, N. Gaspard, A. S. Wahl et al., "Continuous electroencephalography in a surgical intensive care unit," *Intensive Care Medicine*, vol. 40, no. 2, pp. 228–234, 2014.

[9] S. T. Herman, N. S. Abend, T. P. Bleck et al., "Consensus statement on continuous EEG in critically Ill adults and children, part I: Indications," *Journal of Clinical Neurophysiology*, vol. 32, no. 2, pp. 87–95, 2015.

[10] G. B. Young, M. D. Sharpe, M. Savard, E. Al Thenayan, L. Norton, and C. Davies-Schinkel, "Seizure detection with a commercially available bedside EEG monitor and the subhairline montage," *Neurocritical Care*, vol. 11, no. 3, pp. 411–416, 2009.

[11] I. Karakis, G. D. Montouris, J. A. D. Otis et al., "A quick and reliable EEG montage for the detection of seizures in the critical care setting," *Journal of Clinical Neurophysiology*, vol. 27, no. 2, pp. 100–105, 2010.

[12] R. Nitzschke, J. Müller, R. Engelhardt, and G. N. Schmidt, "Single-channel amplitude integrated EEG recording for the identification of epileptic seizures by nonexpert physicians in the adult acute care setting," *Journal of Clinical Monitoring and Computing*, vol. 25, no. 5, pp. 329–337, 2011.

[13] M. A. Hernández-Hernández and J. L. Fernández-Torre, "Color density spectral array of bilateral bispectral index system: Electroencephalographic correlate in comatose patients with nonconvulsive status epilepticus," *Seizure*, vol. 34, pp. 18–25, 2016.

[14] C. A. Williamson, S. Wahlster, M. M. Shafi, and M. B. Westover, "Sensitivity of compressed spectral arrays for detecting seizures in acutely ill adults," *Neurocritical Care*, vol. 20, no. 1, pp. 32–39, 2014.

[15] A. Ntahe, G. Fournis, B. Gohier, and L. Beydon, "Raw EEG characteristics, bispectral index, and suppression ratio variations during generalized seizure in electroconvulsive therapy," *British Journal of Anaesthesia*, vol. 118, no. 6, pp. 955–958, 2017.

25

A Rare but Reversible Cause of Hematemesis: "Downhill " Esophageal Varices

Lam-Phuong Nguyen,[1,2,3] **Narin Sriratanaviriyakul,**[1,2,3] **and Christian Sandrock**[1,2,3]

[1]*Division of Pulmonary, Critical Care, and Sleep Medicine, University of California, Davis, Suite #3400, 4150 V Street, Sacramento, CA 95817, USA*
[2]*Department of Internal Medicine, University of California, Davis, Sacramento, USA*
[3]*VA Northern California Health Care System, Mather, USA*

Correspondence should be addressed to Lam-Phuong Nguyen; lptnguyen@ucdavis.edu

Academic Editor: Kurt Lenz

"Downhill" varices are a rare cause of acute upper gastrointestinal bleeding and are generally due to obstruction of the superior vena cava (SVC). Often these cases of "downhill" varices are missed diagnoses as portal hypertension but fail to improve with medical treatment to reduce portal pressure. We report a similar case where recurrent variceal bleeding was initially diagnosed as portal hypertension but later found to have SVC thrombosis presenting with recurrent hematemesis. A 39-year-old female with history of end-stage renal disease presented with recurrent hematemesis. Esophagogastroduodenoscopy (EGD) revealed multiple varices. Banding and sclerotherapy were performed. Extensive evaluation did not show overt portal hypertension or cirrhosis. Due to ongoing bleeding requiring resuscitation, she underwent internal jugular (IJ) and SVC venogram in preparation for transjugular intrahepatic portosystemic shunt (TIPS), which demonstrated complete IJ and SVC occlusion. She underwent balloon angioplasty with stent placement across SVC occlusion with complete resolution of her varices and resolved hematemesis. "Downhill" varices are extremely rare, though previously well described. Frequently, patients are misdiagnosed with underlying liver disease. High index of suspicion and investigation of alternative causes of varices is prudent in those without underlying liver diseases. Prompt diagnosis and appropriate intervention can significantly improve morbidity and mortality.

1. Introduction

Esophageal varices can be associated with conditions other than liver disease and portal hypertension. There are three different types of esophageal varices, classified based on direction of venous flow: "uphill," "downhill," or idiopathic. The most common type, "uphill," esophageal varices are caused by portal vein hypertension with subsequent collateral, decompressive flow. "Downhill" varices are rare dilated veins resulting from obstruction of the superior vena cava (SVC) leading to redirected blood flow to collateral system [1]. "Downhill" esophageal varices account for 0.4–11% of esophageal varices but less than 0.1% of patients present with hematemesis [2–4]. Often these cases of "downhill" variceal bleed are initially misdiagnosed and thought to be secondary to portal hypertension and/or liver disease. We

report a case where recurrent variceal bleeding was initially misdiagnosed with portal hypertension but later found to have SVC thrombosis.

2. Case Presentation

A 39-year-old African American female with history of diabetes, hypertension, end-stage renal disease (ESRD) on hemodialysis (HD), and recurrent AV fistula thrombosis presented to our institution with recurrent hematemesis. Of note, she was started on dialysis in May of 2012, initially through a tunnel dialysis catheter approximately for one year until her AV fistula matured. She was recently discharged from the intensive care unit one week before for hematemesis and hematochezia. Esophagogastroduodenoscopy (EGD) during previous hospitalization showed 4 columns of large

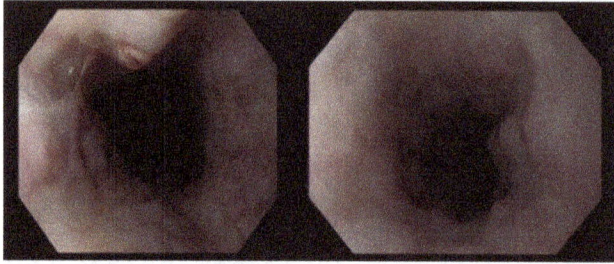

FIGURE 1: Initial EGD with extensive esophageal varices from the mid to distal esophagus.

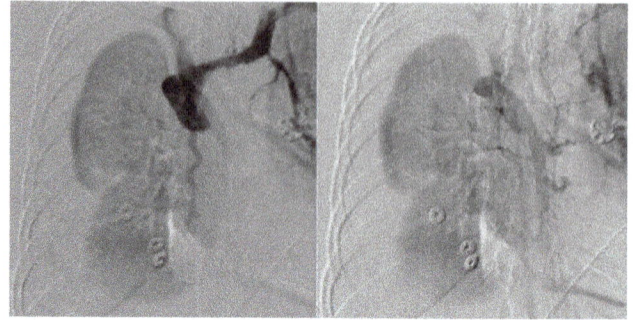

FIGURE 2: SVC venogram with occluded SVC and extensive collateral vessels.

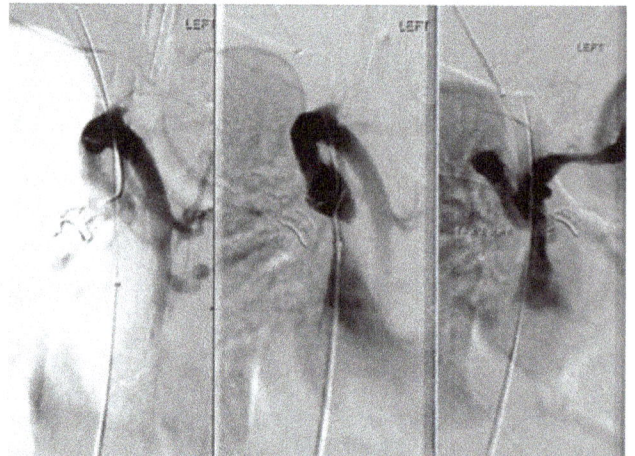

FIGURE 3: SVC venogram showing recannulization and stenting of distal occluded SVC.

esophageal varices 25 cm to the distal esophagus just above the GE junction. There were nipple sign and red wale signs appreciated on the proximal portion of the varices suggesting recent bleeding for which banding and sclerotherapy were performed (Figure 1) with excellent hemostasis. The patient vomited up one cup of bright red blood but denied any associated dizziness, lightheadedness, abdominal pain, or diarrhea. She had been in her usual state of health since recent hospital discharge and denied any history of NSAIDs use, alcohol intake, or smoking history.

Upon presentation, she was afebrile with temperature 37.5°C, blood pressure 150/80 mmHg, heart rate 102–115/min, respiratory rate 16–21/min, and pulsed oximetry 91–100% on room air. Her physical exam was notable for an obese, chronically ill appearing female in no apparent distress. Head and neck exam was notable for facial and upper chest fullness with associated bilateral upper extremities swelling present for several months though the exact duration was unclear to the patient. Cardiac exam revealed evidence of tachycardia, distant heart sounds but no evidence of murmurs. Pulmonary exam was notable for diminished breath sounds at both bases but otherwise without crackles or wheezes. The remainder of her physical exam was unremarkable and without stigmata of liver disease such as telangiectasia, spider nevi, or palmar erythema.

Laboratory studies revealed leukocytosis with a white blood cell count of 18.1×10^9/L with 85% neutrophils, 7% lymphocytes, and 7.5% monocytes as well as hemoglobin of 7.4 g/dL (baseline 11.8 g/dL) and platelets of 127×10^9/L and no atypical lymphocytes. Her blood chemistry test results were notable for blood urea nitrogen of 42 mmol/L, serum creatinine 5.84 mg/dL, albumin 24 g/L, alkaline phosphatase, aspartate aminotransaminase, and alanine aminotransferase which were all within normal limits. Her INR was 1.1 on admission.

She was admitted to the intensive care unit for treatment and further evaluation for recurrent hematemesis of unclear etiology but presumed recurrent variceal bleeding. The patient underwent extensive evaluation including abdominal ultrasound with doppler showing patent main portal veins but evidence to suggest left portal vein portal hypertension. However, her liver CT showed normal hepatic anatomy with patent portal and hepatic veins, though there were extensive varices in the abdominal wall and mesentery. Due to continuous bleeding, requiring ongoing resuscitation and

blood transfusion, a transjugular intrahepatic portosystemic shunt (TIPS) was planned. Internal jugular (IJ) and SVC venogram in preparation for TIPS were performed, which found complete occlusion of her right IJ and SVC (Figure 2). She was subsequently diagnosed with "downhill" esophageal varices due to SVC syndrome and underwent balloon angioplasty with 3 cm × 14 mm Smart stent placement across SVC occlusion (Figure 3) with resolution of her bleeding. Subsequent EGDs later showed complete resolution of her varices (Figure 4).

3. Discussion

"Downhill" esophageal varices account for 0.4–11% of esophageal varices and are commonly due to obstruction of the SVC as a result of direct compression or thrombosis [5]. Bleeding from downhill varices can be extremely rare and there have been less than 20 reported cases in literature. They either are located in the upper esophagus or may involve the entire esophagus depending on the level of SVC obstruction. If obstruction is proximal to the azygos vein, drainage can occur through mediastinal collaterals which resulted in varices limited to the upper portion of the esophagus [3]. If distal to the azygos vein, venous drainage occurs via

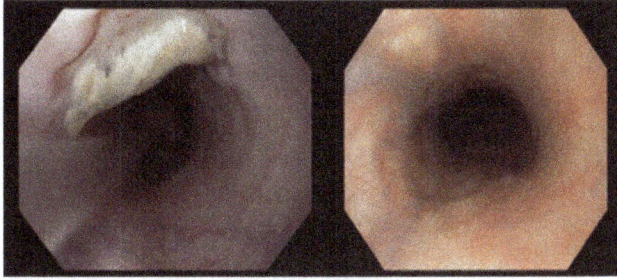

FIGURE 4: One month and four months after IR recannulization and stenting SVC with resolution of varices.

the esophageal plexus leading to varices along the entire esophagus.

There are many reported etiologies of SVC obstruction. Most cases of SVC obstruction are associated with some forms of malignancy including lung, lymphoma, and mediastinal metastases [6, 7]. Nonmalignancy etiologies include pacemaker implantation [8], goiter [9, 10], central venous catheters (dialysis catheter in particular) [11–14], rheumatic heart disease [15], congenital heart disease [16], thymoma [5], and mediastinal fibrosis [17]. There are however no direct association or reported cases linking hypercoagulable state as a contributing cause.

Currently there are no definitive recommendations on screening and management of "downhill" varices. Hemostasis from variceal bleeding is often achieved with endoscopic local intervention such as banding and sclerotherapy [1, 2, 18]. The principle and definitive treatment is to relieve obstruction and revascularize SVC. Percutaneous radiological SVC angioplasty with stent placement had been reported with some success [19]. Underlying primary etiologies of SVC occlusion will need to be addressed and optimized. Finally surgical approach may be indicated for those with tumor causing extrinsic compression such as those with underlying thymoma or goiter.

Exact etiology of our patient's SVC thrombosis remains unclear despite extensive workup. However, she previously had a tunnel central venous dialysis catheter for nearly a year but it was removed two years ago prior to her current presentation. It is possible that her prior TDC catheter could have contributed to the development of her SVC thrombus. Incidences of central venous stenosis and obstruction secondary to dialysis catheter have been reported to be as high as 30% [20, 21]; however, SVC obstruction leading to hematemesis is exceedingly rare and usually occurs after the catheter has been in place for well over 2 years unlike our patient. Our patient's SVC thrombosis could have been present for quite some time prior to her current presentation as the patient was experiencing several months of chest, neck, upper extremities, and facial swelling indicating poor venous return. Her workup included chest imaging which revealed no central or mediastinal masses and serological workups including autoimmune and lupus anticoagulant were all negative. Decision was made to perform angioplasty and stent placement in this case to urgently relieve the SVC obstruction and improve her symptoms, especially in the setting of ongoing hematemesis. Anticoagulation was not initiated after stent placement due to several reasons. First she had recent life-threatening bleeding. Second, there were no hypercoagulable diseases identified. Lastly she was noncomplaint to follow-up and periodically misses her dialysis. Her esophageal varices resolved on subsequent EGD four weeks later. Management of these patients with SVC thrombosis and obstruction can be extremely challenging as there are no current treatment guidelines and it is unclear when or if the stent can be safely removed. We present this case to raise clinician awareness of the alternative causes of varices and the challenges we face in management of these patients. High index of suspicion and investigation of alternative causes of varices is prudent in those without underlying liver diseases, as prompt diagnosis and appropriate intervention can significantly improve outcome.

Abbreviations

EGD: Esophagogastroduodenoscopy
HD: Hemodialysis
IJ: Internal jugular
NSAIDs: Nonsteroidal anti-inflammatory drugs
SVC: Superior vena cava
TIPS: Transjugular intrahepatic portosystemic shunt.

References

[1] S. K. Nayudu, A. Dev, and K. Kanneganti, "'Downhill' esophageal varices due to dialysis catheter-induced superior vena caval occlusion: a rare cause of upper gastrointestinal bleeding," *Case Reports in Gastrointestinal Medicine*, vol. 2013, Article ID 830796, 3 pages, 2013.

[2] M. Areia, J. M. Romãozinho, M. Ferreira, P. Amaro, and D. Freitas, "Downhill varices. A rare cause of esophageal hemorrhage," *Revista Espanola de Enfermedades Digestivas*, vol. 98, no. 5, pp. 359–361, 2006.

[3] B. Felson and A. P. Lessure, "'Downhill' varices of the esophagus," *Diseases of the Chest*, vol. 46, pp. 740–746, 1964.

[4] L. S. Johnson, D. G. Kinnear, R. A. Brown, and D. S. Mulder, "'Downhill' esophageal varices. A rare cause of upper gastrointestinal bleeding," *Archives of Surgery*, vol. 113, no. 12, pp. 1463–1464, 1978.

[5] Y. Inoue, S. Sakai, and T. Aoki, "Downhill oesophageal varices resulting from superior vena cava graft occlusion after resection of a thymoma," *Interactive Cardiovascular and Thoracic Surgery*, vol. 17, no. 3, pp. 598–600, 2013.

[6] T. Shirakusa, A. Iwasaki, and M. Okazaki, "Downhill esophageal varices caused by benign giant lymphoma. Case report and review of downhill varices cases in Japan," *Scandinavian Journal of Thoracic and Cardiovascular Surgery*, vol. 22, no. 2, pp. 135–138, 1988.

[7] Y. Siegel, E. Schallert, and R. Kuker, "Downhill esophageal varices: a prevalent complication of superior vena cava obstruction from benign and malignant causes," *Journal of Computer Assisted Tomography*, vol. 39, no. 2, pp. 149–152, 2015.

[8] N. Basar, K. Cagli, O. Basar et al., "Upper-extremity deep vein thrombosis and downhill esophageal varices: caused by long-term pacemaker implantation," *Texas Heart Institute Journal*, vol. 37, no. 6, pp. 714–716, 2010.

[9] E. L. R. Bédard and J. Deslauriers, "Bleeding 'Downhill' varices: a rare complication of intrathoracic goiter," *Annals of Thoracic Surgery*, vol. 81, no. 1, pp. 358–360, 2006.

[10] K. Monkemuller, K. Monkemuller, D. Poppen, K. Feldmann, and L. J. Ulbricht, "Downhill varices resulting from giant intrathoracic goiter," *Endoscopy*, vol. 42, supplement 2, p. E40, 2010.

[11] A. H. Calderwood and D. S. Mishkin, "Downhill esophageal varices caused by catheter-related thrombosis," *Clinical Gastroenterology and Hepatology*, vol. 6, no. 1, p. e1, 2008.

[12] S. Gopaluni and P. Warwicker, "Superior vena cava obstruction presenting with epistaxis, haemoptysis and gastro-intestinal haemorrhage in two men receiving haemodialysis with central venous catheters: two case reports," *Journal of Medical Case Reports*, vol. 3, article 6180, 2009.

[13] M. W. Greenwell, S. L. Basye, S. S. Dhawan, F. D. Parks, and S. R. Acchiardo, "Dialysis catheter-induced superior vena cava syndrome and downhill esophageal varices," *Clinical Nephrology*, vol. 67, no. 5, pp. 325–330, 2007.

[14] F. A. Hussein, N. Mawla, A. S. Befeler, K. J. Martin, and K. L. Lentine, "Formation of downhill esophageal varices as a rare but serious complication of hemodialysis access: a case report and comprehensive literature review," *Clinical and Experimental Nephrology*, vol. 12, no. 5, pp. 407–415, 2008.

[15] Y. P. Harwani, A. Kumar, A. Chaudhary et al., "Combined uphill and downhill varices as a consequence of rheumatic heart disease: a unique presentation," *Journal of Clinical and Experimental Hepatology*, vol. 4, no. 1, pp. 63–65, 2014.

[16] L. Malloy, M. Jensen, W. Bishop, and A. Divekar, "'Downhill' esophageal varices in congenital heart disease," *Journal of Pediatric Gastroenterology and Nutrition*, vol. 56, no. 2, pp. e9–e11, 2013.

[17] B. Yasar and E. Abut, "A case of mediastinal fibrosis due to radiotherapy and 'downhill' esophageal varices: a rare cause of upper gastrointestinal bleeding," *Clinical Journal of Gastroenterology*, vol. 8, no. 2, pp. 73–76, 2015.

[18] C. Froilán Torres, L. Adán, J. Manuel Suárez, S. Gómez, L. H. Villalba, and R. Plaza Santos, "Therapeutic approach to 'downhill' varices bleeding," *Gastrointestinal Endoscopy*, vol. 68, no. 5, pp. 1010–1012, 2008.

[19] L. Leggio, L. Abenavoli, L. Vonghia et al., "Superior vena cava thrombosis treated by angioplasty and stenting in a cirrhotic patient with peritoneovenous shunt," *Annals of Thoracic and Cardiovascular Surgery*, vol. 14, no. 1, pp. 60–62, 2008.

[20] S. Kundu, "Central venous obstruction management," *Seminars in Interventional Radiology*, vol. 26, no. 2, pp. 115–121, 2009.

[21] A. B. Lumsden, M. J. MacDonald, H. Isiklar et al., "Central venous stenosis in the hemodialysis patient: incidence and efficacy of endovascular treatment," *Cardiovascular Surgery*, vol. 5, no. 5, pp. 504–509, 1997.

26

Circulatory Support with Venoarterial ECMO Unsuccessful in Aiding Endogenous Diltiazem Clearance after Overdose

Erin N. Frazee,[1] Sarah J. Lee,[2] Ejaaz A. Kalimullah,[3] Heather A. Personett,[1] and Darlene R. Nelson[2]

[1] *Hospital Pharmacy Services, Mayo Clinic, 200 1st SW, Rochester, MN 55905, USA*

[2] *Division of Pulmonary and Critical Care Medicine, Mayo Clinic, 200 1st SW, Rochester, MN 55905, USA*

[3] *Department of Emergency Medicine and Division of Pulmonary and Critical Care Medicine, Loyola University Medical Center, 2160 S 1st Avenue, Maywood, IL 60153, USA*

Correspondence should be addressed to Erin N. Frazee; frazee.erin@mayo.edu

Academic Editor: Moritoki Egi

Introduction. In cardiovascular collapse from diltiazem poisoning, extracorporeal membrane oxygenation (ECMO) may offer circulatory support sufficient to preserve endogenous hepatic drug clearance. Little is known about patient outcomes and diltiazem toxicokinetics in this setting. *Case Report.* A 36-year-old woman with a history of myocardial bridging syndrome presented with chest pain for which she self-medicated with 2.4 g of sustained release diltiazem over the course of 8 hours. Hemodynamics and mentation were satisfactory on presentation, but precipitously deteriorated after ICU transfer. She was given fluids, calcium, vasopressors, glucagon, high-dose insulin, and lipid emulsion. Due to circulatory collapse and multiorgan failure including ischemic hepatopathy, she underwent transvenous pacing and emergent initiation of venoarterial ECMO. The peak diltiazem level was 13150 ng/mL (normal 100–200 ng/mL) and it remained elevated at 6340 ng/mL at hour 90. Unfortunately, the patient developed multiple complications which resulted in her death on ICU day 9. *Conclusion.* This case describes the unsuccessful use of ECMO for diltiazem intoxication. Although past reports suggest that support with ECMO may facilitate endogenous diltiazem clearance, it may be dependent on preserved hepatic function at the time of cannulation, a factor not present in this case.

1. Introduction

The American Association of Poison Control Centers reported more than 100,000 cardiovascular medication poisonings in 2011, of which calcium channel blocker (CCB) overdoses were involved in approximately 60% of the fatal events [1]. In both mono- and mixed-exposures of CCBs, diltiazem, a lipophilic, protein-bound, hepatically cleared, nondihydropyridine CCB, carried a significant risk of fatality [2].

Supportive care remains the cornerstone of diltiazem overdose management. Targeted therapies include calcium, high-dose insulin euglycemia, glucagon, lipid emulsion, and cardiac pacing [3]. Enhanced elimination by hemodialysis, hemoperfusion, albumin dialysis, and plasma exchange variably impacts clinical outcomes [3–6]. Because of the inconsistent results of extracorporeal drug removal, there is instead an interest in preservation of endogenous drug clearance mechanisms (i.e., hepatic metabolism) through extracorporeal membrane oxygenation (ECMO-) mediated circulatory support. Little is known about the impact of ECMO on patient outcomes and diltiazem toxicokinetics in this setting.

Herein, we present an unsuccessful case of ECMO use for diltiazem overdose and review the existing literature on circulatory support for nondihydropyridine CCB poisonings.

2. Case Report

A 36-year-old, 68 kg, woman with a history of myocardial bridging syndrome and an unroofing procedure two years prior to admission presented with a two-day history of chest pain for which she self-medicated with 2.4 grams of sustained release (SR) diltiazem over the course of 8

TABLE 1: Vital signs and laboratory measures and events during the admission.

Hours and days after ingestion	Vitals signs and pertinent laboratory values	Events and interventions	Diltiazem level (ng/mL)
8 hours (presentation)	Vitals: HR 77 bpm, BP 102/56 mmHg (MAP 71)	Calcium, glucagon, high-dose insulin, fluids, lipid emulsion, and vasopressors started	—
19 hours	Vitals: HR 78 bpm, supported BP 112/38 mmHg (MAP 53) PAC: CI 5.7 L/min/m^2, SVRi 535 dynes·sec/cm^5/m^2 ABG: pH 6.96, pCO$_2$ 41 mmHg, pO$_2$ 110, HCO$_3$ 9 mmol/L Labs: lactate 8.7 mmol/L; potassium 3.1 mmol/L; glucose 430 mg/dL; AST 79 U/L	PAC placed, transvenously paced at 80 bpm due to interval development of prolonged sinus pauses; methylene blue attempted; CVVH begun	—
23 hours	—	—	1140
25 hours	Immediately before ECMO cannulation: Vitals: HR 96 bpm (paced), supported BP 93/48 mmHg (MAP 63) PAC: CI 4.1 L/min/m^2, SVRi 804 dynes·sec/cm^5/m^2 Labs: lactate >12.2 mmol/L; potassium 2.2 mmol/L; AST 3112 U/L, INR 2.4	V-A ECMO cannulation, total circuit flow 4.8–5.1 L/min (ECMO CI 2.9–3.1 L/min/m^2)	—
39 hours	—	—	9450
44 hours	—	—	7120
51 hours	Hemodynamics: HR 100 (paced; asystolic when pacemaker is off), total ECMO circuit flow 4.6 L/min (ECMO CI 2.7 L/min/m^2) Labs: lactate >18 mmol/L; potassium 4.9 mmol/L	Abdominal compartment syndrome, to operating room for exploration, evacuation of ascites, and temporary closure	13150
71 hours	Labs: lactate 15.4 mmol/L; potassium 8.1 mmol/L; aPTT 63 seconds (heparinized), INR 2.3 TTE: LV EF 10–15% and a severe decrease in right ventricular systolic function; no evidence of tamponade	Persistent elevation in potassium and lactate with increasing abdominal distension; prompted exploration where ischemic small bowel and colon were found along with a large retroperitoneal hematoma; resected and left in discontinuity	2020
90 hours	—	Developed bilateral lower-extremity compartment syndrome requiring fasciotomies	6340
Day 5	—	Underwent abdominal reexploration with creation of an end ileostomy and 3 mucous fistulae	—
Day 7	—	Regained sinus rhythm and downtitrated vasopressors; unable to wean from ECMO	—
Day 8	—	Developed a GI bleed in the setting of refractory thrombocytopenia, anticoagulation for ECMO, and autoanticoagulation from acute liver injury	—
Day 9	—	Transitioned to comfort cares and died	—

HR: heart rate; BP: blood pressure, MAP: mean arterial pressure; PAC: pulmonary artery catheter; CI: cardiac index; SVRi: systemic vascular resistance index; ABG: arterial blood gas; CVVH: continuous venovenous hemofiltration; V-A ECMO: venoarterial extracorporeal membrane oxygenation; AST: aspartate aminotransferase; INR: international normalized ratio; LV EF: left ventricular ejection fraction.

hours. Neither subjective nor objective evidence suggested coingestion. On arrival to the ED, she was mentating appropriately, with a blood pressure (BP) of 102/56 mm Hg and a pulse of 77 beats per minute (bpm) in sinus rhythm (Table 1). She became hypotensive (BP 88/40 mm Hg) and

was administered intravenous (IV) fluids, 5 mg IV glucagon and 3 g of IV calcium gluconate. Hypotension persisted; therefore, a norepinephrine infusion was started. High-dose insulin (1 unit/kg/hr insulin) and a 1.5 mL/kg bolus of lipid emulsion (20% Intralipid) were subsequently given and continued in the ICU (insulin titrated to 10 units/kg/hr within 5 hours of ICU admission; Intralipid infused at 0.5 mL/kg/hr) [7]. At admission to the ICU, she was alert and oriented although increasingly dyspneic. Activated charcoal and gastric lavage were not used given the elapsed time between ingestion and presentation, the patient's nausea and concerns about the risk of aspiration, and her suspected ileus with high vasopressor requirements. Despite escalating norepinephrine doses to 2 mcg/kg/min, with the addition of 1 mcg/kg/min epinephrine, vasopressin at 0.1 units/min, calcium chloride boluses and infusion, and 75 mcg/kg/hr (5 mg/hr) of glucagon, BP remained 80's/30's with a pulse of 60 bpm. Initial ICU laboratory variables showed ionized calcium of 4.4 mg/dL, potassium of 3.4 mmol/L, lactate of 2.72 mmol/L, glucose of 127 mg/dL, and pH of 7.27. She was intubated due to hypoxia secondary to pulmonary edema. Eight hours after ICU admission, she developed frequent prolonged sinus pauses requiring transvenous pacing via a pulmonary artery catheter. She continued to worsen with profound metabolic acidosis requiring continuous venovenous hemofiltration. Charcoal hemoperfusion and albumin dialysis were unavailable for use in this case. Her circulatory collapse was unresponsive to vasopressors and thus two doses of methylene blue (2 mg/kg each) were attempted without a sustained effect. Therefore, she underwent emergent placement of right atrial (40 Fr Medtronic DLP malleable single stage venous cannula, http://www.medtronic.com/) and ascending aorta cannulae (Medtronic EOPA aortic 22 Fr cannula) for initiation of central veno-arterial (V-A) ECMO 13 hours from ICU admission (25 hours after reported ingestion; Table 1). The ECMO circuit was the Cardiohelp device with the HLS Module Advanced 7.0 Bioline heparin-coated portable cardiopulmonary support system (http://www.cardiohelp-us.com/en/home/). The ECMO circuit was primed with 600 cc of Plasmalyte and 1000 U heparin. She was supported for a total of 190 hours.

Peak diltiazem serum concentration was 13150 ng/mL (Figure 1; therapeutic range 100–200 ng/mL; diltiazem concentrations determined with High Performance Liquid Chromatography with Ultraviolet Detection; MEDTOX Scientific, Inc., St. Paul, MN). Desacetyldiltiazem concentrations were not available. Seventy-one hours after ingestion, the diltiazem level decreased to 2020 ng/mL. To confirm downtrend, a diltiazem level 4 days after ingestion was obtained and found to have paradoxically increased to 6340 ng/mL.

Although she received full circulatory support with central V-A ECMO and high-dose vasopressors, she had an extremely low systemic vascular resistance and her course was complicated by global hypoperfusion including organ, limb, and tissue ischemia. She developed multifocal compartment syndrome, thrombocytopenia, uncontrolled gastrointestinal bleeding, and fulminant multiorgan failure leading to a transition to comfort care and death on ICU day 9.

3. Discussion

This report describes the course of a patient who experienced diltiazem SR poisoning and did not survive despite

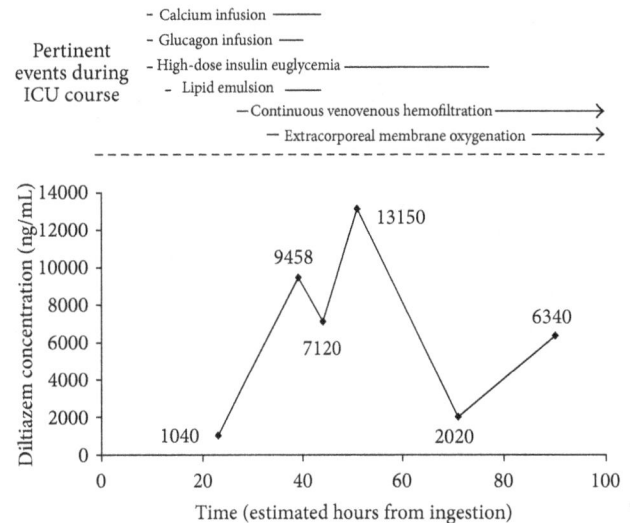

FIGURE 1: Diltiazem serum concentrations and concurrent interventions during ICU course according to suspected time from ingestion based on patient self-report.

maximal medical therapy, transvenous pacing, CVVH, and venoarterial ECMO. She developed profoundly elevated diltiazem serum concentrations and an inconsistent drug decay curve after this overdose. The peak concentration noted was approximately 100-fold greater than the therapeutic range (100–200 ng/mL) and is at the upper limit of what has previously been reported [4–6, 8–11]. No consistent diltiazem elimination rate occurred and levels remained significantly elevated to hour 90 of admission. We hypothesize that the unusually prolonged drug exposure and timing of ECMO initiation relative to the development of hepatic dysfunction may have been critical factors in the patient's outcome.

Although the evidence is limited, circulatory support with ECMO for nondihydropyridine CCB poisonings could theoretically preserve end-organ function and facilitate endogenous hepatic clearance of the drug. Indeed, in 62 critically ill poisoned patients, 12 of whom ingested verapamil or diltiazem, individuals who underwent extracorporeal life support had a significantly better survival than those who did not (86% versus 48%, respectively; P = 0.02) [12]. Three published reports describe the use of ECMO for sustained release nondihydropyridine CCB poisoning in pediatric/neonatal patients. In two patients, CCB poisoning was associated with verapamil in combination with the nonselective beta-blocker propranolol. ECMO cannulation occurred at 4 and 10 hours after intoxication and both patients survived to hospital discharge [13, 14]. The third pediatric case reported is of a 16-year-old female with an acute intentional ingestion of 12 grams of sustained release diltiazem. She received gastric lavage, activated charcoal, and pacing. ECMO began 17 hours after the ingestion and at hour 22 she had evidence of mild hepatic dysfunction with peak AST and ALT of 320 and 197, respectively. After 48 hours of circulatory support, ECMO was terminated due to uncontrolled mediastinal hemorrhage, but the patient was able to survive to discharge [10]. Extracorporeal circulatory support has also infrequently been described in the setting of adult nondihydropyridine CCB intoxications [15–18]. A 41-year-old adult male intentionally ingested multiple medications including verapamil and was successfully managed with 5 hours of percutaneous cardiopulmonary bypass introduced 8 hours after the toxic ingestion [17]. Another case of a polyingestion which included 7.2 g of slow-release verapamil was initiated on ECMO in the emergency department and successfully managed with 6 days of support [15]. Lastly, over ten years at a single center, 17 patients with drug poisoning and shock were placed on extracorporeal life support. Four of these individuals ingested verapamil and received circulatory support within 5 hours of the ingestion. Ten (58%) patients in the overall group developed cannulation-related injuries of the femoral vessels and 13 (76%) patients survived. Two (50%) of the 4 patients with verapamil ingestions survived [16].

Whereas several previous reports have signaled a possible benefit on outcomes with ECMO use for nondihydropyridine CCB poisonings, the patient in this case died despite maximal medical therapy, CVVH to control refractory acidosis and hyperkalemia, and circulatory support with ECMO. Multiple factors may have contributed to this negative clinical outcome. Her course was complicated by delayed mesenteric ischemia which, in the setting of poisonings, has been shown to affect younger patients with fewer risk factors [19]. The diltiazem concentrations seen in this patient were markedly elevated and erratic which suggests that the patient was exposed to sustained toxic levels for a longer period of time than in previous reports. Prior kinetic analyses of SR diltiazem overdoses have demonstrated an elimination half-life of 13–48 hours [5, 10, 11]. Zero order kinetics appear to predominate at concentrations >650 ng/mL with a return to first order elimination below this threshold [6]. Durward and colleagues characterized serial diltiazem levels after overdose in a female patient who received 48 hours of ECMO. The admission diltiazem concentration was approximately 6000 ng/mL. Two rounds of charcoal hemoperfusion were attempted which resulted in temporary reductions in serum diltiazem concentrations with near complete rebound in the 8 hours after each run. By hour 120 after ingestion, her diltiazem concentration was <1000 ng/mL and she survived to be discharged from the hospital. In our case, stability of diltiazem elimination was not achieved and the serum concentration spontaneously rebounded from 2020 ng/mL at hour 71 after ingestion to 6340 ng/mL at hour 90.

The atypical concentration pattern and prolonged exposure we found may have been affected by a number of factors. Diltiazem could have accumulated in the gastrointestinal tract because the patient did not receive gastric decontamination or because of the development of decreased mesenteric perfusion or an ileus. The bowel intervention for mesenteric ischemia may have contributed to the 90-hour rebound in serum concentrations (Table 1). We also cannot exclude the possibility that the 2020 ng/mL serum concentration drawn at 71 hours after ingestion was spurious. The timing of lipid exposure makes it unlikely that an altered volume of distribution associated with this therapy impacted drug levels, but alterations in protein binding may have resulted in heightened serum concentrations of free drug. CVVH

has not been shown to significantly contribute to diltiazem elimination and thus it is unlikely that this concurrent intervention altered the serum levels [20].

In addition to the potential for altered drug absorption and distribution, we also hypothesize that the patient may have experienced altered diltiazem metabolism. It is of particular importance to preserve hepatic perfusion in the case of diltiazem poisonings because the drug undergoes extensive hepatic metabolism via deacetylation and only 1–3% of drug is eliminated unchanged in the urine [20]. Previous reports have either not described liver function at the time of ECMO initiation or demonstrated only mild increases in transaminases. In this case, ECMO began 17 hours from admission (25 hours from ingestion), but there was already significant AST and INR elevation in the absence of therapeutic anticoagulation, suggesting acute ischemic hepatopathy. Mechanical circulatory support to preserve hemodynamics and consequently endogenous drug clearance may have been insufficient to overcome this preexisting organ dysfunction. It is possible that introduction of ECMO prior to the onset of hepatic dysfunction may have resulted in improved perfusion and consequent drug clearance.

This case report of a SR diltiazem overdose describes drug toxicokinetics and the role for ECMO as a therapeutic intervention. We documented prolonged exposure to toxic diltiazem levels and an inconsistent drug decay curve, likely attributable to altered absorption, distribution, and metabolism. Although ECMO may theoretically facilitate endogenous diltiazem clearance, the timing of initiation may be a key determinant in its success. This patient exhibited signs of hepatic failure before ECMO initiation. This may have decreased the likelihood that enhanced circulatory support could facilitate sufficient endogenous drug clearance to offset the risks of the intervention. Future study is indicated to determine if early ECMO initiation in SR diltiazem overdoses improves patient outcomes.

References

[1] A. C. Bronstein, D. A. Spyker, L. R. Cantilena Jr., B. H. Rumack, and R. C. Dart, "2011 Annual report of the American Association of Poison Control Centers' National Poison Data System (NPDS): 29th Annual Report," *Clinical toxicology*, vol. 50, no. 10, pp. 911–1164, 2012.

[2] M. Deters, I. Bergmann, G. Enden et al., "Calcium channel antagonist exposures reported to the Poisons Information Center Erfurt," *European Journal of Internal Medicine*, vol. 22, no. 6, pp. 616–620, 2011.

[3] W. Kerns II, "Management of β-adrenergic blocker and calcium channel antagonist toxicity," *Emergency Medicine Clinics of North America*, vol. 25, no. 2, pp. 309–331, 2007.

[4] M. Belleflamme, P. Hantson, T. Gougnard et al., "Survival despite extremely high plasma diltiazem level in a case of acute poisoning treated by the molecular-adsorbent recirculating

system," *European Journal of Emergency Medicine*, vol. 19, no. 1, pp. 59–61, 2012.

[5] D. M. Roberts, J. A. Roberts, R. J. Boots, R. Mason, and J. Lipman, "Lessons learnt in the pharmacokinetic analysis of the effect of haemoperfusion for acute overdose with sustained-release diltiazem," *Anaesthesia*, vol. 63, no. 7, pp. 714–718, 2008.

[6] K. M. Williamson and G. D. Dunham, "Plasma concentrations of diltiazem and desacetyldiltiazem in an overdose situation," *Annals of Pharmacotherapy*, vol. 30, no. 6, pp. 608–611, 1996.

[7] A. C. Young, L. I. Velez, and K. C. Kleinschmidt, "Intravenous fat emulsion therapy for intentional sustained-release verapamil overdose," *Resuscitation*, vol. 80, no. 5, pp. 591–593, 2009.

[8] R. E. Ferner, O. Odemuyiwa, A. B. Field, S. Walker, G. N. Volans, and D. N. Bateman, "Pharmacokinetics and toxic effects of diltiazem in massive overdose," *Human Toxicology*, vol. 8, no. 6, pp. 497–499, 1989.

[9] F. L. Cantrell and S. R. Williams, "Fatal unintentional overdose of diltiazem with antemortem and postmortem values," *Clinical Toxicology*, vol. 43, no. 6, pp. 587–588, 2005.

[10] A. Durward, A. M. Guerguerian, M. Lefebvre, and S. D. Shemie, "Massive diltiazem overdose treated with extracorporeal membrane oxygenation," *Pediatric Critical Care Medicine*, vol. 4, no. 3, pp. 372–376, 2003.

[11] K. Luomanmäki, E. Tiula, K. T. Kivistö, and P. J. Neuvonen, "Pharmacokinetics of diltiazem in massive overdose," *Therapeutic Drug Monitoring*, vol. 19, no. 2, pp. 240–242, 1997.

[12] R. Masson, V. Colas, J. Parienti et al., "A comparison of survival with and without extracorporeal life support treatment for severe poisoning due to drug intoxication," *Resuscitation*, vol. 83, no. 11, pp. 1413–1417, 2012.

[13] F. De Rita, L. Barozzi, G. Franchi, G. Faggian, A. Mazzucco, and G. B. Luciani, "Rescue extracorporeal life support for acute verapamil and propranolol toxicity in a neonate," *Artificial Organs*, vol. 35, no. 4, pp. 416–420, 2011.

[14] J. Kolcz, J. Pietrzyk, K. Januszewska, M. Procelewska, T. Mroczek, and E. Malec, "Extracorporeal life support in severe propranolol and verapamil intoxication," *Journal of Intensive Care Medicine*, vol. 22, no. 6, pp. 381–385, 2007.

[15] G. Maclaren, W. Butt, P. Cameron, A. Preovolos, R. McEgan, and S. Marasco, "Treatment of polypharmacy overdose with multimodality extracorporeal life support," *Anaesthesia and Intensive Care*, vol. 33, no. 1, pp. 120–123, 2005.

[16] C. Daubin, P. Lehoux, C. Ivascau et al., "Extracorporeal life support in severe drug intoxication: a retrospective cohort study of seventeen cases," *Critical care (London, England)*, vol. 13, no. 4, p. R138, 2009.

[17] M. Holzer, F. Sterz, W. Schoerkhuber et al., "Successful resuscitation of a verapamil-intoxicated patient with percutaneous cardiopulmonary bypass," *Critical Care Medicine*, vol. 27, no. 12, pp. 2818–2823, 1999.

[18] W. G. Hendren, R. S. Schieber, and L. K. Garrettson, "Extracorporeal bypass for the treatment of verapamil poisoning," *Annals of Emergency Medicine*, vol. 18, no. 9, pp. 984–987, 1989.

[19] J. C. Nault, B. Megarbane, J. Theodore et al., "Poisoning-related bowel infarction: characteristics and outcomes," *Clinical Toxicology*, vol. 47, no. 5, pp. 412–418, 2009.

[20] *Diltiazem Full Prescribing Information*, BTA Pharmaceuticals, Bridgewater, NJ, USA, 2010.

27

Use of Early Inhaled Nitric Oxide Therapy in Fat Embolism Syndrome to Prevent Right Heart Failure

Evgeni Brotfain,[1] **Leonid Koyfman,**[1] **Ruslan Kutz,**[1] **Amit Frenkel,**[1]
Shaun E. Gruenbaum,[2] **Alexander Zlotnik,**[1] **and Moti Klein**[1]

[1] *Department of Anesthesiology and Critical Care, General Intensive Care Unit, Soroka Medical Center,
Ben-Gurion University of the Negev, 85102 Beer-Sheva, Israel*
[2] *Department of Anesthesiology, Yale University School of Medicine, New Haven, CT 06511, USA*

Correspondence should be addressed to Evgeni Brotfain; bem1975@gmail.com

Academic Editor: Amit Banga

Fat embolism syndrome (FES) is a life-threatening condition in which multiorgan dysfunction manifests 48–72 hours after long bone or pelvis fractures. Right ventricular (RV) failure, especially in the setting of pulmonary hypertension, is a frequent feature of FES. We report our experience treating 2 young, previously healthy trauma patients who developed severe hypoxemia in the setting of FES. Neither patient had evidence of RV dysfunction on echocardiogram. The patients were treated with inhaled nitric oxide (NO), and their oxygenation significantly improved over the subsequent few days. Neither patient developed any cardiovascular compromise. Patients with FES that have severe hypoxemia and evidence of adult respiratory distress syndrome (ARDS) are likely at risk for developing RV failure. We recommend that these patients with FES and severe refractory hypoxemia should be treated with inhaled NO therapy prior to the onset of RV dysfunction.

1. Introduction

Fat embolism syndrome (FES) is an acute, life-threatening condition characterized by a constellation of symptoms including petechial rash, neurologic dysfunction, thrombocytopenia and anemia, and pulmonary changes [1, 2]. FES is thought to result from intravascular obstruction and injury from intramedullary fat, and symptoms typically develop up to 48–72 hours after long bone fractures, pelvis fractures, or orthopedic surgery [3, 4]. The diagnosis of FES is based on the involvement of multiple organ systems and includes the presence of at least one of major and at least four of minor Gurd's criteria [2].

Patients with FES can rapidly deteriorate within a few hours after the onset of symptoms. Patients may develop acute pulmonary hypertension and subsequent acute right heart failure, cardiovascular collapse, or even death [5, 6]. Early diagnosis and initiation of therapy are essential. Currently,

the therapy is largely supportive, and the optimal treatment for severe FES is debatable.

Here, we describe therapeutic management of refractory hypoxemia due to FES after trauma.

Case 1. A 20-year-old previously healthy man was admitted to our general intensive care unit (ICU) with multiple traumatic injuries after a motor vehicle collision. On admission day, physical examination revealed a right open femur fracture and multiple facial bone fractures (zygoma, maxilla, and nasal bones). The patient was awake and oriented and hemodynamically stable and was oxygenating well on 5 L/min nasal cannula. The patient was transported to the operating room, where he underwent an external fixation of the right femur.

After the procedure, the patient was transported back to the ICU, intubated, and sedated. The following day, he subsequent-ly became severely hypoxic (PO_2/FiO_2 ratio

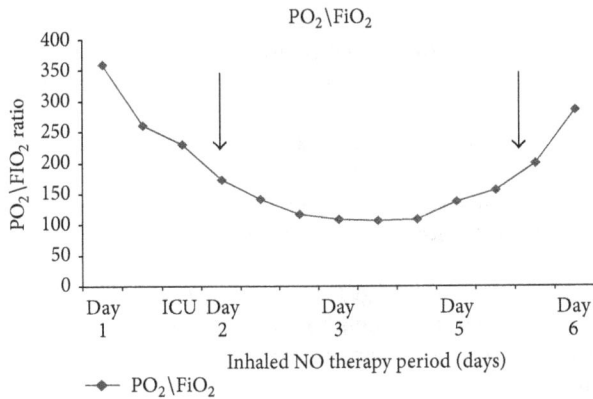

FIGURE 1: Changes in PO_2/FiO_2 ratio during the first patient's ICU stay. Inhaled NO therapy was initiated on the second day of the patient's hospitalization (represented by the first black arrow) due to severe unresponsive persistent hypoxemia (PO_2/FiO_2-110). By the fourth day after hospitalization, the PaO_2/FiO_2 ratio was improving and inhaled NO therapy was discontinued (represented by the second black arrow).

decreasing from 173 to 109, Figure 1) with thrombocytopenia (platelets 70,000/μL), anemia (Hb 6.5 mg/dL), and fever. The patient also developed a petechial rash on his upper body torso. Transthoracic echocardiography without "bubble" study showed mild pulmonary hypertension (systolic pulmonary artery pressure of 46 mmHg) with no evidence of RV dysfunction. A chest x-ray (CXR) showed bilateral diffuse pulmonary infiltrates. After discontinuing all sedating medication the patient remained unconscious. An urgent brain magnetic resonance imaging (MRI) scan showed diffuse cerebral lesions suggestive of FES.

Two days after admission to the ICU, the patient remained intubated and was ventilated by pressure control mechanical ventilation mode (PC-CMV). The patient was hypoxic (O_2 sat <90%) despite sedation with an infusion of fentanyl and midazolam and the following ventilator parameter settings: peak inspiratory pressure (PIP) of 40 cm H_2O, FiO_2 of 1.0, PO_2/FiO_2 ratios of 100–110, positive end-expiratory pressure (PEEP) of 12 cm H_2O, respiratory rate (RR) of 16 breaths/min, I : E ratio of 1:1, and tidal volume (TV) of 6 mL/kg (weight of 90 kg). Inhaled NO therapy was immediately initiated to prevent further cardiovascular deterioration and worsening hypoxemia. The inhaled NO was started at a dose of 20 ppm and titrated up to 46 ppm to maintain O_2 sat >90% on FiO_2 of 0.6. The NO therapy was continued for 4 days with a remarkable improvement in arterial blood oxygenation (PO_2/FiO_2 ratio >200) with the following ventilator parameter settings: PIP of 29 cm H_2O, FiO_2 of 0.5, and PEEP of 8 cm H_2O. Inhaled NO was gradually weaned down and discontinued after two days.

Over the following two weeks since admission to the ICU, the patient's clinical condition improved (Figure 1), and he was successfully extubated. A repeated echocardiography assessment showed complete resolution of his pulmonary hypertension and confirmed normal right and left ventricular functions. The patient's Hb level and platelet count returned

to normal, and the patient's mental status improved to baseline. The patient was discharged from the ICU three weeks after he was admitted.

Case 2. A 21-year-old previously healthy man was admitted to our hospital with an actively bleeding shrapnel wound of the lower extremities, right open femur fracture, and closed left tibia and fibula fractures. After an emergent external fixation of the right femur, primary damage control, and fluid resuscitation, the patient was transported to our ICU intubated.

Two days after ICU admission, the patient developed severe hypoxemia (FiO_2/PO_2 ratio 123, FiO_2 0.7), thrombocytopenia (platelets 50,000 μL), and anemia (Hb 5.5 mg/dL), with a petechial rash on the chest, upper limbs, and abdomen. After discontinuation of sedating drugs the patient remained unconscious with a Glasgow Coma Score (GCS) of 7. Transthoracic echocardiogram revealed an absence of pulmonary hypertension and preserved RV function (RV systolic pressure of 35 mm Hg). A CXR showed diffuse bilateral pulmonary infiltrates. Brain MRI scans revealed cerebral lesions in the deep white matter suggestive of acute FES.

The patient remained intubated and sedated with an infusion of fentanyl and midazolam and was ventilated by PC-CMV with the following ventilator parameter settings: PIP of 42 cm H_2O, FiO_2 of 1.0, PEEP of 15 cm H_2O, I : E ratio of 2:1, TV of 6 mL/kg (weight of 80 kg), and RR of 18 breaths/min. The patient developed persistent hypoxemia (O_2 sat <90%), PO_2/FiO_2 ratio = 120 despite a FiO_2 of 1.0, and inhaled NO therapy was immediately initiated. Inhaled NO was started at a dose of 20 ppm and titrated to 28–30 ppm to maintain O_2 sat >90% on FiO_2 of 0.6. Over the subsequent 72 hours, the patient's oxygenation and respiratory functions remarkably improved (PO_2/FiO_2 ratio of 232, Figure 2) with the following ventilator parameter settings: PIP of 30 cm H_2O, FiO_2 of 0.5, and PEEP of 10 cm H_2O. The NO was weaned down and discontinued. There was no significant cardiovascular compromise observed, and a repeat echocardiogram confirmed normal right and left ventricular functions without evidence of pulmonary hypertension.

Over the next few weeks, the patient had a complete resolution of his hematologic abnormalities, and he was extubated. On discharge, the patient was following commands and opened his eyes spontaneously, but he had residual speech deficits (GCS of 11).

2. Discussion

Acute FES was first described in 1862 by Zenker and systematically defined in 1974 by Guard and Wilson [2]. The diagnosis of FES is based on the presence of specific clinical signs and symptoms. The pathophysiology of FES is thought to result from the systemic embolic effects of large amounts of fat globules and direct free fatty acid toxicity. After a brief asymptomatic period of up to 72 hours, patients develop rapidly progressive, life-threatening signs including respiratory failure, neurological deficits, and right heart failure. Hematologic disturbances, including thrombocytopenia and anemia, and a petechial rash typically follow [2, 4, 5].

PO$_2$\FIO$_2$

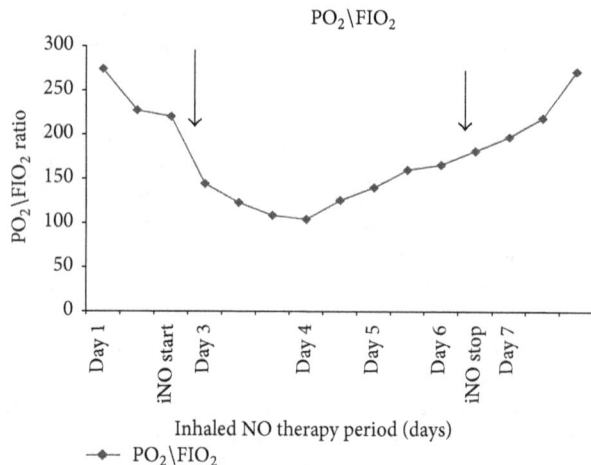

FIGURE 2: Changes in PO$_2$/FiO$_2$ ratio during the second patient's ICU stay. Inhaled NO therapy was initiated on the third day of the patient's hospitalization (represented by the first black arrow) due to severe unresponsive persistent hypoxemia (PO$_2$/FiO$_2$-120). By the sixth day after hospitalization, the PaO$_2$/FiO$_2$ ratio was improving and inhaled NO therapy was discontinued (represented by the second black arrow).

Brain MRI scan findings, although not pathognomonic, are useful for detecting acute involvement of the cerebral deep white mater, basal ganglia, corpus callosum, and cerebellar hemispheres [4].

The risk factors for developing fatal RV dysfunction are poorly understood. Severe adult respiratory distress syndrome (ARDS) or mechanical obstruction to pulmonary artery flow by massive fat embolism (FES) may induce significant pulmonary hypertension and subsequent RV failure [5, 7]. The primary treatment strategy focuses on prevention, early diagnosis, and supportive therapy [4, 6, 8]. Historically, in the setting of severe hypoxemia, anticoagulation, ethylic alcohol, and steroids, hypertonic saline, and inhaled NO have been used without robust evidence.

In both of our cases, FES was diagnosed after a traumatic injury and subsequent early external fixation of a femur fracture. The patients developed ARDS with severe hypoxemia, bilateral diffuse pulmonary infiltrates on CXR, and preserved RV and LV functions. Due to the patients' life-threatening and refractory hypoxia, our primary therapeutic plan was initially aimed at managing the severe respiratory compromise. We suspected that, even in the presence of normal RV function on echocardiogram 72 hours after ICU admission, our patients were likely at risk for developing sudden RV failure due to persistent hypoxemia. In these patients, inhaled NO was used as a rescue therapy in the setting of severe pulmonary compromise and the suspected high risk of developing cardiovascular dysfunction.

Inhaled NO, a potent endogenous vasodilator, has resulted in clinical improvement of oxygenation in severe refractory hypoxemia in patients with ARDS [9–11]. The precise mechanism was based on potential ability of inhaled NO to increase blood flow to well-ventilated lung areas improving intrapulmonary distribution of ventilation and

blood flow ratio (reduce intrapulmonary shunting) [9–11]. However, these studies failed to demonstrate a mortality benefit of NO [9–11]. There is very little evidence in the literature of NO therapy used in patients with FES who developed ARDS. Two studies [12, 13] reported successfully administering inhaled NO in the setting of acute RV failure that developed after massive fat embolism. In Case 1, a 33-year-old man with FES complicated by severe RV systolic pressure (75 mm Hg) responded well to inhaled NO [12]. In Case 2, a 19-month-old girl with severe refractory hypoxemia on FiO$_2$ of 1.0 and significant hemodynamic compromise (dopamine and norepinephrine infusion) caused by acute fat embolism improved with inhaled NO therapy after failing to improve with high frequency mechanical ventilation.

In contrast to prior reports, in which NO therapy was initiated after the presence of RV failure, we initiated therapy before the onset of significant cardiovascular compromise. Our patients were likely at high risk for RV dysfunction due to acute ARDS and severe hypoxemia. After initiation of inhaled NO, neither patient developed cardiovascular dysfunction, and the patients' respiratory condition greatly improved. Furthermore, quicker respiratory improvement due to inhaled NO therapy allowed rapid neurological recovery, which were confirmed by brain MRI scans in both patients.

NO is a safe therapy with a low risk of adverse side effects, including methemoglobinemia and withdrawal symptoms after discontinuation. We recommend that, in patients with FES and severe refractory hypoxemia, inhaled NO therapy could be safely used. Future studies should aim to identify the treatment and preventive effects of inhaled NO therapy in patients with FES who developed pulmonary hypertension and right heart failure.

Authors' Contribution

Evgeni Brotfain and Leonid Koyfman contributed equally to the paper.

References

[1] G. Volpin, A. Gorski, H. Shtarker, and N. Makhoul, "[Fat embolism syndrome following injuries and limb fractures].," *Harefuah*, vol. 149, no. 5, pp. 304–335, 2010.

[2] A. R. Guard and R. E. Wilson, "The fat embolism syndrome," *The Bone & Joint Journal B*, vol. 56, pp. 408–416, 1974.

[3] P. Glover and L. I. Worthley, "Fat embolism," *Critical Care and Resuscitation*, vol. 1, pp. 276–284, 1999.

[4] A. Mellor and N. Soni, "Fat embolism," *Anaesthesia*, vol. 56, no. 2, pp. 145–154, 2001.

[5] N. Shaikh, "Emergency management of fat embolism syndrome," *Journal of Emergencies, Trauma, and Shock*, vol. 2, no. 1, pp. 29–33, 2009.

[6] D. L. Levy, "The fat embolism syndrome: a review," *Clinical Orthopaedics and Related Research*, vol. 2612, pp. 281–286, 1990.

[7] U. Suschner, D. P. Katz, and P. Furst, "Effect of intravenous fat emulsion on lung function in patients with acute respiratory distress syndrome or sepsis," *Critical Care Medicine*, vol. 29, pp. 1569–1574, 2001.

[8] T. M. Dudney and C. G. Elliott, "Pulmonary embolism from amniotic fluid, fat, and air," *Progress in Cardiovascular Diseases*, vol. 36, no. 6, pp. 447–474, 1994.

[9] R. P. Dellinger, J. L. Zimmerman, T. M. Hyers et al., "Inhaled nitric oxide in ARDS: preliminary results of a multicenter clinical trial," *Critical Care Medicine*, vol. 24, article A29, 1996.

[10] B. H. Cuthbertson, P. Dellinger, O. J. Dyar et al., "UK guidelines for the use of inhaled nitric oxide therapy in adult ICUs," *Intensive Care Medicine*, vol. 23, no. 12, pp. 1212–1218, 1997.

[11] A. Afshari, J. Brok, A. M. Møller, and J. Wetterslev, "Inhaled nitric oxide for acute respiratory distress syndrome (ARDS) and acute lung injury in children and adults," *Cochrane Database of Systematic Reviews*, vol. 7, Article ID CD002787, 2010.

[12] T. Miyai, E. Ayala, K. Ravindranath et al., "Inhaled nitric oxide as a rescue therapy in near fatal fat embolism syndrome," *Chest*, vol. 138, p. 139A, 2010.

[13] A. Amigoni, P. Corner, F. Zanella, and A. Pettenazzo, "Successful use of inhaled nitric oxide in a child with fat embolism syndrome," *Journal of Trauma*, vol. 68, no. 3, pp. E80–E82, 2010.

28

An Unusual Case of Refractory Hypoxia on the ICU

Caroline Phillips,[1] Clare Harris,[2] Nathaniel Broughton ⓘ,[1] Thomas Pulimood,[2] and Liam Ring[3]

[1]Department of Anaesthesia and Critical Care, West Suffolk NHS Foundation Trust, Bury St Edmunds, UK
[2]Department of Respiratory Medicine, West Suffolk NHS Foundation Trust, Bury St Edmunds, UK
[3]Department of Cardiology, West Suffolk NHS Foundation Trust, Bury St Edmunds, UK

Correspondence should be addressed to Nathaniel Broughton; nathaniel@doctors.org.uk

Academic Editor: Won S. Park

We present the case of a 68-year-old gentleman who presented with breathlessness and was found to have NSTEMI, pulmonary oedema, and hypoxia. He remained hypoxic despite appropriate treatment and was found to have preserved LV function and raised cardiac output. CT pulmonary angiogram was negative but a cirrhotic liver was incidentally noted and later confirmed via ultrasound. Bedside examination was positive for orthodeoxia, suggesting a diagnosis of hepatopulmonary syndrome (HPS). The finding of significant intrapulmonary shunting on "bubble" echocardiography confirmed the diagnosis. This patient did not have previously diagnosed liver disease and had largely normal LFTs when the diagnosis was first suspected. We discuss HPS in the context of ICU and suggest how it may be screened for using simple tests. There is no correlation between the presence of HPS and severity of liver disease, yet we believe this is the first reported adult case of HPS on the ICU without previously diagnosed cirrhosis.

1. Introduction

Hepatopulmonary syndrome (HPS) is a well-established clinical entity in the context of cirrhotic liver disease and is commonly considered where cirrhotic patients suffer from dyspnoea or hypoxia, also where liver transplantation is being considered. However, it has not previously been reported as a cause of refractory hypoxia in adult patients requiring admission to the Intensive Care Unit (ICU) who do not have a prior diagnosis of liver disease. We describe why HPS might be suspected in hypoxic ICU patients, how it may be screened for using simple bedside assessment, and how a definitive diagnosis can be made.

2. Case Report

A 68-year-old gentleman presented to the Emergency Department (ED) with a six-month history of shortness of breath, which had worsened over the previous five days. He had a past medical history of mild Parkinson's disease, insulin-dependent type II diabetes mellitus, hypertension, and angina. He had recently commenced diuretics in the community for possible cardiac failure. He was a minimal drinker and ex-smoker.

Upon arrival in ED, he was in extremis with a respiratory rate of 30, SpO$_2$ 0.54 on air, improving to 0.72 with the application of 15 L oxygen via a non-rebreathe mask. His blood pressure and heart rate were normal. An arterial blood gas on oxygen showed pH 7.37, PaO$_2$ 5.3 kPa, PaCO$_2$ 6.4 kPa, BE -2.7 mEq/L, and lactate 4.4 mmol/L. There were fine bibasal inspiratory crepitations on auscultation of the chest with chest X-ray (CXR) findings consistent with pulmonary oedema. Laboratory investigations showed a significantly raised troponin T of 141 ng/L on admission, later rising to 1118 ng/L (normal range: <28 ng/L). Other than a mildly elevated CRP of 20 mg/L (normal range: <7 mg/L), blood tests were unremarkable including a normal neutrophil count. His initial ECG showed sinus rhythm with mild lateral ST depression but normal T-waves.

In addition to anticoagulation with aspirin, clopidogrel, and fondaparinux, the patient received glyceryl trinitrate and furosemide infusions in ED. This led to a good diuresis but

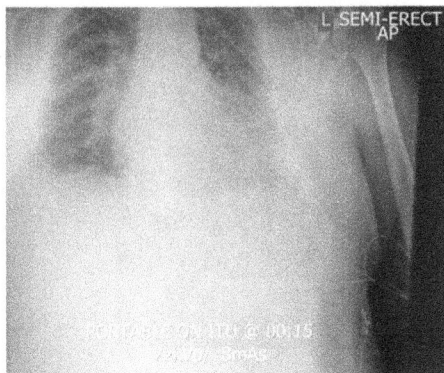

FIGURE 1: Preintubation CXR shortly after ICU admission.

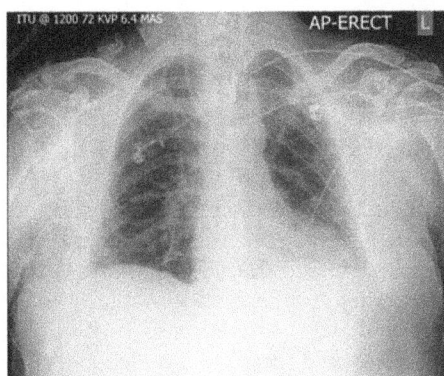

FIGURE 2: Repeat CXR on ICU day 11; ongoing hypoxia despite successful diuresis.

FIGURE 3: Transverse section of upper abdominal viscera; images acquired during CTPA.

FIGURE 4: Screenshot of sequential FiO_2 and SpO_2 values at one-minute intervals upon moving the patient from a semirecumbent to supine position.

persistent hypoxia; PaO_2 improved only to 6.5 kPa despite CPAP of 7 cmH$_2$O. He was, therefore, transferred to the Intensive Care Unit (ICU) for respiratory and circulatory support for a likely non-ST-elevation myocardial infarction (NSTEMI) with hypoxia from presumed cardiogenic pulmonary oedema +/− cardiogenic shock. Lactate had risen to 5.2 mmol/L and base excess deteriorated to −3.2 mEq/L. Non-invasive respiratory support was ineffective and the gentleman required intubation shortly after arrival. A preintubation CXR is shown (Figure 1).

A transthoracic echocardiogram (TTE) showed regional wall motion abnormalities (RWMAs) not present six months earlier, but with normal biventricular size and preserved systolic function. Mild to moderate diastolic dysfunction was found (consistent with chronic hypertension). This suggested the recent myocardial infarction had not resulted in sufficient left ventricular impairment to explain the ongoing hypoxia. Cardiac output monitoring (via LiDCO®) showed a high cardiac output of 8-9 L/min with low vascular resistance; this was also inconsistent with cardiogenic pulmonary oedema and cardiogenic shock.

Despite radiological and clinical resolution of pulmonary oedema the oxygen requirements were largely static; one week after admission he was still requiring FiO_2 0.6 to maintain PaO_2 9-10 kPa; a later CXR is shown (Figure 2). The possibility of a pulmonary embolus was investigated via CT

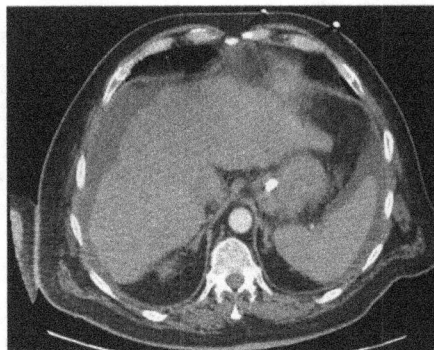

pulmonary angiogram (CTPA). No emboli were visualised in the major pulmonary arteries or their immediate branches; however, poor contrast timing affected imaging of peripheral vessels. The lung parenchyma appeared normal and no pulmonary arteriovenous malformations (AVMs) were seen. Incidental imaging of the upper abdominal viscera showed a nodular and cirrhotic liver with ascites around both the liver and spleen (Figure 3). Subsequent liver ultrasound showed an irregular outline with coarse texture consistent with micronodular cirrhosis. Hepatic vascular flows were normal. Mild finger clubbing was noted during his ICU admission, but no other stigmata of liver disease were present. Of note, this gentleman's liver function tests (LFTs) were largely normal until day seventeen of his admission, except for a stable but mildly raised bilirubin of <35 μmol/L (normal range: 5-17 μmol/L).

In light of the high cardiac output, persistent hypoxia unexplained by cardiac pathology, and a newly noted cirrhotic liver, the possibility of hepatopulmonary syndrome (HPS) was raised. Marked orthodeoxia was demonstrated; the FiO_2 required to achieve fixed SpO_2 rapidly fell from 0.66 to 0.46 upon moving from a semirecumbent to supine posture (Figure 4); however, a test-dose of methylene blue did not improve oxygenation.

A contrast echocardiogram was performed specifically looking for HPS. This showed extensive opacification of the left heart within four to five cardiac cycles, consistent with an intrapulmonary shunt (Figure 5 & supplementary material (available here)); this confirmed the diagnosis.

The ALT first became elevated at 66 IU/L (normal range: <45 IU/L) on day 17 of the patient's admission, progressively rising to 126 IU/L over the next three days. ALP was 213 IU/L on day 20 (normal range: 40–120 IU/L), having also been normal until three days earlier. His bilirubin remained stable

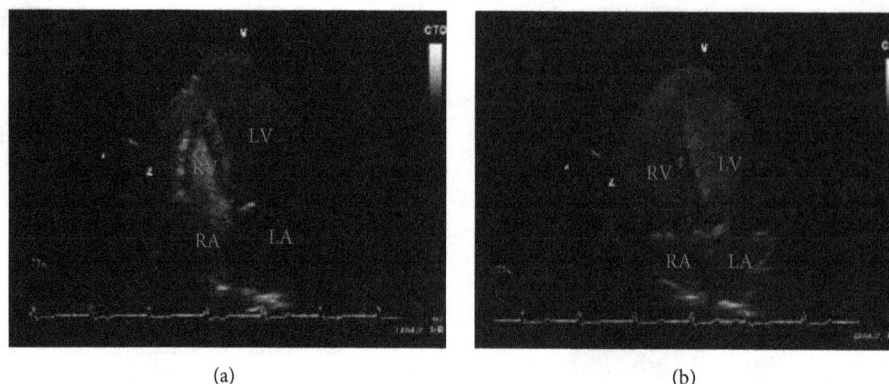

(a)   (b)

FIGURE 5: (a) Contrast/"bubble" TTE at time of injection. (b) Contrast/"bubble" TTE showing extensive opacification of the left heart in 4-5 cardiac cycles.

at <35 μmol/L. An ammonia level was measured on day 19 in view of deterioration in LFTs and a failed sedation hold; the level was 205 μmol/L (normal range: 16–60 μmol/L). Admission INR was not recorded as the patient was not warfarinised; also our institution does not routinely record aspartate aminotransferase (AST); we cannot therefore retrospectively calculate a baseline Bonacini score to assess the likelihood of cirrhosis on admission. Platelet count on admission was 196×10^9/L with ALT 17 IU/L at that time. The INR was later measured at 1.5 when liver disease was suspected; however cirrhosis had already been demonstrated via CT and US imaging.

This gentleman's case was discussed with a tertiary hepatology centre—unfortunately there was no medical therapy that could be offered, and he was not a suitable candidate for liver transplantation given his comorbidities. Following discussion with this gentleman's family, the decision was made to withdraw care.

3. Discussion

3.1. Pseudocardiogenic Hypoxia. This patient was referred to ICU for respiratory and cardiovascular support in the context of an NSTEMI with a large troponin rise and a clinical picture consistent with cardiogenic pulmonary oedema. Given this presentation, left ventricular (LV) impairment and a low cardiac output state might be anticipated. It was therefore surprising to find preserved LV function on echocardiography (despite new RWMAs) alongside a high-output and low-resistance circulation. Whilst the severity of hypoxia at presentation was probably exacerbated by acute pulmonary oedema, the ongoing hypoxia (despite successful diuresis), and consistently hyperdynamic circulation suggested the underlying pathology might be more complicated. Cirrhosis causes systemic vasodilation and therefore reduced systemic vascular resistance [1]. We speculate the LV might have been significantly affected from the presenting NSTEMI and hypoxia; however the abnormally low LV afterload predominated hence the findings of raised output (via LiDCO) and apparent preservation of LV function (via TTE). This may help explain the otherwise contradictory presence of

pulmonary oedema (necessarily requiring vascular congestion) despite a background of hyperdynamic pulmonary flow (secondary to HPS). A unifying theory is a "two-hit" process whereby HPS and hypoxia precipitated a type II infarction leading to acute LV impairment and hospital presentation, the hypoxia later reverting to a sole HPS cause once diuresis was successfully achieved. The disproportionate lactate rise at presentation perhaps supports a hypoxic mechanism.

Differential diagnoses leading to high-output cardiac failure were considered (despite no evidence of chronic fluid overload from TTE); none were consistent with this patient's presentation, with the possible exception of Osler-Weber-Rendu syndrome [2]. Visceral AVMs form in this condition, including in the liver (which may lead to portal hypertension and liver failure) and lung (which may lead to shunting and orthopnoea/platypnoea in severe cases). However, this condition was excluded on the grounds that a CTPA demonstrated no pulmonary AVMs and liver Doppler ultrasound showed normal vascular flow and no hepatic AVMs; there were no cutaneous telangiectasia and no history of GI bleeding/iron-deficiency anaemia, nosebleeds, or haemoptysis. This gentleman did not have a history of alcohol excess or other risk factors for thiamine deficiency which would have led us to consider wet beriberi.

3.2. Hepatopulmonary Syndrome. Hepatopulmonary syndrome is defined by the triad of liver failure, abnormal arterial oxygenation, and intrapulmonary vascular dilatations [3]. The diagnosis is usually made in the context of hypoxaemia in known cirrhosis, when other cardiopulmonary causes have been excluded and pulmonary vasodilatation is demonstrable [4].

HPS has two subtypes; type I is more common and results from diffuse pulmonary vascular dilatation with the normal capillary diameter of 7–15 μm commonly increasing up to 10-fold, and up to 500 μm on occasion [4, 5]. This gross dilatation markedly accelerates pulmonary transit time and impairs the oxygenation of pulmonary capillary blood. This results in functional shunting; this shunt is unique because it partially responds to supplemental oxygen. Type II HPS results from discrete arteriovenous communications (visible on CTPA);

this is true shunt which does not respond to supplemental oxygen [4]. Our patient had type I HPS and we speculate that the poor CTPA contrast timing may have resulted from his abnormal pulmonary haemodynamics.

The precise mechanism underlying type I HPS is uncertain, but vasoactive agents increased in liver disease that dilate the pulmonary circulation (either directly or indirectly) have been identified; these include endotoxin, nitric oxide, and TNF-α. Some limited improvement in oxygenation has been demonstrated following treatment with antibiotics, methylene blue, and pentoxifylline, respectively [6–8]. The observation that pathological vasodilatation of the pulmonary bed may be attenuated without improved oxygenation however suggests a more complex pathophysiology, and recently, impaired hypoxic pulmonary vasoconstriction has been implicated [9].

The diagnosis of HPS does not have to be made in the context of overt or previously diagnosed liver disease. There is, in fact, no relationship between the presence or severity of HPS and the severity of liver disease [3]. In Abrams et al.'s comparison of the diagnostic utility of contrast echocardiography and lung perfusion scan in patients with HPS, they found a similar prevalence of positive contrast echocardiograms (i.e., with intrapulmonary vascular dilatations present) across a range of aetiologies and severities [10]. Similarly Krowka et al. noted that *"severe HPS can occur in patients with mild liver disease"* [11].

Despite this, we are only aware of one adult case having been previously published regarding a patient presenting with hepatopulmonary syndrome without known liver failure (although there are numerous paediatric cases); this recent adult case was not on the ICU [12–16]. Therefore, our patient's case uniquely demonstrates the importance of considering the diagnosis of hepatopulmonary syndrome in cases of unexplained hypoxia in adults on the ICU.

3.3. Orthodeoxia in ICU. Whilst dyspnoea is a typical presenting feature of HPS, other mechanisms for respiratory deterioration exist in patients with liver disease, including anaemia and ascites. Signs of chronic hepatic failure, such as digital clubbing and spider naevi are common in HPS, but nonspecific. The presence of platypnoea-orthodeoxia (in the context of liver disease) is highly specific for HPS [17].

Platypnoea-orthodeoxia is an unusual phenomenon characterised by positional dyspnoea (platypnoea) and hypoxaemia (orthodeoxia) exacerbated in the sitting position/improved in the supine position. Orthodeoxia is defined as a PaO_2 decrease of $\geq 5\%$, or ≥ 4 mmHg (≥ 0.53 kPa) when changing position from supine to upright [18]. Orthodeoxia can most easily be demonstrated in patients on ICU by improved oxygenation upon on laying the patient flat, that is, by reducing FiO_2 whilst achieving constant SpO_2/PaO_2.

There are several causes of platypnoea-orthodeoxia in the general population that can be divided into cardiac, respiratory, abdominal, and autonomic groups. The differential narrows for intubated and ventilated patients to either intracardiac or intrapulmonary shunts. Intracardiac shunting is more common; however, in the context of chronic liver disease, orthodeoxia is highly specific for HPS [17]. Both

intracardiac and intrapulmonary shunts can be identified on contrast echocardiography, making it a good discriminator for the aetiology of platypnoea-orthodeoxia in ICU patients.

HPS preferentially affects basal lung vasculature. Moving from a semirecumbent to supine position will necessarily reduce perfusion to lung bases via gravitational effect. This increases pulmonary circulation to less-affected vascular beds thereby reducing shunt fraction and improving oxygenation; this mechanism is thought to underlie platypnoea-orthodeoxia in the context of HPS [19].

3.4. Role of Contrast Echocardiography. Contrast echocardiography is the use of injected agitated saline to produce bubbles of >15 μm in diameter and then to observe for the presence of microbubbles in the left heart [4]. It can be used to identify both intrapulmonary and intracardiac shunts. An intrapulmonary shunt is defined by microbubbles seen in the left heart after the third beat (and usually before the sixth), due to passage of microbubbles through an abnormally dilated vascular bed. Conversely, visualisation of microbubbles in the left atrium in fewer than three beats is indicative of an intracardiac shunt; no visualisation is consistent with no shunt, as the microbubbles are trapped and absorbed during the first pass through normal pulmonary vasculature [20].

Abrams et al. showed contrast echocardiography to be superior to lung perfusion studies to screen for intrapulmonary vasodilatation in patients with cirrhosis, and it has since been recommended by the European Respiratory Society Task Force of Pulmonary-Hepatic vascular disorders as the first line screening modality for HPS [10, 21]. Abrams et al. noted intrapulmonary vascular dilatation in up to 30% of patients with cirrhosis, although only in 10% was this severe enough to cause hepatopulmonary syndrome [10].

4. Conclusion

Although patients with HPS typically present with hypoxia on the background of chronic liver disease, a presentation with hypoxia (and the complications of hypoxia, as in this case) may be their first. As there is no correlation between the severity of liver failure and the presence of HPS, we advocate the inclusion of HPS into the differential diagnosis for all patients with unexplained hypoxia on ICU. This differential diagnosis should prompt bedside assessment for orthodeoxia; HPS is excluded where orthodeoxia is not found. Patients with unexplained hypoxia will routinely have TTE performed; we advocate this investigation to be extended to contrast echocardiography for patients in whom orthodeoxia has been demonstrated. Should the contrast TTE demonstrate intrapulmonary shunting, a full assessment of liver function should be made.

The first suggestion of liver disease in this case came from the incidental inclusion (and reporting) of the abnormal liver via CTPA. Since a common indication for CTPA in ICU patients is unexplained hypoxia, we speculate whether the imaged field should be *deliberately* extended to the upper abdomen for all CTPA investigations in this cohort. We certainly advocate that where the liver is imaged (either intentionally or not) the appearance should be reported. Abnormal liver appearance in the context of hypoxia should be a further prompt for the bedside assessment of orthodeoxia (and possible consequent contrast TTE).

Any patient in whom HPS is suspected should be discussed with a tertiary centre regarding further assessment and suitability for liver transplantation.

References

[1] G. Fede, G. Privitera, T. Tomaselli et al., "Cardiovascular dysfunction in patients with liver cirrhosis," *Annals of Gastroenterology*, vol. 28, no. 1, pp. 31–40, 2015.

[2] M. E. Begbie, G. M. F. Wallace, and C. L. Shovlin, "Hereditary haemorrhagic telangiectasia (Osler-Weber-Rendu syndrome): A view from the 21st century," *Postgraduate Medical Journal*, vol. 79, no. 927, pp. 18–24, 2003.

[3] M. J. Krowka, "Hepatopulmonary syndromes," *Gut*, vol. 46, no. 1, pp. 1–4, 2000.

[4] V. Ho, "Current concepts in the management of hepatopulmonary syndrome," *Vascular Health and Risk Management*, vol. 4, no. 5, pp. 1035–1041, 2008.

[5] A. Williams, P. Trewby, R. Williams, and L. Reid, "Structural alterations to the pulmonary circulation in fulminant hepatic failure," *Thorax*, vol. 34, no. 4, pp. 447–453, 1979.

[6] A. Rabiller, H. Nunes, D. Lebrec et al., "Prevention of Gram-negative translocation reduces the severity of hepatopulmonary syndrome," *American Journal of Respiratory and Critical Care Medicine*, vol. 166, no. 4, pp. 514–517, 2002.

[7] P. Schenk, C. Madl, S. Rezaie-Majd, S. Lehr, and C. Muller, "Methylene blue improves the hepatopulmonary syndrome," *Annals of Internal Medicine*, vol. 133, no. 9, pp. 701–706, 2000.

[8] J. Zhang, Y. Ling, L. Tang et al., "Pentoxifylline attenuation of experimental hepatopulmonary syndrome," *Journal of Applied Physiology*, vol. 102, no. 3, pp. 949–955, 2007.

[9] F. P. Gómez, J. A. Barberá, J. Roca, F. Burgos, C. Gistau, and R. Rodríguez-Roisin, "Effects of nebulized NG-nitro-L-arginine methyl ester in patients with hepatopulmonary syndrome," *Hepatology*, vol. 43, no. 5, pp. 1084–1091, 2006.

[10] G. A. Abrams, C. C. Jaffe, P. B. Hoffer, H. J. Binder, and M. B. Fallon, "Diagnostic utility of contrast echocardiography and lung perfusion scan in patients with hepatopulmonary syndrome," *Gastroenterology*, vol. 109, no. 4, pp. 1283–1288, 1995.

[11] M. J. Krowka, G. A. Wiseman, O. L. Burnett et al., "Hepatopulmonary syndrome: a prospective study of relationships between severity of liver disease, PaO2 response to 100% oxygen, and brain uptake after 99mTc MAA lung scanning," *CHEST*, vol. 118, no. 3, pp. 615–624, 2000.

[12] A. Puttappa, K. Sheshadri, A. Fabre et al., "Prolonged unexplained hypoxemia as initial presentation of cirrhosis: a case report," *American Journal of Case Reports*, vol. 18, pp. 1–6, 2017.

[13] T. B. Kinane and S. J. Westra, "Case 31-2004: A four-year-old boy with hypoxemia," *The New England Journal of Medicine*, vol. 351, no. 16, pp. 1667–1675, 2004.

[14] B. Jagadisan, S. Krishnamurthy, R. Raghaven et al., "Chronic hypoxemia in a child: thinking outside the box," *Indian Pediatrics*, vol. 51, no. 10, pp. 829–830, 2014.

[15] M. K. Sahu, A. K. Bisoi, N. C. Chander, S. Agarwala, and S. Chauhan, "Abernethy syndrome, a rare cause of hypoxemia: A case report," *Annals of Pediatric Cardiology*, vol. 8, no. 1, pp. 64–66, 2015.

[16] M. L. Govindan, K. W. Kuo, M. G. Mahani, and T. P. Shanley, "Refractory hypoxemia caused by hepatopulmonary syndrome: A case report," *Journal of Medical Case Reports*, vol. 8, no. 1, article no. 418, 2014.

[17] J. B. Seward, B. L. Hayes, H. C. Smith et al., "Playpnea-orthodeoxia: clinical profile, diagnostic work-up, management and report of 7 cases," *Mayo Clinic Proceedings*, vol. 59, no. 4, pp. 221–231, 1984.

[18] G. Rolla, L. Brussino, P. Colagrande et al., "Exhaled nitric oxide and oxygenation abnormalities in hepatic cirrhosis," *Hepatology*, vol. 26, no. 4, pp. 842–847, 1997.

[19] E. D. Robin, D. Laman, B. R. Horn, and J. Theodore, "Platypnea related to orthodeoxia caused by true vascular lung shunts," *The New England Journal of Medicine*, vol. 294, no. 17, pp. 941–943, 1976.

[20] M. J. Krowka, A. J. Tajik, E. R. Dickson, R. H. Wiesner, and D. A. Cortese, "Intrapulmonary vascular dilatations (IPVD) in liver transplant candidates. Screening by two-dimensional contrast-enhanced echocardiography," *CHEST*, vol. 97, no. 5, pp. 1165–1170, 1990.

[21] R. Rodríguez-Roisin, MJ. Krowka, P. Herve et al., "Pulmonary-Hepatic vascular Disorders (PHD)," *European Respiratory Journal*, vol. 24, pp. 861–880, 2004.

29

A Pediatric Case of Diffuse Alveolar Hemorrhage Secondary to Poststreptococcal Glomerulonephritis

Alison Markland,[1] Gregory Hansen,[2] Anke Banks,[3] Rajni Chibbar,[4] and Darryl Adamko[5]

[1] University of Saskatchewan, Saskatoon, SK, Canada
[2] Division of Pediatric Intensive Care, University of Saskatchewan, Saskatoon, SK, Canada
[3] Department of Pediatrics, Cumming School of Medicine, University of Calgary, Calgary, AB, Canada
[4] Department of Laboratory Medicine, University of Saskatchewan, Saskatoon, SK, Canada
[5] Division of Pediatric Respirology, University of Saskatchewan, Saskatoon, SK, Canada

Correspondence should be addressed to Darryl Adamko; darryl.adamko@usask.ca

Academic Editor: Mehmet Doganay

This report summarizes a case of a 4-year-old girl with poststreptococcal glomerulonephritis and diffuse alveolar hemorrhage, an atypical presentation in this age group and type of vasculitic disease. We propose that her rapid improvement in clinical status was due to her treatment, continuous renal replacement therapy (CRRT). This mechanism would have impacted recovery by removing factors such as endothelial microparticles, superantigens, and immune complexes that have been postulated as the pulmonary-renal link. This may be an interesting avenue of exploration going forward given the lack of evidence in treating such conditions and emergence of CRRT.

1. Introduction

Diffuse alveolar hemorrhage (DAH) can be a life-threatening complication following numerous causes including respiratory infection, vasculitic diseases, or malignancy. Of the vasculitides in children, DAH is most commonly associated with granulomatosis and polyangiitis or antiglomerular basement membrane (anti-GBM) vasculitis. However, association of poststreptococcal glomerulonephritis (PSGN) with DAH is extremely rare; of the five cases reported only one was pediatric. In this report, we discuss a second case of a young child presenting with severe respiratory distress and significant hemoptysis who dramatically improved with continuous renal replacement therapy (CRRT).

2. Case

A 4-year-old female presented to the Pediatric Emergency Department at Royal University Hospital in Saskatoon, SK, Canada, with 4 days of worsening cough and increased work of breathing and one day of anuria. Her initial vital signs showed a temperature of 37.5 degrees Celsius, pulse rate of 125 beats per minutes, blood pressure of 114/58 mmHg, respiratory rate of 70 breaths per minute, and oxygen saturation of 95% on 30 litres of high flow oxygen with 21% FiO2. On exam, she had bilateral periorbital edema, crusted nasal discharge, and pallor. Rash and purpura were absent. She had nasal flaring, intercostal retractions, and coarse crackles bilaterally although more prominent on the right.

She had cough, sore throat, and rhinorrhea at a walk-in clinic approximately one-week prior and was given a prescription for amoxicillin. She also had iron deficiency anemia six months prior and started oral iron supplementation. She otherwise had no significant past medical history, significant travel history, or recent infectious contacts. Her mother, however, did have a history of treated tuberculosis (TB). Her immunizations were up to date.

Initial laboratory investigations revealed white blood cell count 9.08×10^9/L, decreased hemoglobin 60 g/L, and normal platelet count of 349×10^9/L. Her urea (16.9 mmol/L) and creatinine (46 umol/L) were elevated. She had a slightly elevated CRP (34.5 mg/L), normal glucose (6.7 mmol/L), normal sodium (142 mmol/L), high potassium (5.9 mmol/L),

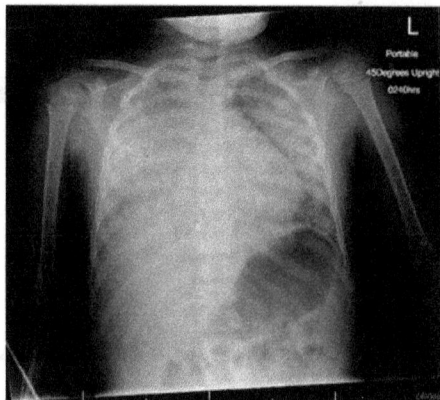

FIGURE 1: Radiograph on day of admission. Radiograph showing dense consolidation of the right lung obscuring the cardiothymic silhouette and tracheal deviation towards the right. Bilateral consolidation with associated air bronchograms.

mildly elevated chloride (112 mmol/L), and a low bicarbonate (15 mmol/L). Her D-dimer was 929 ug/L, APTT was low-normal (22 seconds), and fibrinogen was normal (3.42 g/L). Her urinalysis demonstrated leukocyte esterase 500 WBC/uL, protein 1.5 g/L, and blood 250 RBC/uL, with negative nitrites. Urine microscopy revealed leukocytes 20–50 WBC/HPF, erythrocytes 11–20 RBC/HPF, and granular casts 3–5/LPF.

She was transferred to the Pediatric Intensive Care Unit (PICU) after over 250 mL of hemoptysis. Her initial arterial gas showed a normal anion gap metabolic acidosis with concomitant respiratory acidosis (pH 7.25, carbon dioxide 43 mmHg, bicarbonate 18 mmol/L, and corrected anion gap 13.5). Her first chest X-ray showed bilateral consolidations with air bronchograms, consistent with diffuse pulmonary hemorrhage (Figure 1). She was initiated on bilevel positive airway pressure, but she continued to deteriorate with worsening respiratory acidosis (arterial pH 7.01, carbon dioxide 73 mmHg, and bicarbonate 18 mmol/L). She was intubated and shortly thereafter required high frequency oscillation ventilation (HFOV).

With our suspected diffuse alveolar hemorrhage, an upper gastrointestinal bleed (GI) was considered in the differential diagnosis. We elected not to pursue investigations of the GI tract, because her initial management in the PICU after intubation was revealing. A nasogastric tube was promptly inserted which did not indicate any evidence of gastric blood. More importantly, initial tracheal aspirates from closed inline suctioning revealed bright red blood, with subsequent aspirates suggesting a mixture of bright red and congealed blood. With her microcuffed endotracheal tube inflated and routinely monitored (q12 hrs) for minimum inflation pressures, risks for significant aspiration should have been mitigated.

She received two transfusions of packed red blood cells to correct the anemia. Given her worsening clinical status and anuria, CRRT was initiated. This led to a rapid improvement in her electrolyte abnormalities. Further investigations revealed positive perinuclear anti-neutrophil cytoplasmic

antibody (p-ANCA) with anti-myeloperoxidase antibody IgG 30, and negative cytoplasmic ANCA (c-ANCA) anti-proteinase 3 antibody IgG 2. Both complements C3 (0.18 g/L) and C4 (0.10 g/L) were low. Anti-glomerular basement membrane (GBM), anti-phospholipid, and antinuclear antibodies were negative.

Although vasculitis was strongly suspected due to the constellation of pulmonary and renal findings, infectious causes were also considered. Nasopharyngeal swab for rhinovirus was positive. Blood, urine, and lower respiratory cultures were negative. *Mycobacterium tuberculosis* polymerase chain reaction (PCR), acid fast bacilli stain, *Bordetella*, *Mycoplasma pneumoniae*, and *Hantavirus* PCR were also negative.

A renal biopsy was performed which demonstrated enlarged glomeruli with diffuse endocapillary hypercellularity with numerous neutrophils and closure of glomerular capillaries (Figure 2). There was endothelial cell swelling but no areas of glomerular capillary wall necrosis or cellular crescents. On immunofluorescent histology, C3 stain showed glomeruli with finely granular 3+, irregular diffuse staining of capillary walls, and mesangium (Starry sky pattern) and IgG demonstrated 1-2+ focal segmental, granular capillary wall staining. There was no immunopositivity with IgA antibody. Electron microscopy confirmed the increased numbers of endocapillary and infiltrative inflammatory cells in the glomerular tuft as well as swelling of endothelial cells. Scattered mesangial, subendothelial deposits were present. However, the classical subepithelial "hump like" deposits were rare. The case was also reviewed by pediatric nephropathologist to confirm the diagnosis of PIGN and to rule out C3 nephropathy. Following the biopsy, a streptozyme test was done which was positive with a titre of 1 : 100.

High dose methylprednisolone therapy was initiated under the suspicion of vasculitis following renal biopsy. Upon receiving the results of the biopsy 3 days after admission, corticosteroid was stopped and emphasis was given to supportive treatment. Her chest X-ray improved greatly by day 5 in hospital (Figure 3) and she was successfully weaned off HFOV and CRRT. She subsequently developed systemic hypertension, which was managed with captopril and amlodipine. At the age of 4 years she was too young for pulmonary function tests at our institution, and a CT chest did not seem warranted given her clinical improvement.

She was evaluated in pulmonary and nephrology follow-up clinics 3 months after discharge. There was no further history of cough, shortness of breath, or anemia and the CXR completely cleared. Her C3 and C4 normalized and her blood pressure remained normotensive. She will receive long-term monitoring for respiratory and renal impairment, but she is expected to have a complete recovery.

3. Discussion

Herein, we present a case of a child suffering DAH in the setting of PSGN. PSGN leading to pulmonary disease has been described in only a few cases and is exceedingly rare in the pediatric population [1–7]. This case highlights a unique presentation of PSGN with DAH, signs of fluid overload, AKI,

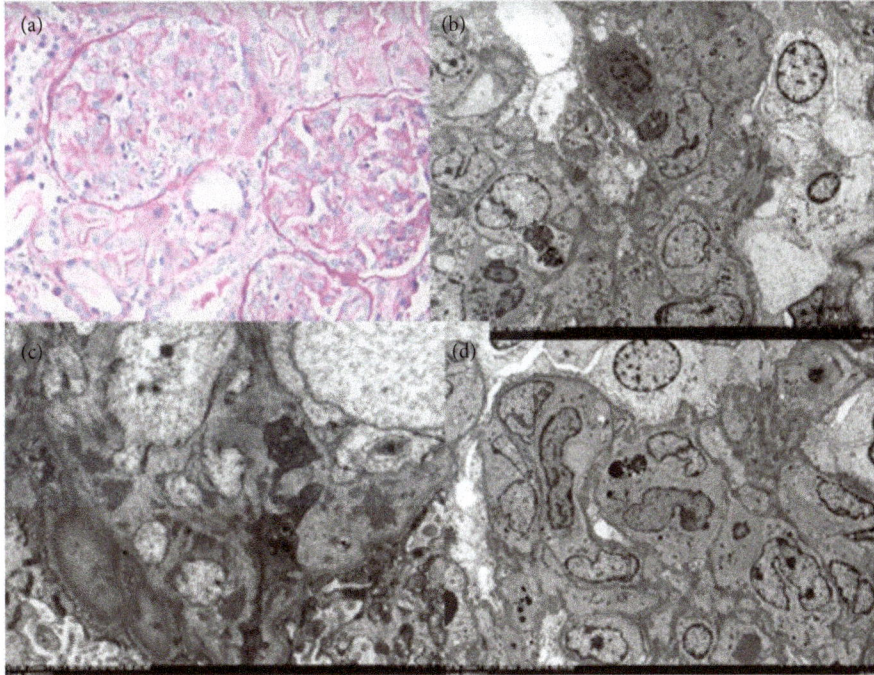

FIGURE 2: Renal biopsy. (a) Acute diffuse proliferative glomerulonephritis with intracapillary neutrophils and closure of glomerular capillaries and infiltration of capillaries. (b) and (c) Portion of glomerus shows intracapillary inflammatory cells, swelling of endothelial cells, mesangium, and subendothelial and (d) rare subepithelial dense deposits.

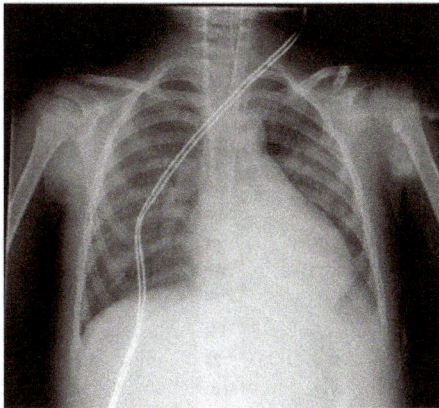

FIGURE 3: Follow-up radiograph. Improvement in pulmonary disease from previous image five days following admission and treatment. Mild perihilar consolidation persists with basal atelectasis.

severe respiratory compromise that quickly resolved with a short course of systemic corticosteroids, and CRRT.

Poststreptococcal glomerulonephritis is globally the most common cause of acute nephritis in children [8]. Following streptococcal infection of the respiratory tract or skin with a nephritogenic strain of Group A beta hemolytic *Streptococcus*, kidney injury may occur. The putative mechanism favored for glomerulonephritis following streptococcal infection is immune complex formation deposition in the glomerulus. However, the exact pathophysiology is largely unknown with proposed mechanisms including trapping of

circulating immune complex versus in situ immune complex formation [9–11]. Diagnosis of PSGN is made with evidence of streptococcal infection either by documented culture or antibody titers in the presence of acute nephritis. Although renal biopsy is not routinely part of the diagnostic formulation in PSGN, it may be useful if there is no documented evidence of streptococcal infection or in cases of recurrence [12]. On histological exam, focal segmental proliferative or mesangioproliferative patterns are the typical types of glomerular injury documented. C3 dominant staining with subepithelial "humps" and subendothelial deposits are commonly seen [13].

The common link between lung and kidney disease is likely related to similar cellular morphology of the vessels with a similar response to immune disorders. In the case of immune mediated hemorrhage in the lung, the hypotheses for vessel leak are (1) vessel injury from neutrophil activation (e.g., through antineutrophil antibodies (ANCA associated vasculitis, AAV)), (2) immune complex deposition with activation of complement, anaphylatoxin, and mast cells, or (3) abnormal lymphocyte inflammation and injury [14–16]. For example, infection with *Staph. aureus* or *Streptococcus* species is associated with exacerbation of AAV kidney disease. These organisms can act as superantigens, which activate T cells to injury vessels. High circulating endothelial microparticles (EMP) have been identified in children with other nephritic syndromes such as Henoch-Schönlein purpura [17]. High EMP concentrations may also induce significant lung pathology, including pulmonary edema, neutrophil recruitment, and endothelial-alveolar barrier compromise [18]. The mechanism of pulmonary hemorrhage in our case is unknown but we suggest that her biopsy would be in keeping with a form of AAV, though the role of superantigen is another factor to consider.

The patient in the previously reported that pediatric case of PSGN related DAH also required treatment in the intensive care unit and was similarly treated with corticosteroids for a brief period [2]. However, she was not ill enough to require CRRT or HFOV. It is difficult to say whether corticosteroids had an impact on resolution of symptoms and prognosis, as supportive therapy alone is the mainstay of treatment, with no evidence that other therapies offer a therapeutic advantage [19]. It is possible that the steroids were not necessary and this was the natural course of disease. In contrast, one case report by De Torrente et al. indicated that corticosteroids were necessary to treat pulmonary hemorrhage with poststreptococcal glomerulonephritis in an adult [20].

While it is plausible that the steroid pulse may have altered her clinical trajectory, we also propose the potential positive therapeutic effect of continuous renal replacement therapy (CRRT) on diffuse alveolar hemorrhage. Recently, a CRRT model utilizing a filter pore size of 200 μm significantly reduced EMP concentrations over a short duration [21]. We used a 69 CRRT hemofilter (Baxter Gambro). Removal of factors like EMP, anti-neutrophil antibodies, immune complexes, or superantigens could have been the important factor expediting recovery. Future directions of research may involve investigation of the use of CRRT in pulmonary-renal syndrome.

Prognosis for pediatric patients following PSGN is good. Only 10% of pediatric patients affected by PSGN will go on to have persistent hematuria or proteinuria; fewer still will have chronic kidney disease [22]. Prognosis for children with DAH is less predictable. Pulmonary hemorrhage from anti-GBM vasculitis has led to long-term deficits in pulmonary function, but recurrence of DAH has been reported. Patients with DAH secondary to idiopathic pulmonary hemosiderosis, however, are reported to have long standing deficits in lung function and higher mortality [23].

4. Conclusion

Presented above is a case of a 4-year-old in significant distress due to DAH resulting from PSGN. This presentation is rare and has been described in only one other instance in a child. This atypical presentation was followed by a rapid improvement in clinical presentation and symptoms following CRRT. We propose that CRRT impacted recovery by removing factors such as EMP, superantigens, and immune complexes that have been postulated as the pulmonary-renal link. This may be an interesting avenue of exploration going forward given the lack of evidence in treating such conditions.

References

[1] J. L. Niles, E. P. Böttinger, G. R. Saurina et al., "The syndrome of lung hemorrhage and nephritis is usually an ANCA-associated condition," *JAMA Internal Medicine*, vol. 156, no. 4, pp. 440–445, 1996.

[2] N. Gilboa, S. McIntire, L. Hopp, and D. Ellis, "Acute noncrescentic poststreptococcal glomerulonephritis presenting with pulmonary hemorrhage," *Pediatric Nephrology*, vol. 7, no. 2, pp. 147–150, 1993.

[3] Y. Thangaraj, I. Ather, H. Chataut et al., "Diffuse alveolar hemorrhage as a presentation of acute poststreptococcal glomerulonephritis," *American Journal of Medicine*, vol. 127, no. 9, pp. e15–e17, 2014.

[4] M. Santagati, T. Spanu, M. Scillato et al., "Rapidly fatal hemorrhagic pneumonia and group A streptococcus serotype M1," *Emerging Infectious Diseases*, vol. 20, no. 1, pp. 98–101, 2014.

[5] M. Yoshida, H. Yamakawa, M. Yabe et al., "Diffuse alveolar hemorrhage in a patient with acute poststreptococcal glomerulonephritis caused by impetigo," *Internal Medicine*, vol. 54, no. 8, pp. 961–964, 2015.

[6] K. S. Chugh, V. K. Gupta, P. C. Singhal, and S. Sehgal, "Case report: poststreptococcal crescentic glomerulonephritis and pulmonary hemorrhage simulating Goodpasture's syndrome," *Annals of Allergy, Asthma & Immunology*, vol. 47, no. 2, pp. 104–106, 1981.

[7] H.-Y. Sung, H. L. Chang, M.-J. Shin et al., "A case of poststreptococcal glomerulonephritis with diffuse alveolar hemorrhage," *Journal of Korean Medical Science*, vol. 22, no. 6, pp. 1074–1078, 2007.

[8] J. R. Carapetis, A. C. Steer, E. K. Mulholland, and M. Weber, "The global burden of group A streptococcal diseases," *The Lancet Infectious Diseases*, vol. 5, no. 11, pp. 685–694, 2005.

[9] T. M. Eison, B. H. Ault, D. P. Jones, R. W. Chesney, and R. J. Wyatt, "Post-streptococcal acute glomerulonephritis in children: clinical features and pathogenesis," *Pediatric Nephrology*, vol. 26, no. 2, pp. 165–180, 2011.

[10] K. Lange, A. A. Azadegan, G. Seligson, R. C. Bovie, and H. Majeed, "Asymptomatic poststreptococcal glomerulonephritis in relatives of patients with symptomatic glomerulonephritis. Diagnostic value of endostreptosin antibodies," *Child Nephrology and Urology*, vol. 9, no. 1-2, pp. 11–15, 1988.

[11] Z. Bircan, M. Kervancioğlu, F. Demir, S. Katar, and H. Onur, "Frequency of microscopic hematuria in acute poststreptococcal glomerulonephritis," in *Pediatc Nephrol*, vol. 13, pp. 269–270, 1999.

[12] R. Coppo, B. Gianoglio, M. G. Porcellini, and S. Maringhini, "Frequency of renal diseases and clinical indications for renal biopsy in children (report of the italian national registry of renal biopsies in children)," *Nephrology Dialysis Transplantation*, vol. 13, no. 2, pp. 293–297, 1998.

[13] N. Kambham, "Postinfectious glomerulonephritis," *Advances in Anatomic Pathology*, vol. 19, no. 5, pp. 338–347, 2012.

[14] D. Kluth and A. Rees, "Anti-glomerular basement membrane disease," *Journal of the American Society of Nephrology*, vol. 10, pp. 2446–2453, 1999.

[15] P. S. Mehler, M. W. Brunvand, M. P. Hutt, and R. J. Anderson, "Chronic recurrent goodpasture's syndrome," *American Journal of Medicine*, vol. 82, no. 4, pp. 833–835, 1987.

[16] E. J. Fitzsimons and C. F. Lange, "Hybridomas to specific streptococcal antigen induce tissue pathology in vivo; autoimmune mechanisms for post-streptococcal sequelae," *Autoimmunity*, vol. 10, no. 2, pp. 115–124, 1991.

[17] I. Dursun, R. Düsünsel, H. M. Poyrazoglu et al., "Circulating endothelial microparticles in children with Henoch-Schönlein

A Pediatric Case of Diffuse Alveolar Hemorrhage Secondary to Poststreptococcal...

127

purpura; preliminary results," *Rheumatology International*, vol. 31, no. 12, pp. 1595–1600, 2011.

[18] J. C. Densmore, P. R. Signorino, J. Ou et al., "Endothelium-derived microparticles induce endothelial dysfunction and acute lung injury," *Shock*, vol. 26, no. 5, pp. 464–471, 2006.

[19] S. Roy III, W. M. Murphy, and B. S. Arant Jr., "Poststreptococcal crescenteric glomerulonephritis in children: comparison of quintuple therapy versus supportive care," *Journal of Pediatrics*, vol. 98, no. 3, pp. 403–410, 1981.

[20] A. De Torrente, M. M. Popovtzer, S. J. Guggenheim, and R. W. Schrier, "Serious pulmonary hemorrhage, glomerulonephritis, and massive steroid therapy," *Annals of Internal Medicine*, vol. 83, no. 2, pp. 218-219, 1975.

[21] A. H. Abdelhafeez, P. M. Jeziorczak, T. R. Schaid et al., "Clinical CVVH model removes endothelium-derived microparticles from circulation," *Journal of Extracellular Vesicles (JEV)*, vol. 3, no. 1, p. 23498, 2014.

[22] R. G. Van De Voorde, "Acute poststreptococcal glomerulonephritis: the most common acute glomerulonephritis," *Pediatrics in Review*, vol. 36, no. 1, pp. 3–13, 2015.

[23] K. H. Soergel and S. C. Sommers, "Idiopathic pulmonary hemosiderosis and related syndromes," *American Journal of Medicine*, vol. 32, no. 4, pp. 499–511, 1962.

30

Severe Uncompensated Metabolic Alkalosis due to Plasma Exchange in a Patient with Pulmonary-Renal Syndrome: A Clinician's Challenge

Mohsin Ijaz,[1] Naeem Abbas,[2] and Dmitry Lvovsky[1]

[1]*Division of Pulmonary and Critical Care Medicine, Department of Medicine, Bronx Lebanon Hospital Center, 1650 Selwyn Avenue, Suite 12F, Bronx, NY 10457, USA*
[2]*Department of Medicine, Bronx Lebanon Hospital Center, 1650 Selwyn Avenue, Suite 10C, Bronx, NY 10457, USA*

Correspondence should be addressed to Mohsin Ijaz; doctor.mohsin@hotmail.com

Academic Editor: Mehmet Doganay

Metabolic alkalosis secondary to citrate toxicity from plasma exchange is very uncommon in patients with normal renal function. In patients with advanced renal disease this can be a fatal event. We describe a case of middle-aged woman with Goodpasture's syndrome treated with plasma exchange who developed severe metabolic alkalosis. High citrate load in plasma exchange fluid is the underlying etiology. Citrate metabolism generates bicarbonate and once its level exceeds the excretory capacity of kidneys, the severe metabolic alkalosis ensues. Our patient presented with generalized weakness, fever, and oliguria and developed rapidly progressive renal failure. Patient had positive serology for antineutrophilic cytoplasmic antibodies myeloperoxidase (ANCA-MPO) and anti-glomerular basement membrane antibodies (anti-GBM). Renal biopsy showed diffuse necrotizing and crescentic glomerulonephritis with linear glomerular basement membrane staining. Patient did not respond to intravenous steroids. Plasma exchange was started with fresh frozen plasma but patient developed severe metabolic alkalosis. This metabolic alkalosis normalized with cessation of plasma exchange and initiation of low bicarbonate hemodialysis. ANCA-MPO and anti-GBM antibodies levels normalized within 2 weeks and remained undetectable at 3 months. Patient still required maintenance hemodialysis.

1. Introduction

Anti-glomerular basement membrane antibody disease is a rare but well-recognized cause of glomerulonephritis. The incidence is reported to be one case per one million population [1]. About 60–70% of the affected patients present with pulmonary involvement in the form of alveolar hemorrhage [2]. In the setting of advanced renal failure, metabolic alkalosis (MA) is an uncommon phenomenon. Citrate is used as an anticoagulant for plasma exchange fluid and its in vivo conversion into bicarbonate leads to the metabolic alkalosis and its attendant complications. Double positive (serum positive for anti-GBM and ANCA-MPO) Goodpasture's disease is associated with worse renal outcomes and tobacco smoking increases chances of relapse of disease [2]. Aggressive treatment strategies in the form of immunosuppressive medications and plasmapheresis are the

mainstay of treatment [3]. Failure to respond to conservative management can lead to the need for hemodialysis (HD).

2. Case Presentation

A 54-year-old woman presented with generalized body aches, weakness, back pain, and fever of one-week duration. She had medical history of hypertension, depression, osteoarthritis, and smoking. Patient felt generalized weakness and had decrease in urine output, with dysuria and dark colored urine.

On admission, she was hemodynamically stable, alert, coherent, and oriented. Cardiovascular examination showed normal heart sounds, with no murmur, rub, or gallops. Respiratory examination revealed equal bilateral air movements with no adventitious sounds. Abdomen was soft, nontender with no organomegaly. Neurological examination showed

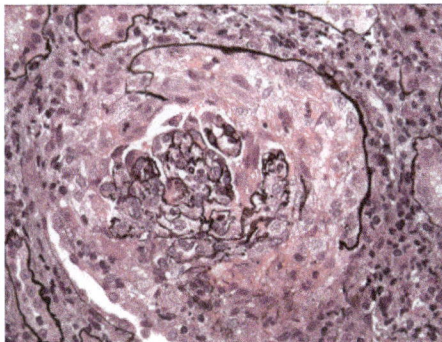

FIGURE 1: Diffuse necrotizing and crescentic glomerulonephritis.

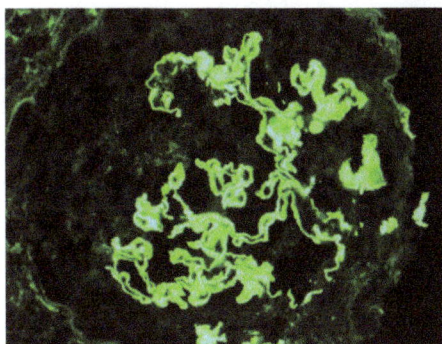

FIGURE 2: Immunofluorescence stain with linear glomerular basement membrane staining for IgG.

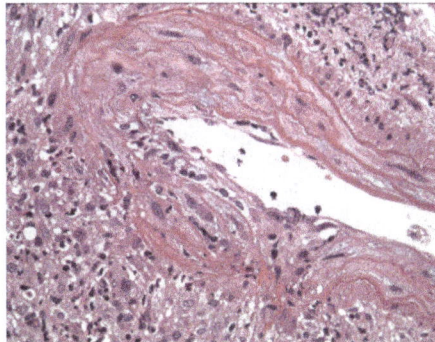

FIGURE 3: Medium caliber vessel shows transmural arteritis with disruption of the elastic and focal fibrinoid necrosis.

intact cranial nerves with no motor or sensory deficit. There was no leg edema or cutaneous manifestation of vasculitis.

Patient was noted to be in rapidly progressing acute renal failure and anemia. Autoimmune work-up revealed positive ANCA-MPO and anti-GBM antibody. Renal sonogram showed normal sized kidneys and no signs of obstruction. Renal biopsy showed diffuse necrotizing and crescentic glomerulonephritis (GN) with linear GBM staining consistent with acute, severe anti-GBM nephritis; ANCA associated focal necrotizing vasculitis; moderate tubular atrophy; interstitial fibrosis (Figures 1, 2, 3, and 4). She was given pulse intravenous methylprednisolone therapy (1000 mg daily) for three days and later on switched to tapering doses of oral prednisone. Patient was given trial of cyclophosphamide which was abandoned because of intolerance due to recalcitrant nausea and vomiting and gross hematuria.

In the next few days, she developed sudden shortness of breath, cough with hemoptysis, and hypoxia with oxygen saturation dropping down to 84% on ambient air, with crackles at lung bases bilaterally. She had acute hypoxic respiratory failure requiring orotracheal intubation and mechanical ventilation with full sedation. Computerized tomography (CT) of the chest revealed ground glass opacities and interstitial changes bilaterally (Figure 5). Given the acute onset of hypoxia, with no obvious source and explanation, bronchoscopy was performed which showed diffuse alveolar hemorrhage (Figure 6). Bronchoalveolar lavage was negative for any bacterial growth.

The patient was started on plasma exchange with fresh frozen plasma and hemodialysis for nonresolving acute renal failure. During the process of plasmapheresis with fresh frozen plasma, her laboratory data were noted to be significant for severe MA and respiratory alkalosis with pH ranging up to 7.67, HCO_3^- level going up to 34, and low ionized calcium of 0.94. Metabolic component of alkalosis was predominant from the high citrate load given during plasmapheresis (Table 1). All these parameters were reversed with cessation of plasmapheresis. The patient was continued on low bicarbonate HD. There was appropriate response in the level of anti-GBM and ANCA-MPO level, but no sustained improvement in renal function was noted and patient ended up in receiving long term HD.

3. Discussion

Goodpasture's syndrome is a rare disorder of acute glomerulonephritis and alveolar hemorrhage due to autoantibodies binding to the alveolar and glomerular basement membranes. It affects mainly young individuals, men being more commonly affected, and the majority of them are smokers [3]. Slightly fewer than half of them can present with pulmonary symptoms such as shortness of breath, hypoxia, and hemoptysis. Alveolar hemorrhage can be readily and reliably diagnosed by bronchoalveolar lavage. The renal outcome heavily depends on the initial serum creatinine and end-stage renal disease requiring hemodialysis or renal transplantation occurs in up to 42% of the individuals [2].

Serum anti-GBM antibody is a very specific marker of the disease and its level is correlated with the severity of the disorder. About 10%–40% of Goodpasture's syndrome patients will also have serum ANCA antibodies. The recognition of ANCA is very important as this group of patients is more likely to have treatable disease than others who have only anti-GBM antibodies [2]. Plasma exchange remains the modality of choice. The other options are corticosteroids and other immunosuppressive agents such as cyclophosphamide [4].

MA is frequently encountered in the inpatient setting. It may result in severe tissue hypoxia from compensatory alveolar hypoventilation and left shift of the oxyhemoglobin curve. The other dreaded complication is cardiac arrhythmias

(a)   (b)

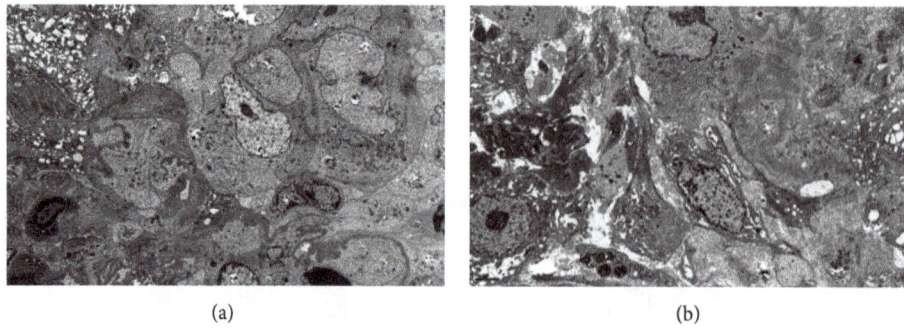

FIGURE 4: Electron microscopy shows all of the glomeruli sampled revealing global involvement by cellular crescents. Focal areas of GBM rupture associated with fibrin extravasation are noted. No immune deposits are identified. Tubules show degenerative changes and the interstitium contains patchy moderate inflammation.

TABLE 1: Laboratory parameters (on admission day and later on after initiation of hemodialysis and plasmapheresis).

Parameters	On admission	Day 1	Day 2	Day 4	Day 5	Day 6	Day 7	Day 9	Day 12
pH	7.31	7.42	7.56	7.61	7.68	7.47	7.51	7.50	7.47
PCO_2 (mmHg)	52	39	28	26.4	20.9	25.2	39.3	38	41.2
PO_2 (mmHg)	40	129	320	162	129	99	198	216	192
Sodium (mEq/mL)	145	143	143	141	138	138	131	138	138
Potassium (mEq/mL)	4.4	4.3	2.9	3.8	4.4	4.4	3.9	2.9	2.8
Bicarbonate (mEq/mL)	21	26	34	27	28	17	23	29	25
Chloride (mEq/mL)	102	103	101	105	108	108	92	96	93
BUN (mg/dL)	29	49	13	35	17	17	56	24	41
Creatinine (mg/dL)	2.8	8.7	2.7	4.5	2.3	2.3	7.8	4.7	6.3
Hematocrit %	27.4	17.6	24.8	25.8	25	25	24.2	22	22.8
ANCA-MPO		>8				22.8			3.1
Anti-GBM antibody		7.4				2.8			1

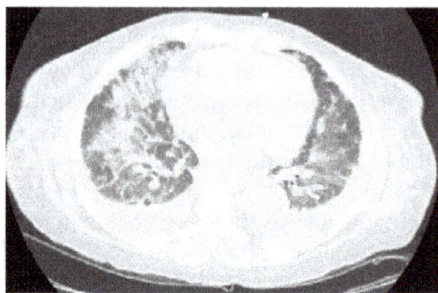

FIGURE 5: CT chest showing bilateral alveolar infiltrates and ground glass opacities.

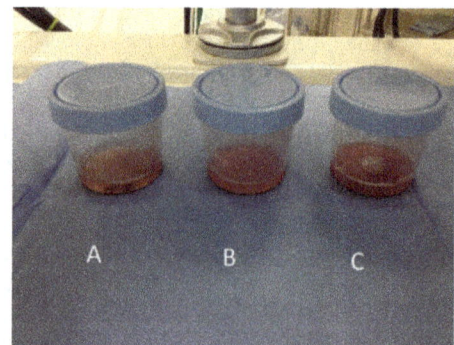

FIGURE 6: Bronchoalveolar fluid showed evidence of diffuse alveolar hemorrhage (A–C).

from alkalemia, associated low serum ionized calcium, and hypokalemia [5]. Severe MA with pH more than 7.55 is an emergent condition. In one study, Wilson et al. showed that a rising pH was associated with increased mortality (41% with pH 7.55 to 7.56, 47% with pH 7.57 to 7.59, 65% with pH 7.6 to 7.64, and 80% with pH 7.65 to 7.7) [6].

Plasma exchange is a well-established tool for the management of various immune and nonimmune conditions. Plasmapheresis is thought to remove the large molecular weight antibodies and proinflammatory markers. The development of MA in the context of plasma exchange has been described in many conditions such as systemic lupus erythematous, Goodpasture's syndrome, and ANCA vasculitis, suggesting that the underlying pathology is with plasma exchange rather than the underlying medical condition for which plasmapheresis is being used [7–9]. Three molecules of bicarbonate are generated from one molecule of citrate. Our patient was anuric and so unable to eliminate excess bicarbonate generated from citrate. Modifications in the plasma exchange protocol like albumin solution or cryoprecipitate with no citrate load, rather than fresh frozen plasma (FFP) which requires citrate for anticoagulation purpose, can prevent this complication. Citrate induced MA in individuals with renal insufficiency can be managed by HD following therapeutic plasma exchange. The overall mortality reported with plasmapheresis is 0.03–0.05 [10]. The most common complications reported are cardiac and respiratory [10].

There are two main mechanisms for the development of MA in the setting of advanced renal disease. Exogenous mechanism occurs in the form of ingestion or treatment with base therapy. Endogenous pathway acts in the form of HCO_3^- reclamation in the tubules in the setting of hypovolemia or loss of Na^+, Cl^-, or H^+, usually due to diuretics therapy or vomiting [11]. FFP is anticoagulated with sodium citrate at 14 g/dL. The metabolism of sodium citrate ($C_6H_5O_7Na_3$) to CO_2 and H_2O finally yields 3 molecules of $NaHCO_3$ [12]. The renal tubules have the extraordinary capacity to absorb the citrate and metabolic alkalosis slows down the net reabsorption of citrate. All the excreted citrate metabolizes to CO_2 which is about 15% of total renal production of CO_2 [13].

Pearl and Rosenthal [9] described that MA can be prevented if 3 percent of albumin or cryoprecipitate rather than FFP is used as replacement for the removal of patient plasma. Hsu et al. [5] used normal bicarbonate hemodialysate of 25 to 28 mEq/L to successfully treat the severe MA secondary to plasma exchange. Plasmapheresis has been recommended for the treatment of anti-GBM disease, with the aim of removing circulating pathogenic antibodies. It results in rapid reduction of the anti-GBM levels as observed in our case [1]. In 2007, the American Society for Apheresis guidelines recommend that all patients with anti-GBM antibody, not already on dialysis, should undergo intensive plasma exchange for at least 14 days or until anti-GBM antibodies become undetectable [14].

Our patient had similar clinical course. She developed severe MA with attendant biochemical parameters, which fortunately resolved with cessation of plasmapheresis. However, her renal failure did not improve, despite the undetectable anti-GBM antibody level, and is currently on HD.

4. Conclusions

Patients with advanced renal dysfunction with impaired excretory capacity undergoing plasma exchange with FFP anticoagulated with citrate require more frequent monitoring of acid base disturbance. These patients are prone to develop MA if subjected to high citrate load, which will metabolize to bicarbonate. Certain modifications in the plasmapheresis protocol such as albumin solution or cryoprecipitate with no citrate load can prevent the development of MA. The clinician should be able to identify this severe metabolic disorder, which if left untreated or unattended can lead to very sinister outcomes including the tissue hypoxia, neuromuscular excitability, and fatal arrhythmia.

Abbreviations

ANCA-MPO: Antineutrophilic cytoplasmic antibodies myeloperoxidase
anti-GBM: Anti-glomerular basement membrane antibodies
MA: Metabolic alkalosis
GN: Glomerulonephritis
CT: Computerized tomography
FFP: Fresh frozen plasma.

Disclosure

All authors have confirmed that the paper is not under consideration for review at any other journal.

Authors' Contribution

All authors have made contributions to the paper and have reviewed it before submission.

References

[1] T. Lahmer and U. Heemann, "Anti-glomerular basement membrane antibody disease: a rare autoimmune disorder affecting the kidney and the lung," *Autoimmunity Reviews*, vol. 12, no. 2, pp. 169–173, 2012.

[2] R. Lazor, L. Bigay-Gamé, V. Cottin et al., "Alveolar hemorrhage in anti-basement membrane antibody disease: a series of 28 cases," *Medicine*, vol. 86, no. 3, pp. 181–193, 2007.

[3] J. B. Levy, A. N. Turner, A. J. Rees, and C. D. Pusey, "Long-term outcome of anti-glomerular basement membrane antibody disease treated with plasma exchange and immunosuppression," *Annals of Internal Medicine*, vol. 134, no. 11, pp. 1033–1042, 2001.

[4] F. Dammacco, S. Battaglia, L. Gesualdo, and V. Racanelli, "Goodpasture's disease: a report of ten cases and a review of the literature," *Autoimmunity Reviews*, vol. 12, no. 11, pp. 1101–1108, 2013.

[5] S. C. Hsu, M. C. Wang, H. L. Liu, M. C. Tsai, and J. J. Huang, "Extreme metabolic alkalosis treated with normal bicarbonate hemodialysis," *American Journal of Kidney Diseases*, vol. 37, no. 4, pp. e3.1–e3.4, 2001.

[6] R. F. Wilson, D. Gibson, A. K. Percinel et al., "Severe alkalosis in critically ill surgical patients," *Archives of Surgery*, vol. 105, no. 2, pp. 197–203, 1972.

[7] X. Chen and N. Chen, "Plasma exchange in the treatment of rapidly progressive glomerulonephritis," *Contributions to Nephrology*, vol. 181, pp. 240–247, 2013.

[8] M. B. Marques and S. T. Huang, "Patients with thrombotic thrombocytopenic purpura commonly develop metabolic alkalosis during therapeutic plasma exchange," *Journal of Clinical Apheresis*, vol. 16, no. 3, pp. 120–124, 2001.

[9] R. G. Pearl and M. H. Rosenthal, "Metabolic alkalosis due to plasmapheresis," *The American Journal of Medicine*, vol. 79, no. 3, pp. 391–393, 1985.

[10] M. H. Mokrzycki and A. A. Kaplan, "Therapeutic plasma exchange: complications and management," *American Journal of Kidney Diseases*, vol. 23, no. 6, pp. 817–827, 1994.

[11] M. E. Ostermann, Y. Girgis-Hanna, S. R. Nelson, and J. B. Eastwood, "Metabolic alkalosis in patients with renal failure," *Nephrology Dialysis Transplantation*, vol. 18, no. 11, pp. 2442–2448, 2003.

[12] S. von Vietinghoff, F. C. Luft, and R. Kettritz, "A 77 year-old haemodialysis patient with unexpected alkalosis," *Nephrology Dialysis Transplantation*, vol. 20, no. 11, pp. 2569–2570, 2005.

[13] S. B. Baruch, R. L. Burich, C. K. Eun, and V. F. King, "Renal metabolism of citrate," *The Medical Clinics of North America*, vol. 59, no. 3, pp. 569–582, 1975.

[14] Z. M. Szczepiorkowski, N. Bandarenko, H. C. Kim et al., "Guidelines on the use of therapeutic apheresis in clinical practice—evidence-based approach from the Apheresis Applications Committee of the American Society for Apheresis," *Journal of Clinical Apheresis*, vol. 22, no. 3, pp. 106–175, 2007.

31

The No-Win Resuscitation: Ventricular Septal Rupture and Associated Acute Aortic Occlusion

Jan-Thorben Sieweke,[1] Jens Vogel-Claussen,[2] Andreas Martens,[3] Jörn Tongers,[1] Andreas Schäfer,[1] Johann Bauersachs,[1] and L. Christian Napp ⓘ[1]

[1]Cardiac Arrest Center, Department of Cardiology and Angiology, Hannover Medical School, Hannover, Germany
[2]Institute for Diagnostic and Interventional Radiology, Hannover Medical School, Hannover, Germany
[3]Department of Cardiothoracic, Transplantation and Vascular Surgery, Hannover Medical School, Hannover, Germany

Correspondence should be addressed to L. Christian Napp; napp.christian@mh-hannover.de

Academic Editor: Chiara Lazzeri

A 66-year-old patient was admitted under continuous resuscitation for pulseless electrical activity. After return of spontaneous circulation ECG showed signs of acute inferior ST-elevation myocardial infarction, and echocardiography showed acute right ventricular failure with a dilated right ventricle. Carotid pulses were present in the absence of femoral pulses. Subsequent computed tomography demonstrated inferior myocardial infarction with ventricular septal rupture and thrombotic occlusion of the thoracic aorta, resulting in a heart-brain-circulation with loss of perfusion downstream of the aortic arch. *Teaching Points*. The present case prototypically demonstrates the fatal consequence of acute ventricular septal rupture and the eminent value of computed tomography and palpation of carotid in addition to femoral pulses in resuscitated patients. It is, to the best of our knowledge, the first description of an acute aortic occlusion in a patient with acute ventricular septal rupture.

1. Introduction

Prognosis of out-of-hospital cardiac arrest remains poor [1], despite loads of efforts in emergency and critical care medicine. Major goals to improve outcome are early return of spontaneous circulation (ROSC) with only minimal no-flow-time prior to and during cardiopulmonary resuscitation (CPR), and early detection of the cause of arrest, paralleled by optimal post-resuscitation care. Efficacy of chest compressions and ROSC are usually monitored by palpation of pulses, commonly femoral pulses, in addition to capnography. However, in selected cases palpation of femoral pulses only is not reliable, either with coexisting peripheral artery disease or with rare conditions as in our case. After ROSC a dedicated diagnostic and therapeutic program has to be started to improve outcomes. At this stage the diagnostic pathway should also include computed tomography (CT), as already practiced by an increasing number of large centers, for determining the cause of arrest

and to uncover important comorbidities. In our case the CT scan inadvertently uncovered a fatal diagnosis.

2. Case Presentation

A 66-year-old female patient, who was hospitalized in a psychiatric clinic, suddenly developed dysarthria and anisocoria with subsequent loss of consciousness. Without palpable pulses immediate bystander CPR was performed and the patient was transferred to our hospital. On the way CPR of the ventilated patient was continued with a mechanical resuscitation device (LUCAS 2, Physio-Control™). After 45 minutes of CPR for pulseless electrical activity spontaneous circulation returned as assessed by a palpable carotid pulse, however femoral pulses were absent, precluding cannulation for mechanical circulatory support (MCS). ECG showed ST-segment elevation in leads II, III, aVF, and V6 (Figure 1). Fast-track echocardiography demonstrated severe dysfunction of the dilated right ventricle. Pericardial effusion and severe

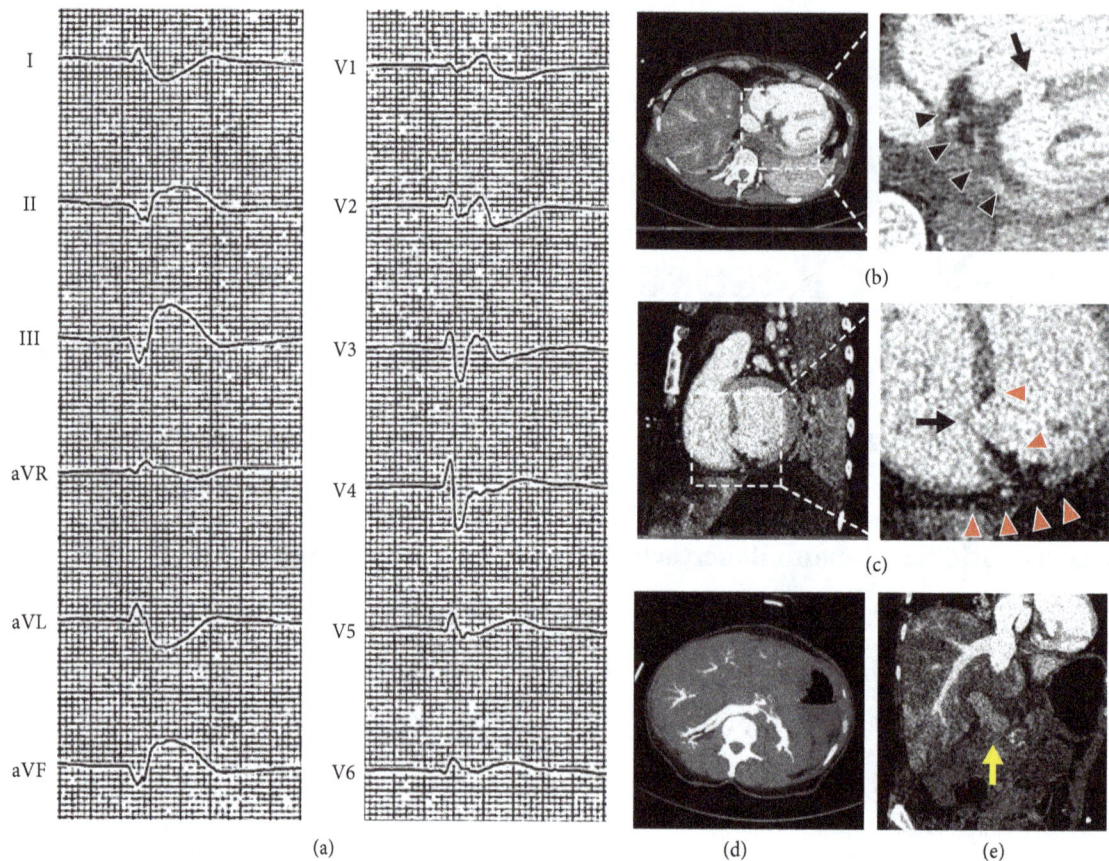

(a)   (b)   (c)   (d)   (e)

FIGURE 1: **Signs and consequences of ventricular septal rupture due to acute myocardial infarction.** (a) ECG. ST-segment elevation in leads II, III, aVF, and V6. (b) to (e): Computed tomography. (b) Transverse plane. Acute inferior myocardial infarction (black arrowheads) and ventricular septal rupture (black arrow), both associated with dilation of the right ventricle and retrograde flow of contrast agent into the liver veins due to acute right heart failure. (c) Sagittal plane. Ventricular septal rupture (black arrow) due to acute myocardial infarction with extensive microvascular obstruction (red arrowheads). (d) Transverse plane, arterial phase after intravenous injection of contrast agent. Contrast is seen in renal and hepatic veins as a sign of severe venous congestion. (e) Sagittal oblique plane, late phase after injection of contrast agent. Hepatic veins, hepatic parenchyma, and the portal vein (yellow arrow) are still opacified due to backward failure of the right heart.

aortic regurgitation were absent. Medical history comprised an infrarenal aortic aneurysm. Acute aortic dissection Stanford Type A, De Bakey I with involvement of the right coronary artery was suspected. As percutaneous MCS was not possible without femoral pulses and since Type-A-dissection would have prompted emergency surgery, the heart team decided for immediate computed tomography (CT), which showed no signs of Type A aortic dissection, pulmonary embolism, intracerebral bleeding, or carotid stenosis, but severe ubiquitous aortic calcification. Main findings were as follows: a large ventricular septal rupture with classical radiological signs of acute myocardial infarction (Figure 1), signs of severe backward failure with contrast agent being observed in hepatic veins, renal veins (Figure 1), the portal vein and the inferior vena cava (Figure 1), and thrombotic occlusion of the descending aorta just distal to the left subclavian artery (Figure 2). The latter was probably facilitated by massive left-to-right shunt and associated severe forward failure. Shortly after the CT scan the patient had to be resuscitated again, but due to futility with subtotal body ischemia without any option for MCS or emergent surgery resuscitation was terminated.

3. Discussion

Acute ventricular septal rupture is one of the most dangerous complications of myocardial infarction [2, 3]. In patients with large septal defects and conservative management, mortality is unacceptably high with rates up to 100% [4]. Therefore, those patients are classic candidates for urgent surgery, and recently results of interventional closure are even more encouraging, with survival rates reaching over 50% [5]. In this context CT has emerged as the gold standard for assessment of anatomy before treatment [4].

Our patient had an acute ventricular septal rupture due to acute inferior myocardial infarction resulting in right ventricular failure and low cardiac output syndrome. In such cases MCS is an important option as a bridge to surgery or intervention [6, 7], which was not feasible due to proximal aortic occlusion. The massive left-to-right shunt maybe does not solely explain aortic occlusion. Additional plaque rupture of a diseased aorta or local dissection associated with CPR may have been the initial injury triggering local thrombosis. Alternatively, classic aortic dissection Stanford Type B, De

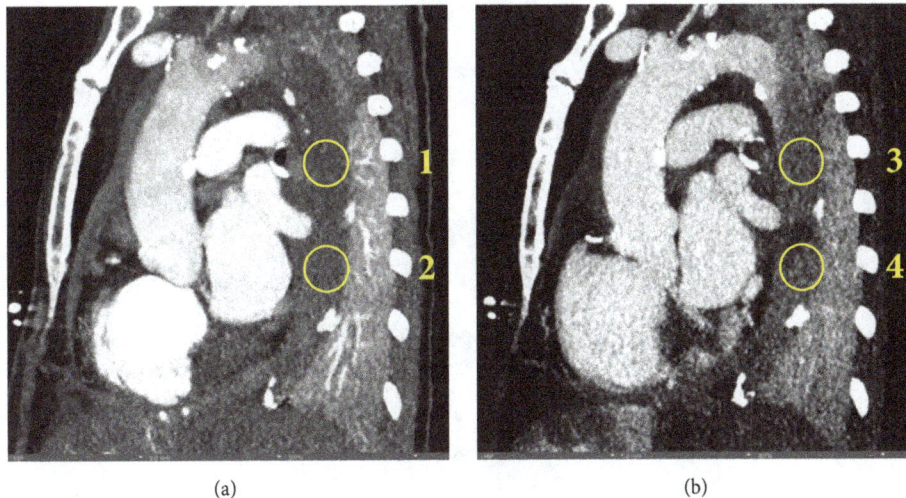

(a)								(b)

FIGURE 2: **Acute aortic occlusion.** Computed tomography. (a) Sagittal plane, arterial phase after intravenous injection of contrast agent. The descending aorta is not filled with contrast (circle 1: 70 HU, circle 2: 73 HU). Note the severe calcification of the aorta. (b) Sagittal plane, late phase after intravenous injection of contrast. While few contrast enters the proximal part of the thrombus (apposition zone, circle 3: 105 HU), it does not reach the already more solid parts of the thrombus (circle 4: 78 HU). HU: Hounsfield Units.

Bakey III may have been present subsequently resulting in thrombosis. Furthermore, tissue embolization from septal rupture could have been the initial trigger for thrombus formation. However, CT findings were consistent with a very large thrombus without signs of aortic dissection or tissue embolism, thus suggesting that low cardiac output was the predominant determinant of the developing occlusion. Unfortunately, confirmation of those findings would have required autopsy, which was declined by the patient's family. In addition efficacy of mechanical CPR may have been limited in this particular patient due to the left-to-right shunt, which could have been a reason for low flow in the aorta triggering subsequent thrombosis.

Notwithstanding, the absence of femoral pulses in the presence of carotid pulses after CPR should prompt a CT scan, as in our case. Fast-track echocardiography in the emergency room after ROSC did not uncover the VSR in our patient, maybe due to the very basal position of the defect. Without aortic occlusion, the patient would have had a chance to survive - with the use of MCS, septal closure, coronary intervention, and appropriate post-cardiac arrest care. Irrespective of the outcome in this single case, CT would have been a prerequisite for treatment planning.

To the best of our knowledge, the present case is the first to illustrate an acute occlusion of the descending aorta in a patient after out-of-hospital cardiac arrest. It corroborates the extraordinary role of palpating all major pulses and echocardiography during cardiac arrest management, as well as the value of computed tomography after ROSC, either to search for therapeutic options or to detect fatal situations in order to terminate therapy.

References

[1] B. Grunau, J. C. Reynolds, F. X. Scheuermeyer et al., "Comparing the prognosis of those with initial shockable and non-shockable rhythms with increasing durations of CPR: Informing minimum durations of resuscitation," *Resuscitation*, vol. 101, pp. 50–56, 2016.

[2] B. M. Jones, S. R. Kapadia, N. G. Smedira et al., "Ventricular septal rupture complicating acute myocardial infarction: A contemporary review," *European Heart Journal*, vol. 35, no. 31, pp. 2060–2068, 2014.

[3] P. Sulzgruber, F. El-Hamid, L. Koller et al., "Long-term outcome and risk prediction in patients suffering acute myocardial infarction complicated by post-infarction cardiac rupture," *International Journal of Cardiology*, vol. 227, pp. 399–403, 2017.

[4] M. C. Hamilton, J. C. Rodrigues, R. P. Martin, N. E. Manghat, and M. S. Turner, "The In Vivo Morphology of Post-Infarct Ventricular Septal Defect and the Implications for Closure," *JACC: Cardiovascular Interventions*, vol. 10, no. 12, pp. 1233–1243, 2017.

[5] P. A. Calvert, J. Cockburn, D. Wynne et al., "Percutaneous closure of postinfarction ventricular septal defect in-hospital outcomes and long-term follow-up of UK experience," *Circulation*, vol. 129, no. 23, pp. 2395–2402, 2014.

[6] M. B. Ancona, L. Regazzoli, A. Mangieri, F. Monaco, M. De Bonis, and A. Latib, "Post-infarct ventricular septal rupture: early Impella implantation to delay surgery and reduce surgical risk," *Cardiovascular Intervention and Therapeutics*, vol. 32, no. 4, pp. 381–385, 2017.

[7] L. C. Napp, C. Kühn, and J. Bauersachs, "ECMO in cardiac arrest and cardiogenic shock," *Herz*, vol. 42, no. 1, pp. 27–44, 2017.

32

Venovenous Extracorporeal Membrane Oxygenation for Negative Pressure Pulmonary Hemorrhage in an Elderly Patient

Kenichiro Ishida, Mitsuhiro Noborio, Nobutaka Iwasa, Taku Sogabe, Yohei Ieki, Yuki Saoyama, Kyosuke Takahashi, Yumiko Shimahara, and Daikai Sadamitsu

Traumatology and Critical Care Medical Center, National Hospital Organization, Osaka National Hospital, 2-1-14 Hoenzaka, Chuo-ku, Osaka 540-0006, Japan

Correspondence should be addressed to Kenichiro Ishida; kenichiro1224@gmail.com

Academic Editor: Chiara Lazzeri

The patient in this case report was an 88-year-old male. Acute upper airway obstruction by food led to transient cardiac arrest, and negative pressure pulmonary hemorrhage (NPPH) occurred 1 hour after the foreign body obstruction. Using venovenous extracorporeal membrane oxygenation (ECMO) for severe acute respiratory distress syndrome resulting from NPPH, his respiratory state was recovered and hemoptysis stopped. NPPH is a life-threatening disease, the rapid recognition of which is required to initiate appropriate therapy. Although active hemorrhage might be a contraindication for ECMO, our experience showed this to be an effective treatment option. Moreover, our experience suggests that the application of ECMO to elderly patients should be considered on a case-by-case basis.

1. Introduction

Negative pressure pulmonary edema (NPPE) and hemorrhage (NPPH) are uncommon problems resulting from upper airway obstruction [1]. A previous report showed that NPPE and NPPH resolve rapidly with short-term ventilatory support [2]. However, NPPE and NPPH can lead to life-threatening respiratory insufficiency requiring extracorporeal membrane oxygenation (ECMO) [3]. Although active hemorrhage might be a contraindication for ECMO, it is considered for life-threatening acute respiratory distress syndrome (ARDS) when the underlying condition is reversible despite optimal ventilatory support [4]. Age is an important prognosis-related factor [5–7]. However, the application of ECMO to older patients is not contraindicated [8, 9]. This paper presents our experience of successful treatment with venovenous (VV) ECMO for NPPH following foreign body obstruction.

2. Case Presentation

The patient was an 88-year-old male. He had chronic heart failure, but his activity of daily living level was independent. When he presented to our hospital for a regular follow-up appointment, he lost consciousness suddenly during lunch at a restaurant in the hospital. Cardiac arrest occurred and bystander cardiopulmonary resuscitation (CPR) was performed by a layperson. Medical staff rushed to the scene, and the initial rhythm at the time of cardiac arrest was nonshockable. Advanced cardiac life support was started immediately. The oral cavity was occluded by rice and a piece of laver; therefore, manual ventilation was impossible. Thus, the foreign body was removed using Magill forceps. The trachea was intubated and spontaneous circulation was resumed after two cycles of chest compression. The patient was taken to the intensive care unit (ICU) for further resuscitation. On admission to the ICU, the patient's blood

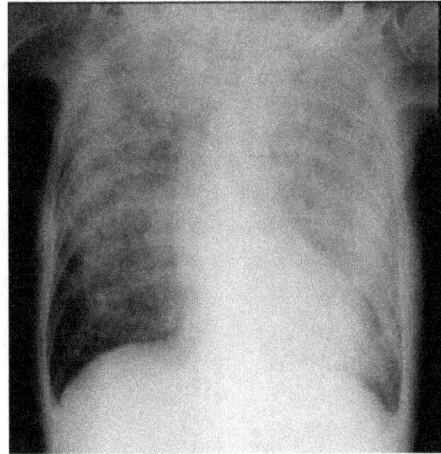

FIGURE 1: A chest radiograph on admission to the intensive care unit showed diffuse bilateral infiltrates, consistent with pulmonary edema and hemorrhage.

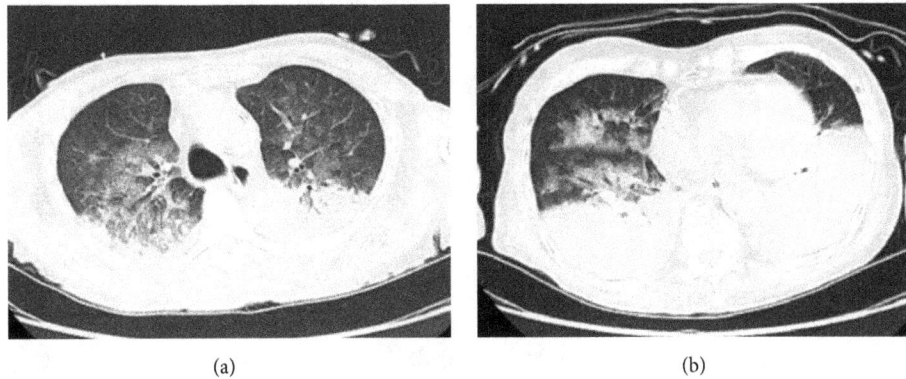

(a)   (b)

FIGURE 2: A thoracic computed tomography scan demonstrated bilateral parenchymal consolidation in gravity-dependent areas and ground glass-appearing opacities of lung parenchyma (a). Bilateral atelectasis was observed in the lower lung fields (b).

pressure was 170/105 mmHg, his heart rate was 90 bpm, his peripheral oxygen saturation level was 88% with 10 L/min of oxygen via a bag valve mask, and he was in a coma.

The patient was responsive to verbal commands immediately after admission to the ICU. However, copious frothy blood-tinged secretions were suctioned from his endotracheal tube 1 hour after the foreign body obstruction. No food was found in the secretions. A chest X-ray showed bilateral infiltrates (Figure 1), compatible with pulmonary hemorrhage. Thoracic computed tomography (CT) showed bilateral parenchymal consolidation in gravity-dependent areas and ground glass-appearing opacities of lung parenchyma (Figure 2). His hemodynamic status was maintained with inotropes, but no abnormality in cardiac function was detected on echocardiography. His respiratory status had promptly deteriorated with hypoxemia, compatible with severe ARDS. The ventilator settings had to be elevated (biphasic positive airway pressure) from 20/10 cmH$_2$O to 28/20 cmH$_2$O. Fractional inspired oxygen was increased from 60% to 100%, but hypoxemia persisted (PaO$_2$ 54 mmHg). Arterial hypercapnia (PaCO$_2$ 55 mmHg) also persisted. Therefore, VV ECMO (Capiox emergent bypass system; Terumo Inc., Tokyo, Japan) was used for the treatment of ARDS resulting from pulmonary hemorrhage 5 hours after onset of the latter.

After systemic anticoagulation with 5000 U of heparin delivered intravenously, ECMO was initiated at a flow rate of 2.4 L/min with an 18 Fr drainage cannula in the right femoral vein and a 15 Fr reinfusion cannula in the internal jugular vein. A continuous heparin infusion (400 U/h) was applied to maintain an activated clotting time (ACT) of 160–200 seconds. ACT was measured every 2 hours and a platelet transfusion was required due to gradual progression of thrombopenia. Moreover, red blood cells were transfused to maintain hemoglobin of 12 g/dL and hematocrit of 40%. The ventilator was then set to a lung-protective strategy with a positive end-expiratory pressure of 10 cmH$_2$O. On admission and hospital day 1, a flexible bronchoscopy revealed fresh blood in the entire tracheobronchial tree (Figure 3). Cytology was negative for hemosiderin-laden macrophages. Tests for autoimmune markers, including anti-neutrophil cytoplasmic antibodies, were negative. NPPH was diagnosed based on these results. The patient was successfully decannulated after 2 days of ECMO support and weaned off ventilator support

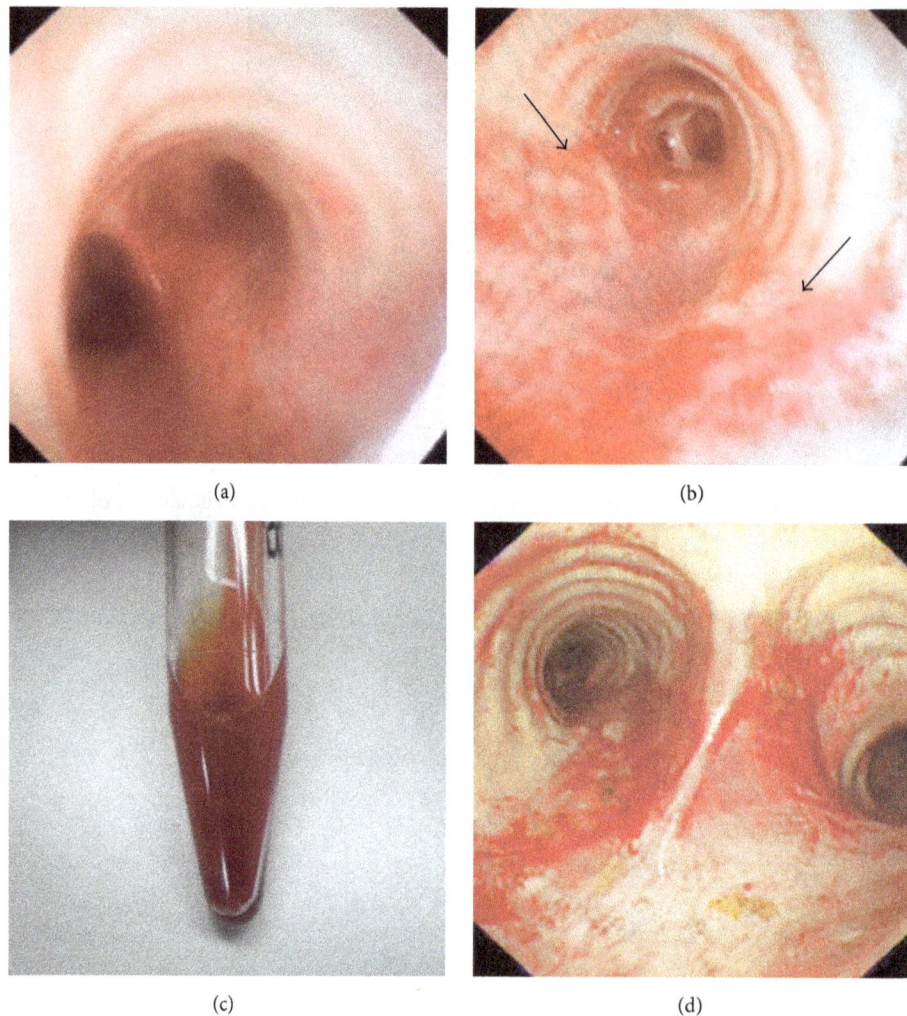

FIGURE 3: Flexible bronchoscopy on the day of admission revealed fresh blood in the entire tracheobronchial tree (a), and a copious frothy blood-tinged secretion was suctioned form the throat (b, c). Tracheobronchial tree on hospital day 1 (d).

within the next 6 days. Hemoptysis decreased progressively and stopped 2 days after ECMO. The only ECMO-related complication was slight thrombus formation in the right jugular and femoral veins, which required continuous heparin infusion after ECMO.

On hospital day 9, the patient was weaned from mechanical ventilation and extubated. However, reintubation was required because of respiratory deterioration due to chronic heart failure related to his underlying illness on hospital day 13. Thereafter, tracheostomy was performed and he was weaned from mechanical ventilation. The length of the ICU stay was 20 days. The patient was alert with no respiratory support or supplementary oxygen and was transferred to a rehabilitation hospital following ICU discharge.

3. Discussion

This report raises two important issues. First, NPPH is a reversible disease, but it can be a life-threatening complication of acute upper airway obstruction. Second, ECMO usage

is feasible and effective for elderly patients in the clinical setting of pulmonary hemorrhage.

NPPE and NPPH are uncommon problems resulting from upper airway obstruction [1]. Although the mechanisms of these diseases remain uncertain, it has been postulated that increased microvascular pressure and pulmonary capillary permeability, and mechanical disruption of the alveolar capillary membrane, are related to intrathoracic pressure, which results in NPPE and NPPH [10–12]. Acute upper airway obstruction by food led to transient cardiac arrest in our patient. A copious frothy blood-tinged secretion was suctioned from the endotracheal tube 1 hour after the foreign body obstruction was removed. No food was found in the secretions. There were episodes of pulmonary hemorrhage after the upper airway obstruction and negative cytology and autoimmune marker test results, indicating NPPH, not aspiration pneumonia. Several factors may be associated with the onset of NPPH. First, there might be markedly negative intrathoracic pressure during inspiratory effort against airway obstruction. Second, transient cardiac arrest and chest compression during CPR might influence microvascular congestion and hemorrhage. Moreover, capillaries might become fragile in patients of advanced age.

A previous report showed that NPPE and NPPH resolved rapidly with short-term ventilatory support [2]. However, NPPE and NPPH can lead to life-threatening respiratory insufficiency requiring ECMO [3]. In our patient, the ventilator settings had to be raised to maintain the PaO_2 after the onset of NPPH. However, hypoxemia persisted due to a ventilation-perfusion imbalance resulting from pulmonary hemorrhage and atelectasis. The treatment of NPPE and NPPH is supportive. NPPH is a life-threatening disease, the rapid recognition of which is required to initiate appropriate therapy.

ECMO treatment is considered for life-threatening ARDS when the underlying condition is reversible despite optimal ventilatory support [4]. We initiated ECMO for early-onset NPPH because it was considered reversible. We initially hesitated to initiate ECMO in our elderly patient due to reports showing that the length of mechanical ventilation, severity of multiple organ failure, and immune status of the patients were prognosis-related factors during ECMO. Moreover, age is an important prognosis-related factor [5–7]. However, the application of ECMO to elderly patients is not contraindicated [8, 9]. In our elderly patient, a good result was expected because his underlying condition was considered reversible and he did not have multiple comorbidities.

To safely maintain the ECMO circuit, systemic anticoagulation is required. On the other hand, bleeding is a serious complication of ECMO. The application of ECMO to hemorrhagic patients is not contraindicated and ECMO treatment for hemorrhagic patients—such as those with pulmonary hemorrhage, intracranial hemorrhage, and multiple trauma—has been reported [13–16]. Although the optimal anticoagulation management that minimizes bleeding during ECMO treatment of pulmonary hemorrhage patients is unknown, several methods—such as heparin-free ECMO or the use of nafamostat mesilate as an alternative anticoagulation agent to reduce the risk of bleeding—have been reported [13–15]. In our patient, a continuous heparin infusion was adapted to maintain an ACT of 160–200 seconds. At that time, red blood cell and platelet transfusions were required. Hemoptysis decreased progressively and stopped 2 days after ECMO without uncontrollable bleeding. Changing anticoagulation agents and interventional radiology as a hemostatic option were considered in case of refractory bleeding. ECMO usage was feasible and effective for our elderly patient in the clinical setting of pulmonary hemorrhage.

4. Conclusions

In summary, we reported our experience of VV ECMO for NPPH following foreign body obstruction. NPPH is a life-threatening disease, the rapid recognition of which is required to initiate appropriate therapy. Although active hemorrhage might be a contraindication for ECMO, our experience showed this to be an effective treatment option. Moreover, our experience suggests that the application of ECMO to elderly patients should be considered on a case-by-case basis.

References

[1] T. A. Tami, F. Chu, T. O. Wildes, and M. Kaplan, "Pulmonary edema and acute upper airway obstruction," *The Laryngoscope*, vol. 96, no. 5, pp. 506–509, 1986.

[2] M. S. Koh, A. A. L. Hsu, and P. Eng, "Negative pressure pulmonary oedema in the medical intensive care unit," *Intensive Care Medicine*, vol. 29, no. 9, pp. 1601–1604, 2003.

[3] D. Marino, M. Baggi, G. Casso, and A. Pagnamenta, "Near-fatal acute postobstructive pulmonary oedema requiring extraporal membrane oxygenation," *Intensive Care Medicine*, vol. 36, no. 2, pp. 365–366, 2010.

[4] G. J. Peek, M. Mugford, R. Tiruvoipati et al., "Efficacy and economic assessment of conventional ventilatory support versus extracorporeal membrane oxygenation for severe adult respiratory failure (CESAR): a multicentre randomised controlled trial," *The Lancet*, vol. 374, no. 9698, pp. 1351–1363, 2009.

[5] M. Schmidt, E. Zogheib, H. Rozé et al., "The PRESERVE mortality risk score and analysis of long-term outcomes after extracorporeal membrane oxygenation for severe acute respiratory distress syndrome," *Intensive Care Medicine*, vol. 39, no. 10, pp. 1704–1713, 2013.

[6] F. Pappalardo, M. Pieri, T. Greco et al., "Predicting mortality risk in patients undergoing venovenous ECMO for ARDS due to influenza A (H1N1) pneumonia: the ECMOnet score," *Intensive Care Medicine*, vol. 39, no. 2, pp. 275–281, 2013.

[7] T. B. Enger, A. Philipp, V. Videm et al., "Prediction of mortality in adult patients with severe acute lung failure receiving venovenous extracorporeal membrane oxygenation: a prospective observational study," *Critical Care*, vol. 18, no. 2, article R67, 2014.

[8] P. Mendiratta, X. Tang, R. T. Collins, P. Rycus, T. V. Brogan, and P. Prodhan, "Extracorporeal membrane oxygenation for respiratory failure in the elderly: a review of the extracorporeal life support organization registry," *ASAIO Journal*, vol. 60, no. 4, pp. 385–390, 2014.

[9] W. H. Cho, D. W. Kim, H. J. Yeo et al., "Clinical characteristics of respiratory extracorporeal life support in elderly patients with severe acute respiratory distress syndrome," *Korean Journal of Critical Care Medicine*, vol. 29, no. 4, pp. 266–272, 2014.

[10] R. D. Fremont, R. H. Kallet, M. A. Matthay, and L. B. Ware, "Postobstructive pulmonary edema: a case for hydrostatic mechanisms," *Chest*, vol. 131, no. 6, pp. 1742–1746, 2007.

[11] J. B. West and O. Mathieu-Costello, "Stress failure of pulmonary capillaries: role in lung and heart disease," *The Lancet*, vol. 340, no. 8822, pp. 762–767, 1992.

[12] J. B. West, K. Tsukimoto, O. Mathieu-Costello, and R. Prediletto, "Stress failure in pulmonary capillaries," *Journal of Applied Physiology*, vol. 70, no. 4, pp. 1731–1742, 1991.

[13] W. Hohenforst-Schmidt, A. Petermann, A. Visouli et al., "Successful application of extracorporeal membrane oxygenation due to pulmonary hemorrhage secondary to granulomatosis with polyangiitis," *Drug Design, Development and Therapy*, vol. 7, pp. 627–633, 2013.

[14] G. J. Hwang, S. H. Sheen, H. S. Kim et al., "Extracorporeal membrane oxygenation for acute life-threatening neurogenic pulmonary edema following rupture of an intracranial aneurysm,"
Journal of Korean Medical Science, vol. 28, no. 6, pp. 962–964,
2013.

[15] M. Arlt, A. Philipp, S. Voelkel et al., "Extracorporeal membrane
oxygenation in severe trauma patients with bleeding shock,"
Resuscitation, vol. 81, no. 7, pp. 804–809, 2010.

[16] D. Kimura, S. Shar, M. Briceno-Medina et al., "Management of
massive diffuse alveolar hemorrhage in a child with systemic
lupus erythematosu," *Journal of Intensive Care*, vol. 3, no. 1,
article 10, 2015.

33

An Atypical Case of Myxedema Coma with Concomitant Nonconvulsive Seizure

Pratik Patel,[1] Mikhael Bekkerman,[1,2] Cristina Varallo-Rodriguez,[1] and Rajendra Rampersaud[3]

[1]Department of Medicine, St. John's Riverside Hospital, 967 N. Broadway, Yonkers, NY 10701, USA
[2]Lake Erie College of Osteopathic Medicine, 1858 W Grandview Blvd, Erie, PA 16509, USA
[3]Pulmonary and Critical Care, St. John's Riverside Hospital, 967 N. Broadway, Yonkers, NY 10701, USA

Correspondence should be addressed to Rajendra Rampersaud; raj_rampersaud@hotmail.com

Academic Editor: Chiara Lazzeri

Hypothyroidism is a prevalent condition in the general population that is treatable with appropriately dosed thyroid hormone replacement medication. Infrequently, patients will present with myxedema coma, characterized by hypothermia, hypotension, bradycardia, and altered mental status in the setting of severe hypothyroidism. Myxedema coma has also been known to manifest in a number of unusual and dangerous forms. Here, we present the case of a woman we diagnosed with an uncharacteristic expression of myxedema coma and nonconvulsive seizure complicated by a right middle cerebral artery infarct.

1. Introduction

Hypothyroidism is a result of the inability of the thyroid gland to produce thyroid hormone sufficient enough to satisfy the requirements of peripheral tissues. Overt hypothyroidism is prevalent in the United States, hovering at 3.2–3.7% of the populations studied [1]. Clinical features of hypothyroidism can vary depending on a number of factors including age of onset and the severity of the disease and most commonly present as fatigue, lethargy, weakness, weight gain, cold intolerance, hair loss, depression, and xerosis. Measuring thyroid stimulating hormone (TSH) levels is the most appropriate method of diagnosing hypothyroidism. A thyroxine (T4) level should further be obtained if an abnormality is detected in the patient's TSH. A low level of T4 together with an elevated TSH confirms a diagnosis of hypothyroidism [2]. Severe hypothyroidism can manifest as myxedema coma, a rare, but frequently fatal disease characterized classically by hypothermia, bradycardia, hypotension, altered mental status, and cold intolerance. Several studies have shown that myxedema coma can present atypically, without the most common symptoms and clinical findings [3–7]. It is important for clinicians to be aware of the uncommon presentations of myxedema coma in order to avoid preventable complications.

2. Case Presentation

A 70-year-old woman with a past medical history of hypothyroidism, coronary artery disease, cerebrovascular accident with right-sided weakness, and hypertension presented to the emergency department for altered mental status. Earlier that day, she had an appointment for a screening colonoscopy with her gastroenterologist. During the procedure, she was given propofol at 50 mg for sedation. The colonoscopy was complicated by stool in the rectum, and it was subsequently aborted. It was noted that her mental status was not improving after cessation of propofol, and thus the patient was sent to the emergency department. Vitals on arrival were notable for tachycardia at 120 bpm, temperature of 96.8°F (36°C), and blood pressure of 146/83 mm Hg. On examination, the patient was awake with her eyes open, but she was not responding to verbal stimuli. She reacted verbally and withdrew her extremities in response to pain, and her extremities were held in flexion. She scored an 11 on the NIH Stroke Scale. An ECG in the emergency department demonstrated normal sinus

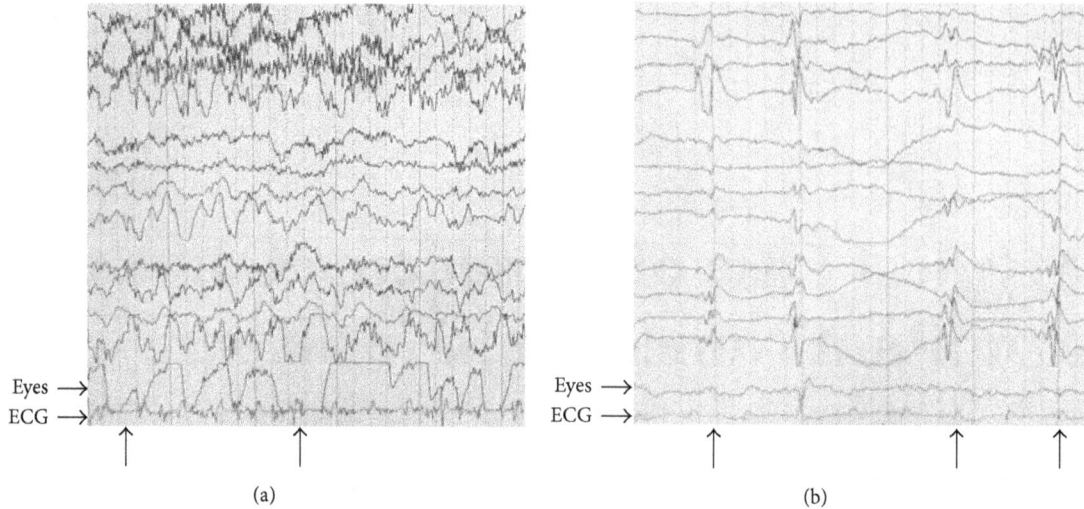

FIGURE 1: Electroencephalogram (EEG) displaying seizure-like activity at initial presentation (a) and at 10 days after admission (b). Arrows denote paroxysmal discharges.

rhythm and a right bundle branch block. Laboratory studies on arrival revealed hyponatremia, hypokalemia, an elevated blood urea nitrogen (BUN) and creatinine, elevated glucose (298), elevated lactic acid (3.1), and an elevated thyroid stimulating hormone (TSH) at 175.0 mIU/mL. A CT of the head revealed no overt hemorrhage. An echocardiogram and magnetic resonance angiography study were performed to rule out a possible ischemic event, both of which resulted in no significant abnormalities. The patient was given an electroencephalogram (EEG), during which she developed left arm myoclonus. The EEG showed paroxysmal bursts of discharges suspect for complex partial seizures and wave complexes near the end of recording, suggesting nonconvulsive status epilepticus (Figure 1). The patient's son reported that she has no previous history of seizure activity. The patient received lorazepam 3 mg and placed on levetiracetam 1,500 mg and valproate 500 mg.

The patient was transferred to the intensive care unit and intubated the following day for airway protection after initiation of a midazolam drip. Due to the uncertain nature of her condition, we examined a broader differential diagnosis before we were confident with myxedema coma. The consulting endocrinologist initially began treatment with levothyroxine 25 mcg IV and hydrocortisone 100 mg three times daily. The midazolam drip was discontinued to assess the mental status of the patient, but the patient remained unarousable despite not being on any sedation medication. The nonconvulsive status epilepticus was treated with fosphenytoin 500 mg every 12 hours, lacosamide 200 mg twice a day, and levetiracetam 2000 mg twice a day. Approximately one week later, the patient's status epilepticus terminated and was noted with EEG. To assess for adrenal gland functionality, ACTH and AM cortisol levels were measured. The patient's ACTH level was found to be 49.9 pg/mL and her AM cortisol level was noted at 27.1 mcg/dL, not suggestive of any adrenal gland dysfunction. The patient remained intubated in the ICU for two weeks in a comatose state with occasional left

sided myoclonus and bilateral upper and lower extremity nonpitting edema. She was unresponsive to verbal or painful stimuli. The patient's TSH and free thyroxine (T4) levels as measured in the ICU initially trended down but began to rise again after two weeks (Table 1).

The diagnosis of myxedema coma was made based on the patient's clinical presentation and a score of 65 on the diagnostic scoring system published in 2014 by Popoveniuc et al. [8]. The typical characteristics of myxedema coma, including bradycardia, hypotension, and hypothermia, were absent in this case. However, a score of >60 using these criteria is reported to be diagnostic of myxedema coma with a sensitivity of 100%. The patient's dose of levothyroxine was increased to 50 mcg IV, 25 mcg IM, and 25 mcg of liothyronine (T3) in the ICU and subsequently levothyroxine was increased to 50 mcg bid IV and 50 mcg of liothyronine due to the later increase in the patient's TSH levels.

A repeat CT of the head was performed after 14 days in the ICU, which revealed a large, nonhemorrhagic middle cerebral artery (MCA) infarct that was not present on admission (Figure 2). On the same hospital day, the patient became arousable, and she was able to follow basic verbal commands. She had marked weakness of the left lower extremity and absent motor function of the left upper extremity. A tracheostomy was performed due to depressed respiratory function and inability to wean off ventilator support. The patient was scheduled to undergo a percutaneous endoscopic gastrostomy (PEG) tube insertion and subsequent transfer to a long-term rehabilitation facility to help improve her motor function as well as her respiratory function.

3. Discussion

Myxedema coma is a rare endocrine emergency due to the advent of rapid TSH ELISA testing but has been reported to occur with an incidence of 220,000 per year in western countries [9]. The mortality rate is reported to be 60%. It

TABLE 1: Measured TSH and free thyroxine (T4) levels during hospitalization. Normal values for TSH range between 0.358 and 3.74 mIU/mL and free T4 range between 0.76 and 1.46 ng/dL.

Day of hospitalization	1	3	5	9	11	13	17
TSH level (mIU/mL)	175.00	35.70	7.53	20.10	18.10	30.90	50.70
Free T4 level (ng/dL)	0.58	0.75	0.56	0.37	0.38	0.47	0.69

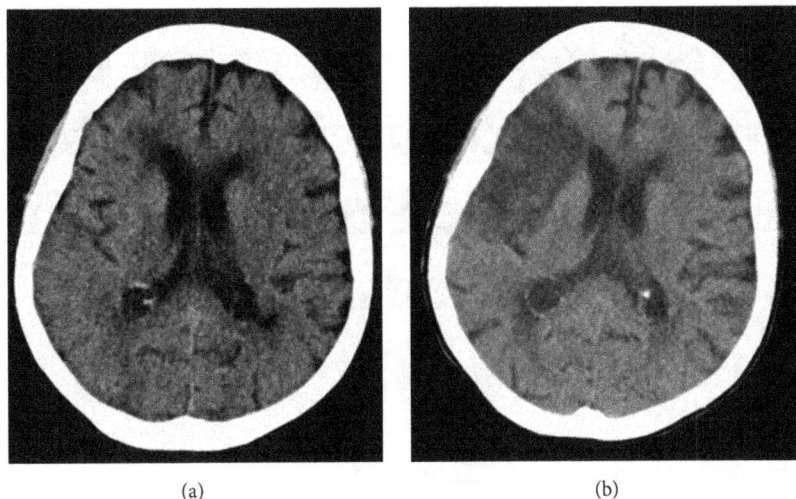

(a)   (b)

FIGURE 2: CT scan of the head performed on admission (a) compared to one performed after 14 days in the ICU (b) shows development of a large right MCA infarct.

typically presents as a state of severe hypothyroidism with cold intolerance, hypothermia, hypoventilation, hypercapnia, bradycardia, and cardiomegaly. Oftentimes there is a precipitating factor such as infection, trauma, medication, CVA, or a metabolic abnormality [8]. In our case, the precipitating factor was likely the propofol administration during the patient's colonoscopy. The patient's myxedema coma together with her epileptic activity likely resulted in cerebral vasoconstriction and subsequently hypoperfusion to her brain, precipitating the right middle cerebral artery infarction. It is important to suspect myxedema coma in patients with a history of hypothyroidism presenting with altered mental status after a known precipitating event and to begin empiric treatment with large doses of synthetic T4 (200–400 mcg) and T3 promptly to avoid complications [3]. A swift diagnosis can be critical to a patient's prognosis. There are several published criteria available that allow physicians to make the diagnosis of myxedema coma [8, 10]. Additionally, we recommend ruling out seizure in a patient that presents in a newly onset obtunded or comatose state due to risk of cerebral hypoperfusion and ischemic infarct.

Competing Interests

The authors declare that there is no conflict of interests regarding the publication of this paper.

References

[1] Y. Aoki, R. M. Belin, R. Clickner, R. Jeffries, L. Phillips, and K. R. Mahaffey, "Serum TSH and total T4 in the United States population and their association with participant characteristics: National Health and Nutrition Examination Survey (NHANES 1999–2002)," *Thyroid*, vol. 17, no. 12, pp. 1211–1223, 2007.

[2] M. T. McDermott, "In the clinic. Hypothyroidism," *Annals of Internal Medicine*, vol. 151, no. 11, Article ID ITC61, 2009.

[3] A. Majid-Moosa, J. M. Schussler, and A. Mora, "Myxedema coma with cardiac tamponade and severe cardiomyopathy," *Proceedings (Baylor University. Medical Center)*, vol. 28, no. 4, pp. 509–511, 2015.

[4] J. Y. Ahn, H.-S. Kwon, H. C. Ahn, and Y. D. Sohn, "A case of myxedema coma presenting as a brain stem infarct in a 74-year-old Korean woman," *Journal of Korean Medical Science*, vol. 25, no. 9, pp. 1394–1397, 2010.

[5] S. Dixit, M. K. Dutta, and M. Namdeo, "A rare case of myxedema coma with Neuroleptic Malignant Syndrome (NMS)," *Journal of Clinical and Diagnostic Research*, vol. 9, no. 5, pp. VD01–VD3, 2015.

[6] D. Chaudhari, V. Gangadharan, and T. Forrest, "Heart failure presenting as myxedema coma: case report and review article," *Tennessee Medicine*, vol. 107, no. 2, pp. 39–41, 2014.

[7] D. Chaudhari, V. Gangadharan, and T. Forrest, "Heart failure presenting as myxedema coma: case report and review article," *Tennessee Medicine*, vol. 106, no. 5, pp. 39–40, 2013.

[8] G. Popoveniuc, T. Chandra, A. Sud et al., "A diagnostic scoring system for myxedema coma," *Endocrine Practice*, vol. 20, no. 8, pp. 808–817, 2014.

[9] J. C. Galofré and R. V. García-Mayor, "Densidad de incidencia del coma mixedematoso," *Endocrinologia*, vol. 44, pp. 103–104, 1997.

[10] Y. V. Chiong, E. Bammerlin, and C. N. Mariash, "Development of an objective tool for the diagnosis of myxedema coma," *Translational Research*, vol. 166, no. 3, pp. 233–243, 2015.

34

Double Bolus Alteplase Therapy during Cardiopulmonary Resuscitation for Cardiac Arrest due to Massive Pulmonary Embolism Guided by Focused Bedside Echocardiography

Hafiz B. Mahboob [1,2] **and Bruce W. Denney**[1,2]

[1] *University of Nevada School of Medicine, Reno, NV, USA*
[2] *Renown Regional Medical Center, Reno, NV, USA*

Correspondence should be addressed to Hafiz B. Mahboob; hmahboob@medicine.nevada.edu

Academic Editor: Chiara Lazzeri

Massive pulmonary embolism (PE) frequently leads to cardiac arrest (CA) which carries an extremely high mortality rate. Although available, randomized trials have not shown survival benefits from thrombolytic use. Thrombolytics however have been used successfully during resuscitation in clinical practice in multiple case reports and in retrospective studies. Recent resuscitation guidelines recommend using alteplase for PE related CA; however they do not offer a standardized treatment regimen. The most consistently applied approach is an intravenous bolus of 50 mg tissue plasminogen activator (t-PA) early during cardiopulmonary resuscitation (CPR). There is no consensus on the subsequent dosing. We present a case in which two 50 mg boluses of t-PA were administered 20 minutes apart during CPR due to persistent hemodynamic compromise guided by bedside echocardiogram. The patient had an excellent outcome with normalization of cardiac function and no neurologic sequela. This case demonstrates the benefit of utilizing bedside echocardiography to guide administration of a second bolus of alteplase when there is persistent hemodynamic compromise despite achieving return of spontaneous circulation after the initial bolus, and there is evidence of persistent right ventricle dysfunction. Future trials are warranted to help establish guidelines for thrombolytic use in cardiac arrest to maximize safety and efficacy.

1. Introduction

Cardiac arrest due to PE is a lethal condition [1–5]. Thrombolytics have been used successfully, mostly late in CPR after initial unresponsiveness to traditional advanced cardiac life support (ACLS) [6–11]. Recent resuscitation guidelines advocate using alteplase in PE related cardiac arrest [12–17]. There are no clear guidelines or protocols for the administration of thrombolytics during CPR. We present an approach of double bolus therapy during CPR guided by focused bedside echocardiography. This case suggests the potential benefit of using bedside echocardiography to guide the administration of a second bolus of alteplase given the excellent outcome in this case.

2. Case Report

A 56-year-old, previously healthy Caucasian female presented to the emergency department (ED) with acute, severe shortness of breath and pleuritic chest pain for two hours with pulse of 140/min and respiratory rate of 30/min. She had undergone total right knee replacement surgery two weeks prior. She was taking aspirin 81 mg twice daily but no other medications and had no other medical history. She was brought in via ambulance in severe respiratory distress, diaphoretic, and a room air oxygen saturation of 70% and complained "I cannot breathe." There was some bruising at the surgical site and a small right knee effusion, but the surgical site was well healed with no erythema

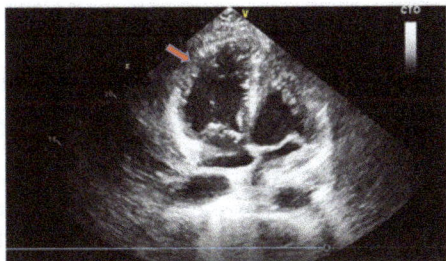

FIGURE 1: Transthoracic echocardiogram obtained before administration of t-PA: apical views showing a severely dilated right ventricle (RV) with reduced right ventricular systolic function. RV free wall is hypokinetic and RV apical wall is hypercontractile (arrow; McConnell sign). Left ventricular size and systolic function are normal.

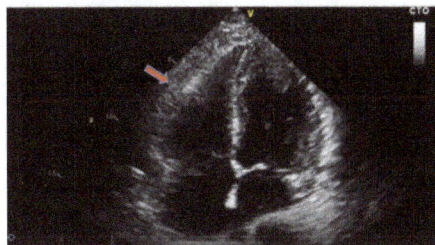

FIGURE 2: Transthoracic echocardiogram 24 hours after t-PA administration: showing improvement in RV size (arrow) and function but still dilated.

or purulence. Her electrocardiogram (ECG) showed sinus tachycardia without any acute ischemic changes.

She was immediately given 5000 units of intravenous heparin due to the high suspicion of pulmonary embolism. Her oxygen saturations remained around 70–79% despite receiving 100% oxygen (15 L) via nonrebreather mask. Arterial blood gas (ABG) on 100% oxygen showed (pH 6.8, pCO2 58.6, and PaO2 188) severe acidosis with an elevated A-a gradient of 334.8 mmHg. Patient was emergently intubated due to persistent respiratory distress, increased work of breathing, continued air hunger, and worsening respiratory acidosis with hypercapnia despite being on 100% oxygen via nonrebreather mask. She was given etomidate and succinylcholine and intubated without difficulty.

Shortly after intubation, she underwent cardiac arrest with pulseless electrical activity (PEA). Immediate CPR was started. She received 50 mEq intravenous (IV) sodium bicarbonate, 1 mg of IV epinephrine, and 1 mg of IV atropine with four cycles of chest compression during first round of resuscitation. Emergent bedside echocardiogram was performed at the first pulse check and showed a severely dilated right ventricle (RV), with reduced right ventricular systolic function and normal left ventricular (LV) size and systolic function. These findings were suggestive of a massive PE (Figure 1 and videos 1, 2). The first bolus of alteplase 50 mg IV was given at the fifth minute into CPR with ongoing chest compression. She had return of spontaneous circulation (ROSC) one minute following the t-PA bolus. However, she went into cardiac arrest again, approximately at 15 minutes into the code with recurrent PEA. During the second round of resuscitation, she received 1 mg of epinephrine with three cycles of chest compression and had ROSC after four minutes of CPR.

However, despite achieving the ROSC, she was hypotensive and therefore norepinephrine infusion was started. Echocardiogram was still showing persistent evidence of RV dysfunction with normal LV function. Given her persistent hemodynamic compromise with recurrent cardiac arrest, the decision was made to administer a second bolus of 50 mg alteplase, which was given at 24 minutes into the code. She developed PEA for a third time approximately at 29 minutes into the code. During third round of resuscitation, she received 1 mg of epinephrine and had ROSC. She required CPR for a total of 32 minutes, with three rounds of resuscitation and 2 IV boluses of 50 mg alteplase, 20 minutes apart. Her chest X-ray at this point showed bilateral perihilar opacities with mild cardiomegaly, consistent with pulmonary edema. Her other laboratory findings are summarized in the table (Table 1).

After the third round of CPR, she also received a transfusion of two units of packed red blood cells via Belmont rapid infuser due to anemia. Bicarbonate infusion was initiated due to severe acidosis. Full dose heparin anticoagulation was started per postthrombolytics protocol. Some ecchymosis and swelling were noticed at the recent knee surgical site but she did not develop any significant bleeding complications after thrombolytic therapy. Venous Doppler ultrasound was done later which was positive for deep venous thrombosis in the gastrocnemius and popliteal veins of the right lower extremity. She was then transferred to the intensive care unit where bronchoscopy showed small pink frothy septum consistent with pulmonary edema but no evidence of aspiration.

Repeat echocardiogram the next day showed improvement in RV size and function (Figure 2 and video 3). She remained on vasopressor support, bicarbonate infusion, and epoprostenol (continuous inhalation at a rate of 360 mcg/hour) due to hypotension, acidosis, and hypoxia, respectively, which were titrated off over 24 hours.

Subsequent computed tomography angiogram of the chest performed eighty-four hours after CA showed segmental PE in right middle and left lower lobe with scattered air space opacities, atelectasis, and pleural effusions (Figure 3).

She had an excellent outcome without any neurologic sequelae or any bleeding complications. She was liberated from mechanical ventilation on hospital day 3 and supplemental oxygen was gradually weaned from high flow nasal cannula to room air by the time of discharge. Apixaban was initiated on hospital day 3. She was discharged home on hospital day 5, ambulating independently, on room air and on apixaban. On 3 months' follow-up, she had complete normalization of right ventricular size and systolic function without any residual pulmonary hypertension (Figures 4(a) and 4(b) and videos 4, 5).

TABLE 1: Patient characteristics.

Variable	Value	Target range
Pulse	140/minute	60–100/minute
Respiratory rate	34–50/minute	12–14/minute
Blood pressure	109/67 mmHg	120/80 mmHg
Temperature	97°F	97–99°F
Oxygen saturation		
Room air	70%	88–100%
100% oxygen	70–79%	88–100%
ABG on 15 L oxygen nonrebreather (NRB)		
Ph	6.8	7.4
pO2	188 mmHg	100 mmHg
pCO2	58.6 mmHg	40 mmHg
HCO3	9.2 mmol/L	25 mmHg
Laboratory data		
WBC	4.5×10^9/L	$4-10 \times 10^9$/L
Neutrophil	73%	50–60%
Hemoglobin	7.2 g/dl	12–14 g/dl
Hematocrit	22.83%	35–45%
Platelets	133×10^9/L	$130-450 \times 10^9$/L
Sodium	140 mEq/L	135–145 mEq/L
Potassium	4.5 mEq/L	3.6–5 mEq/L
Chloride	96 mEq/L	98–110 mEq/L
CO2	19 mEq/L	25 mEq/L
BUN	17 mg/dL	25 mg/dL
Creatinine	0.96 mg/dL	1.0 mg/dL
Anion gap	15 mEq/L	10–12 mEq/L
Lactic acid	4.4 mmol/L	<2.0 mmol/L
Troponin	4.2 ng/mL	<0.03 ng/mL
Calcium	6.6 mg/dL	8 mg/dL
Ionized calcium	<1.0 mmol/L	1.1 mmol/L
AST	372 U/L	45 U/L
ALT	214 U/L	40 U/L
ALP	156 U/L	100 U/L
T. bilirubin	1.0 mg/dL	1.0 mg/dL
CPK	203 IU/L	50 IU/L

ABG: arterial blood gas.

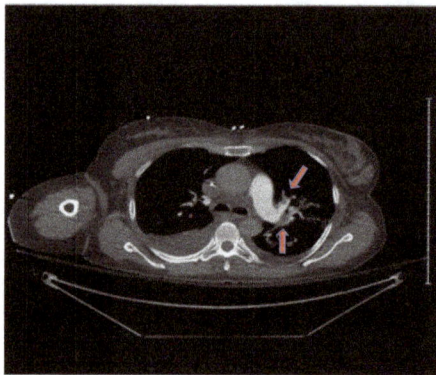

FIGURE 3: CT angiogram showing pulmonary embolism (arrow).

3. Discussion

Pulmonary embolism is the third most frequent cardiovascular disease in the United States (US) and has an extremely high morbidity and mortality [1–3]. Massive pulmonary embolism can cause cardiac arrest in 41% of cases and this is the major predictor of PE related mortality, which ranges from 65% to 95% [4, 5]. Pulmonary embolism is responsible for 2% to 15% of unexpected sudden deaths [4, 5], 2% of all cardiac arrests (CA) cases, and 6.5% of CA cases of extracardiac origin [5]. Moreover, in clinical setting, pulmonary embolism is often not suspected and is underestimated as a cause of acute cardiopulmonary collapse [18, 19].

Massive PE causes sudden increase in pulmonary vascular resistance (PVR) and mean pulmonary arterial pressure (mPAP) which is proportional to degree of obstruction in patients without preexisting pulmonary vascular disease [1]. It leads to increased RV wall tension and RV failure [20]. Eventually it leads to obstructive cardiogenic shock due to decrease in LV preload [21]. Presence of RV hypokinesis in patients with acute PE is associated with significantly increased mortality and a 14% risk for having a recurrent PE

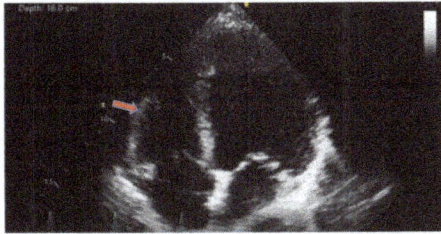

(a) Transthoracic echocardiogram after 3 months, showing interval normalization of RV size (arrow) and function and normalization of the right ventricular systolic pressure with an estimate of 19 mmHg

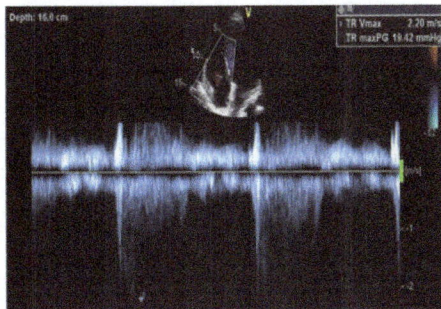

(b) Transthoracic echocardiogram after 3 months, showing interval normalization of RV size (arrow) and function and normalization of the right ventricular systolic pressure with an estimate of 19 mmHg

FIGURE 4

[2, 22, 23]. Massive PE can cause acute myocardial infarction (AMI) [24]. Massive PE can also lead to various types of cardiac arrhythmias including PEA, asystole, and ventricular fibrillation [25–30].

Traditional ACLS and CPR have been the common practice for PE related cardiac arrest [31, 32]. Vasopressor support and anticoagulation are used as well. However, only heparinization will not affect the clot burden and hemodynamic insult acutely. Systemic thrombolytic agents can minimize clot burden by clot lysis and can decrease the risk of recurrent Pes, and therefore long term pulmonary hypertension [33]. However, majority of benefit from thrombolytic therapy in patients with pulmonary embolism is limited to hemodynamic compromise [34], and fibrinolytics are not recommended in normotensive patients [35]. Catheter guided clot lysis can be considered in case of contraindication to systemic thrombolysis. Surgical embolectomy is reserved for unstable patients who have failed maximal medical treatment or in case of contraindication to thrombolytics [36].

Unfortunately, there are no strong prospective studies to show a survival benefit for the use of fibrinolytic drugs in cardiac arrest due to massive PE. Two available randomized control trials have failed to show a statistically significant outcome [37, 38]. However, these studies had various limitations such as late administration of thrombolytics and small sample size. Overall, in clinical practice, systemic thrombolytic therapy is less frequently used for a multitude of reasons; they include (a) limited evidence, (b) risk of bleeding with high dose of thrombolytics [39], (c) especially

having ongoing CPR [40], and (d) lack of specific guidelines regarding thrombolytic dosing and timing.

Thrombolytic therapy also carries 9–22% risk of major bleeding, including a 1–5% risk of intracranial hemorrhage [2, 33, 40–42]. A nonrandomized study suggested a relative contraindication to thrombolytic use for CPR duration > 10 minutes. This study analyzed use of thrombolytics in cardiac arrest due to AMI and concluded that thrombolysis could safely be applied to patients who undergo a CPR of <10 min. They did not include patients with CPR > 10 mins in their study [37]. Janata et al. in their study showed that CPR duration of >10 min did not have any impact on major bleeding complications in patients receiving thrombolytic therapy [6].

There have been numerous cases reported in American and European literature, where thrombolysis (various formulations and regimens) was used in confirmed PE or clinically suggestive history of PE related cardiac arrest cases. Thrombolytic therapy has showed very favorable outcomes even when administered late during the CPR and as slow infusions after a prolonged CPR [6–11, 24–26]. Even though the available evidence for the utility of thrombolytics in such instances is of low quality, but due to the extremely high mortality of PE related cardiac arrest and frequently reported success with thrombolytics, its use is being advocated in recent resuscitation guidelines [12–17].

Unfortunately, there is no consensus regarding the dosage and timing of thrombolytics during resuscitation. The American Heart Association (AHA) recommends a two-hour infusion of 100 mg of alteplase in those with hemodynamic compromise. However, they do not clearly address the issue of cardiac arrest [15]. The European Resuscitation Council (ERC) and European Society of Cardiology (ESC) recommend a dose of 100 mg alteplase over 2 hours or 0.6 mg/kg over 15 minutes, though again they do not specifically address the approach in cardiac arrest [12]. The British Thoracic Society in 2003 recommended a 50 mg bolus of IV alteplase, which is the regimen most frequently used in recent published literature [10, 14, 16, 17].

However, there is no existing consensus or established guidance for subsequent approach. Surgical embolectomy or catheter guided interventions can be considered for unstable patients or those who have failed maximal medical treatment [34, 36]. Fengler and Brady in their review suggested administering a second bolus of alteplase [43].

We used focused bedside echocardiogram in our patient, as she was hemodynamically unstable and was experiencing recurrent cardiac arrest. Based on our echocardiogram findings of persistent RV dysfunction and dilatation with persistent hemodynamic compromise, we administered second bolus of t-PA with excellent outcome. This emphasizes the potential implacability of echocardiography for decision-making in such situations.

Echocardiography has limited sensitivity and specificity for the diagnosis of acute PE [44]. However, transthoracic echocardiography can be helpful to identify acute PE related right ventricular dysfunction [45]. Echocardiographic findings of RV strain include dilation of RV, flattened interventricular septum (D-sign of interventricular septal shift), and the classic sign of RV apical wall hypercontractility with hypokinesis of the RV free wall and base termed as "McConnell" sign [45–47]. McConnell sign is only 77% sensitive but has a specificity of 94% for acute PE, as RV failure due to chronic pulmonary hypertension typically shows global hypokinesis [47].

Presence of RV strain has more than twofold increase in risk of early mortality compared with patients with no signs of RV strain [34]. Use of echocardiography in diagnosis and management of hemodynamically unstable patients have also been recommended by the ESC [48]. A recent study showed that the average time from beginning of CPR to get a suitable echo image was 3.9 minutes (17 seconds to 10 minutes) [49].

We used focused echocardiography to guide repeat alteplase bolus administration, as our patient remained hemodynamically unstable, despite successful ROSC after initial alteplase bolus. Fortunately, despite prolonged CPR, our patient had an excellent outcome with no cardiac or neurologic sequela. At three months' follow-up, the patient had complete normalization of right RV function without any residual pulmonary hypertension (Figures 4(a) and 4(b) and videos 4, 5).

4. Conclusion

Recent resuscitation guidelines recommend using thrombolytic therapy during resuscitation in cases of CA due to massive PE [1, 15–19]. Most consistently applied approach is 50 mg intravenous alteplase early during CPR. There is no existing consensus on subsequent approach. We present a case of double bolus alteplase guided by focused bedside echocardiography. Echocardiographic evidence of persistent RV dysfunction and dilatation in the setting of persistent hemodynamic instability, recurrent arrest, or even failure to achieve ROSC with initial bolus may warrant the administration of second bolus of alteplase. Future well-designed trials are needed to establish guidelines for thrombolytic therapy in CA to maximize safety and efficacy.

Acknowledgments

The authors want to thank Mokshya Sharma M.D., Charles D. Graham M.D., Ahmed Waseem M.D., and Asad Javed M.D. for their help in preparation and review of this manuscript. They would also like to thank Troy Wiedenbeck M.D. and Dirk Vandergon M.D. for their help in reviewing echocardiographic material. They would also like to acknowledge permission of patient to publish this case.

References

[1] C. Gerges, N. Skoro-Sajer, and I. M. Lang, "Right ventricle in acute and chronic pulmonary embolism (2013 grover conference series)," *Pulmonary Circulation*, vol. 4, no. 3, pp. 378–386, 2014.

[2] S. Z. Goldhaber, L. Visani, and M. de Rosa, "Acute pulmonary embolism: clinical outcomes in the International Cooperative Pulmonary Embolism Registry (ICOPER)," *The Lancet*, vol. 353, no. 9162, pp. 1386–1389, 1999.

[3] C. Bergamo, "Thrombolysis for pulmonary embolism and risk of all-cause mortality, major bleeding, and intracranial hemorrhage: A meta-analysis: Chatterjee S, Chakraborty A, Weinberg A, et al. JAMA 2014;311(23):2414-21.," *The Journal of Emergency Medicine*, vol. 47, no. 5, p. 618, 2014.

[4] M. Gallerani, R. Manfredini, L. Ricci et al., "Sudden death from pulmonary thromboembolism: Chronobiological aspects," *European Heart Journal*, vol. 13, no. 5, pp. 661–665, 1992.

[5] M. Kuisma and A. Alaspaa, "Out-of-hospital cardiac arrests of non-cardiac origin. Epidemiology and outcome," *European Heart Journal*, vol. 18, no. 7, pp. 1122–1128, 1997.

[6] K. Janata, M. Holzer, I. Kürkciyan et al., "Major bleeding complications in cardiopulmonary resuscitation: the place of thrombolytic therapy in cardiac arrest due to massive pulmonary embolism," *Resuscitation*, vol. 57, no. 1, pp. 49–55, 2003.

[7] T. Zhu, K. Pan, and Y. Wang, "Successful resuscitation with thrombolysis of pulmonary embolism due to thrombotic thrombocytopenic purpura during cardiac arrest," *The American Journal of Emergency Medicine*, vol. 33, no. 1, pp. 132–132.e4, 2015.

[8] T. Hsin, F. W. Chun, and H. L. Tao, "Ultra-long cardiopulmonary resuscitation with thrombolytic therapy for a sudden cardiac arrest patient with pulmonary embolism," *The American Journal of Emergency Medicine*, vol. 32, no. 11, pp. 1443.e3–1443.e4, 2014.

[9] R. Gupta, A. Jindal, and H. Cranston-D'Amato, "Benefits of thrombolytics in prolonged cardiac arrest and hypothermia over its bleeding risk," *International Journal of Critical Illness & Injury Science*, vol. 4, no. 1, p. 88, 2014.

[10] Q. Yin, X. Li, and C. Li, "Thrombolysis after initially unsuccessful cardiopulmonary resuscitation in presumed pulmonary embolism," *The American Journal of Emergency Medicine*, vol. 33, no. 1, pp. 132.e1–132.e2, 2015.

[11] M. Sharifi, Z. Vajo, S. Javadpoor et al., "Pulseless electrical activity in pulmonary embolism treated with thrombolysis (from the "PEAPETT" study)," *The American Journal of Emergency Medicine*, vol. 34, no. 10, pp. 1963–1967, 2016.

[12] S. V. Konstantinides, A. Torbicki, and G. Agnelli, "2014 ESC Guidelines on the diagnosis and management of acute pulmonary embolism: The Task Force for the Diagnosis and Management of Acute Pulmonary Embolism of the European Society of Cardiology (ESC)Endorsed by the European Respiratory Society (ERS)," *European Heart Journal*, vol. 35, no. 43, pp. 3033–3073, 2014.

[13] J. Soar, G. D. Perkins, G. Abbas et al., "European Resuscitation Council guidelines for resuscitation 2010 section 8. Cardiac arrest in special circumstances: electrolyte abnormalities, poisoning, drowning, accidental hypothermia, hyperthermia, asthma, anaphylaxis, cardiac surgery, trauma, pregnancy, electrocution," *Resuscitation*, vol. 81, no. 10, pp. 1400–1433, 2010.

[14] E. J. Lavonas, I. R. Drennan, A. Gabrielli et al., "Part 10: special circumstances of resuscitation: 2015 American Heart Association guidelines update for cardiopulmonary resuscitation and emergency cardiovascular care," *Circulation*, vol. 132, no. 18, supplement 2, pp. S501–S518, 2015.

[15] M. R. Jaff, M. S. McMurtry, S. L. Archer et al., "Management of massive and submassive pulmonary embolism, iliofemoral deep vein thrombosis, and chronic thromboembolic pulmonary hypertension: a scientific statement from the american heart association," *Circulation*, vol. 123, no. 16, pp. 1788–1830, 2011.

[16] British Thoracic Society Standards of Care Committee Pulmonary Embolism Guideline Development Group, "British Thoracic Society guidelines for the management of suspected acute pulmonary embolism," *Thorax*, vol. 58, no. 6, pp. 470–483, 2003.

[17] G. O'Connor, G. Fitzpatrick, A. El-Gammal, and P. Gilligan, "Double Bolus Thrombolysis for Suspected Massive Pulmonary Embolism during Cardiac Arrest," *Case Reports in Emergency Medicine*, vol. 2015, Article ID 367295, 5 pages, 2015.

[18] P. D. Stein, "Silent pulmonary embolism," *JAMA Internal Medicine*, vol. 160, no. 2, pp. 145-146, 2000.

[19] W. Bougouin, E. Marijon, B. Planquette et al., "Factors Associated with Pulmonary Embolism-Related Sudden Cardiac Arrest," *Circulation*, vol. 134, no. 25, pp. 2125–2127, 2016.

[20] P. Pruszczyk, A. Bochowicz, A. Torbicki et al., "Cardiac troponin T monitoring identifies high-risk group of normotensive patients with acute pulmonary embolism," *CHEST*, vol. 123, no. 6, pp. 1947–1952, 2003.

[21] J. C. Lualdi and S. Z. Goldhaber, "Right ventricular dysfunction after acute pulmonary embolism: Pathophysiologic factors, detection, and therapeutic implications," *American Heart Journal*, vol. 130, no. 6, pp. 1276–1282, 1995.

[22] J. S. Alpert, R. Smith, C. J. Carlson, I. S. Ockene, L. Dexter, and J. E. Dalen, "Mortality in Patients Treated for Pulmonary Embolism," *Journal of the American Medical Association*, vol. 236, no. 13, pp. 1477–1480, 1976.

[23] R. L. Miller, S. Das, T. Anandarangam et al., "Association between right ventricular function and perfusion abnormalities in hemodynamically stable patients with acute pulmonary embolism," *CHEST*, vol. 113, no. 3, pp. 665–670, 1998.

[24] C. Toprak, A. Avci, B. Ozturkeri, M. M. Tabakci, and G. Kahveci, "PE with ST-segment elevation in leads V1 -3 and AVR treated successfully by catheter directed high-dose bolus thrombolytic therapy during CPR," *The American Journal of Emergency Medicine*, vol. 32, no. 12, pp. 1557–1557.e3, 2014.

[25] M. Marzegalli, P. Rietti, M. A. Chirico et al., "Heart arrest in acute pulmonary embolism: An anatomo-clinical study," *Giornale Italiano Di Cardiologia*, vol. 24, pp. 21–26, 1994.

[26] I. Kürkciyan, G. Meron, F. Sterz et al., "Pulmonary embolism as a cause of cardiac arrest: presentation and outcome," *JAMA Internal Medicine*, vol. 160, no. 10, pp. 1529–1535, 2000.

[27] C. Deasy, J. E. Bray, K. Smith, L. R. Harriss, S. A. Bernard, and P. Cameron, "Out-of-hospital cardiac arrests in young adults in Melbourne, Australia-Adding coronial data to a cardiac arrest registry," *Resuscitation*, vol. 82, no. 10, pp. 1302–1306, 2011.

[28] O. C. Akinboboye, E. J. Brown Jr., R. Queirroz et al., "Recurrent pulmonary embolism with second-degree atrioventricular block and near syncope," *American Heart Journal*, vol. 126, no. 3, pp. 730–732, 1993.

[29] P. Koutkia and T. J. Wachtel, "Pulmonary embolism presenting as syncope: Case report and review of the literature," *Heart & Lung: The Journal of Acute and Critical Care*, vol. 28, no. 5, pp. 342–347, 1999.

[30] E. P. Hess, R. L. Campbell, and R. D. White, "Epidemiology, trends, and outcome of out-of-hospital cardiac arrest of noncardiac origin," *Resuscitation*, vol. 72, no. 2, pp. 200–206, 2007.

[31] P. D. Stein and F. Matta, "Thrombolytic therapy in unstable patients with acute pulmonary embolism: Saves lives but underused," *American Journal of Medicine*, vol. 125, no. 5, pp. 465–470, 2012.

[32] B. W. Lin, D. H. Schreiber, G. Liu et al., "Therapy and outcomes in massive pulmonary embolism from the Emergency Medicine Pulmonary Embolism in the Real World Registry," *The American Journal of Emergency Medicine*, vol. 30, no. 9, pp. 1774–1781, 2012.

[33] S. M. Arcasoy and J. W. Kreit, "Thrombolytic therapy of pulmonary embolism: A comprehensive review of current evidence," *CHEST*, vol. 115, no. 6, pp. 1695–1707, 1999.

[34] M. Ten Wolde, M. Söhne, E. Quak, M. R. Mac Gillavry, and H. R. Büller, "Prognostic value of echocardiographically assessed right ventricular dysfunction in patients with pulmonary embolism," *JAMA Internal Medicine*, vol. 164, no. 15, pp. 1685–1689, 2004.

[35] S. Konstantinides, A. Geibel, M. Olschewski et al., "Association between thrombolytic treatment and the prognosis of hemodynamically stable patients with major pulmonary embolism: Results of a multicenter registry," *Circulation*, vol. 96, no. 3, pp. 882–888, 1997.

[36] C. Schmid, S. Zietlow, T. O. F. Wagner, J. Laas, and H. G. Borst, "Fulminant pulmonary embolism: Symptoms, diagnostics, operative technique, and results," *The Annals of Thoracic Surgery*, vol. 52, no. 5, pp. 1102–1107, 1991.

[37] B. W. Böttige, H. Böhrer, A. Bach, J. Motsch, and E. Martin, "Bolus injection of thrombolytic agents during cardiopulmonary resuscitation for massive pulmonary embolism," *Resuscitation*, vol. 28, pp. 45–54, 1994.

[38] R. B. Abu-Laban, J. Christenson, G. D. Innes et al., "Tissue plasminogen activator in cardiac arrest with pulseless electrical activity," *The New England Journal of Medicine*, vol. 346, pp. 1522–1528, 2002.

[39] U. Klinge, B. Klosterhalfen, C. Tons et al., "A bleeding complication as a consequence of bolus lysis after resuscitation," in *Deutsche Medizinische Wochenschrift*, vol. 116, pp. 1293-1294, 1991.

[40] A. N. Tenaglia, R. M. Califf, R. J. Candela et al., "Thrombolytic therapy in patients requiring cardiopulmonary resuscitation," *American Journal of Cardiology*, vol. 68, no. 10, pp. 1015–1019, 1991.

[41] J.-L. Diehl, G. Meyer, J. Igual et al., "Effectiveness and safety of bolus administration of alteplase in massive pulmonary embolism," *American Journal of Cardiology*, vol. 70, no. 18, pp. 1477–1480, 1992.

[42] E. Hamel, G. Pacouret, D. Vincentelli et al., "Thrombolysis or heparin therapy in massive pulmonary embolism with right ventricular dilation: Results from a 128-patient monocenter registry," *CHEST*, vol. 120, no. 1, pp. 120–125, 2001.

[43] B. T. Fengler and W. J. Brady, "Fibrinolytic therapy in pulmonary embolism: an evidence-based treatment algorithm," *The American Journal of Emergency Medicine*, vol. 27, no. 1, pp. 84–95, 2009.

[44] M. Miniati, S. Monti, L. Pratali et al., "Value of transthoracic echocardiography in the diagnosis of pulmonary embolism: results of a prospective study in unselected patients," *American Journal of Medicine*, vol. 110, no. 7, pp. 528–535, 2001.

[45] P. MacCarthy, A. Worrall, G. McCarthy, and J. Davies, "The use of transthoracic echocardiography to guide thrombolytic therapy during cardiac arrest due to massive pulmonary embolism," *Emergency Medicine Journal*, vol. 19, no. 2, pp. 178-179, 2002.

[46] J. A. Lodato, R. P. Ward, and R. M. Lang, "Echocardiographic predictors of pulmonary embolism in patients referred for helical CT," *Journal of Echocardiography*, vol. 25, no. 6, pp. 584–590, 2008.

[47] M. V. McConnell, S. D. Solomon, M. E. Rayan, P. C. Come, S. Z. Goldhaber, and R. T. Lee, "Regional right ventricular dysfunction detected by echocardiography in acute pulmonary embolism," *American Journal of Cardiology*, vol. 78, no. 4, pp. 469–473, 1996.

[48] S. V. Konstantinides, A. Torbicki, G. Agnelli et al., "Erratum: 2014 ESC Guidelines on the diagnosis and management of acute pulmonary embolism (European Heart Journal (2014) 35 (3033-73) DOI 10.1093/eurheartj/ehu283," *European Heart Journal*, vol. 36, no. 39, p. 2666, 2015.

[49] P. Varriale and J. M. Maldonado, "Echocardiographic observations during inhospital cardiopulmonary resuscitation," *Critical Care Medicine*, vol. 25, no. 10, pp. 1717–1720, 1997.

35

Use of High-Flow Nasal Cannula Oxygen Therapy in a Pregnant Woman with Dermatomyositis-Related Interstitial Pneumonia

Tomohiro Shoji, Takeshi Umegaki, Kota Nishimoto, Natsuki Anada, Akiko Ando, Takeo Uba, Munenori Kusunoki, Kanako Oku, and Takahiko Kamibayashi

Department of Anesthesiology, Kansai Medical University Hospital, Osaka, Japan

Correspondence should be addressed to Takeshi Umegaki; umegakit@hirakata.kmu.ac.jp

Academic Editor: Mabrouk Bahloul

A 33-year-old pregnant woman was referred to our hospital with respiratory distress at 30 weeks of gestation. Chest computed tomography (CT) scans revealed pulmonary infiltrates along the bronchovascular bundles and ground-glass opacities in both lungs. Despite immediate treatment with steroid pulse therapy for suspected interstitial pneumonia, the patient's condition worsened. Respiratory distress was slightly alleviated after the initiation of high-flow nasal cannula (HFNC) oxygen therapy (40 L/min, FiO$_2$ 40%). We suspected clinically amyopathic dermatomyositis (CADM) complicating rapidly progressive refractory interstitial pneumonia. In order to save the life of the patient, the use of combination therapy with immunosuppressants was necessary. The patient underwent emergency cesarean section and was immediately treated with immunosuppressants while continuing HFNC oxygen therapy. The neonate was treated in the neonatal intensive care unit. The patient's condition improved after 7 days of hospitalization; by this time, she was positive for myositis-specific autoantibodies and was diagnosed with interstitial pneumonia preceding dermatomyositis. This condition can be potentially fatal within a few months of onset and therefore requires early combination immunosuppressive therapy. This case demonstrates the usefulness of HFNC oxygen therapy for respiratory management as it negates the need for intubation and allows for various treatments to be quickly performed.

1. Introduction

High-flow nasal cannula (HFNC) oxygen therapy is widely used in the management of acute respiratory failure and also has applications in cases with acute exacerbation of interstitial pneumonia (IP) [1–3]. Although pregnant patients with IP rarely develop concurrent complications of polymyositis (PM) or dermatomyositis (DM), the prompt diagnosis of PM/DM in these patients is critical due to the high risk of potentially fatal outcomes to both the mother and the fetus [4–6]. This case report describes the use of HFNC oxygen therapy without intubation in a 33-year-old pregnant woman who developed progressive IP complicated by DM at 28 weeks of gestation. The patient was successfully treated with combination immunosuppressive therapy.

2. Case Report

A 33-year-old pregnant woman was admitted to our hospital due to respiratory distress at 30 weeks of gestation. The patient had previously undergone three vaginal deliveries. A review of family history revealed that the patient's paternal grandmother had rheumatoid arthritis and the patient's father had unspecified IP. The patient first experienced respiratory distress in her 28th week of gestation; her condition deteriorated two weeks later, and she was transported to our hospital via ambulance. Upon admission, the patient was lucid and afebrile (36.5°C). The respiratory and hemodynamic levels are revealed in Table 1. She had blood pressure of 88/49 mmHg, a heart rate of 86 bpm, a respiratory rate of 18 breaths/minute, and peripheral oxygen saturation (SpO$_2$) on room air of 90%. Fine crackles were noted in both lower lung fields.

Laboratory examination revealed slight elevations in white blood cell count (11,900/μl), serum C-reactive protein concentration (2.65 mg/dl), and aldolase level (7.1 U/l). Serum KL-6 level was highly elevated at 986 U/ml. An arterial blood gas test showed poor oxygenation with arterial oxygen partial pressure (PaO$_2$) on room air of 61.7 mmHg.

TABLE 1: The respiratory and hemodynamic levels from hospital admission to ICU discharge.

Variables	Oxygen therapy	SpO$_2$ (%)	PaO$_2$ (mmHg)	Respiratory rate (min^{-1})	Systolic blood pressure (mmHg)
Hospital admission	Room air	90	61.7	18	88
ICU admission	HFNC 40 L/min, FiO2 0.40	94	64.5	28	111
ICU day 2	HFNC 40 L/min, FiO2 0.40	95	73.5	19	94
ICU day 3	HFNC 40 L/min, FiO2 0.40	95	73.3	17	124
ICU day 4	HFNC 40 L/min, FiO2 0.40	96	89.3	17	122

ICU: intensive care unit; SpO$_2$: oxygen saturation of peripheral artery; PaO$_2$: partial pressure of arterial oxygen; HFNC: high-flow nasal cannula; FiO2: fraction of inspiratory oxygen.

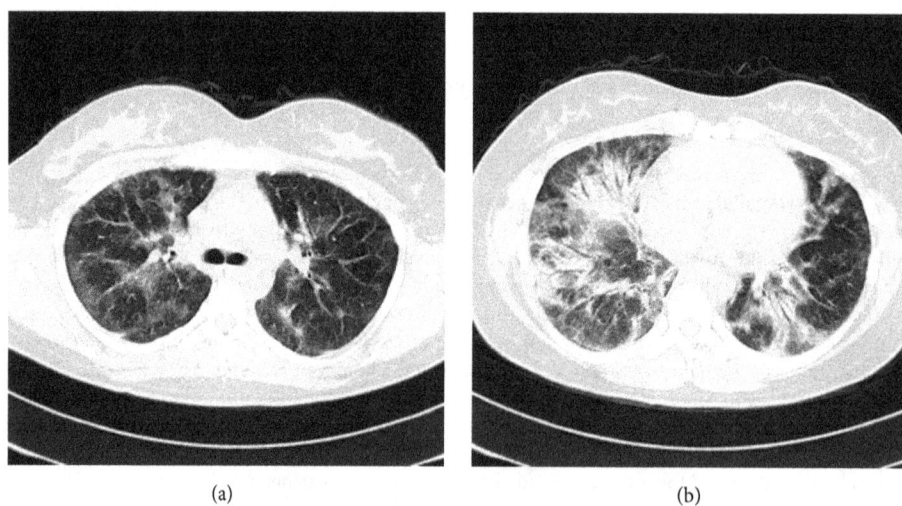

(a)   (b)

FIGURE 1: Chest CT scans showing the patient's middle (a) and lower (b) lung fields upon admission. Bilateral pulmonary infiltrates along the peripheral bronchovascular bundles and ground-glass opacities with a panlobular distribution were observed.

Although the patient had eczema and ulceration on the dorsal surface of both hands on the first day of hospitalization, she did not present with Gottron's sign or muscle weakness, which are characteristic of DM. Chest computed tomography (CT) scans (Figure 1) revealed pulmonary infiltrates along the bronchovascular bundles and panlobular ground-glass opacities in both lungs. N-terminal (NT) pro-B-type natriuretic peptide (BNP) level was at 258.8 pg/ml without renal dysfunction. Cardiac dysfunction was not revealed except for slight dilatation of the left ventricle. The differential diagnosis included idiopathic IP and IP complicated by a collagen disease such as DM. Due to the rapid progression of respiratory distress within a short period of time, the patient was given intravenous methylprednisolone pulse therapy (1 g/day) from the first day of hospitalization. Despite this

treatment, the patient's condition worsened on the second day of hospitalization, and she developed orthopnea (grade V based on the Hugh-Jones classification). As a result, HFNC oxygen therapy was initiated at 30 L/min with a fraction of inspired oxygen (FiO$_2$) of 0.30 according to the instructions of the intensivists and anesthesiologists. However, this did not improve respiratory distress with SpO$_2$ remaining at 90%. HFNC oxygen parameters were increased to 40 L/min with FiO$_2$ at 0.40, and respiratory distress began to improve (SpO$_2$: 92–94%).

Due to the rapid disease progression and resistance to steroid treatment, we suspected IP complicated by PM/DM or clinically amyopathic DM (CADM), which is a form of DM without overt signs of myositis. Accordingly, we deemed it necessary to begin immunosuppressive therapy. At 30 weeks

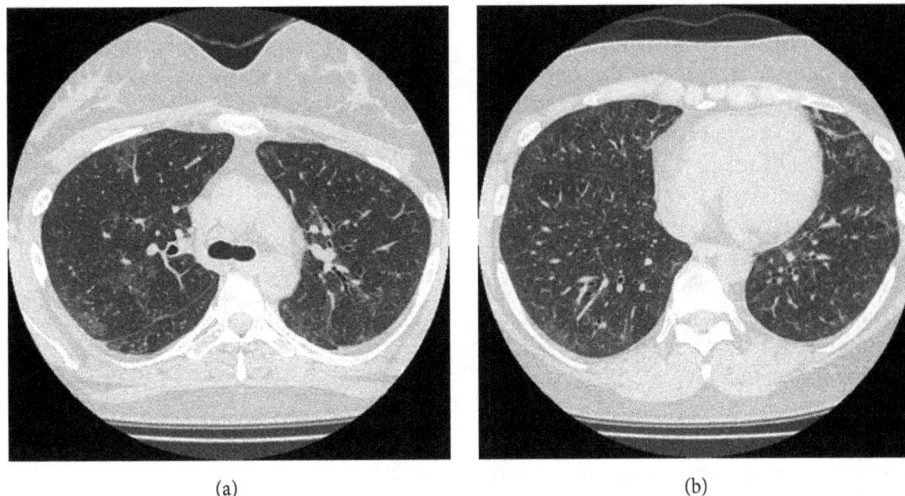

(a)   (b)

FIGURE 2: Chest CT scans showing the patient's middle (a) and lower (b) lung fields after two months from the initiation of treatment. The pulmonary infiltrates had disappeared.

of gestation, the fetal body weight was over 1500 g, and it was determined that the neonate could be treated at the neonatal intensive care unit after delivery. HFNC oxygen therapy was continued, and an emergency cesarean section without use of tocolytics was performed under spinal anesthesia. The neonate weighed 1550 g, and the Apgar scores at one minute and five minutes after birth were 8 and 9, respectively. Tracheal intubation was not required during the procedure. A chest X-ray indicated that the pulmonary infiltrates had spread further. Due to this exacerbation of IP, we began treatment with ciclosporin (0.2 g/day) from the third day of hospitalization. On the following day, we observed newly formed heliotrope rash on both upper eyelids and keratotic rash along the surface of the fingers of both hands. Chest CT scans confirmed that the infiltrates had expanded since the patient was admitted, and cyclophosphamide pulse therapy (1 g/month) was added to the patient's regimen on the fifth day of hospitalization.

With HFNC oxygen therapy (40 L/min, FiO_2: 0.40), respiratory distress was alleviated (SpO_2: 93–96%). Three days after the cesarean section (fifth day of hospitalization), the patient was transferred from the intensive care unit to a general ward. On the seventh day of hospitalization, the results of analysis of a blood sample taken on the day of admission showed that the patient had positive titers for autoantibodies against aminoacyl tRNA synthetase (ARS), including anti-Jo-1 antibodies. Due to the presence of anti-ARS antibodies, we excluded the possibility of CADM. The patient's respiratory condition further improved, and the parameters of HFNC oxygen therapy were reduced to 30 L/min with FiO_2 at 0.30. A chest CT scan taken after 18 days of hospitalization indicated a new case of pneumomediastinum, but the interstitial shadows in the lung field had substantially receded. The patient was discharged after 47 days of hospitalization. Following 2 months of treatment, chest CT scans showed that the pneumomediastinum and the interstitial shadows had disappeared (Figure 2). During

that time, the patient complained of polyarthralgia. Together with the other symptoms of heliotrope rash, elevated aldolase level, elevated C-reactive protein concentration, and positive titers for anti-ARS antibodies, the inclusion of arthralgia fulfilled the diagnostic criteria for DM as stipulated by Japan's Ministry of Health, Labour and Welfare based on Tanimoto et al. [7]. The final diagnosis was IP preceding DM with delayed manifestation of specific cutaneous findings without overt signs of myositis.

3. Discussion

This case provided valuable findings that the use of HFNC oxygen therapy was able to contribute to the alleviation of respiratory distress in rapidly progressive IP. To the best of our knowledge, this report describes the first case of rapidly progressive IP where hypoxia was successfully prevented in both the mother and the fetus without intubation.

It has been reported that the use of HFNC oxygen therapy in acute respiratory failure cases did not result in lower intubation rates relative to oxygen therapy delivered through a face mask and noninvasive positive-pressure ventilation, but it was associated with more ventilator-free days and a higher survival rate [3]. In addition, HFNC oxygen therapy allows for patients to eat, drink, and move around without the need to interrupt treatment [8]. Our case did not require intubation throughout the cesarean section procedure and immunosuppressive therapy, which allowed her to have meals, converse with others, and interact with her child. In addition to alleviating respiratory distress, the use of HFNC oxygen therapy may have reduced the patient's feelings of anxiety and improved her quality of life during hospitalization. This form of respiratory management should therefore be considered for other similar cases in the future.

The association between the prognosis of IP patients with DM and the degree of myositis disease activity has been previously documented, and the early use of immunosuppressants should be employed in cases with rapidly progressive IP [5]. When refractory IP is complicated by PM/DM or CADM, the pulmonary tissue may become irreversibly damaged. As a result, the condition may become resistant to combination immunosuppressive therapy and eventually lead to death after only several months [5, 9, 10]. As our patient's respiratory condition continued to worsen despite immediate steroid pulse therapy, we suspected refractory IP complicated by PM/DM or CADM, and the early use of immunosuppressive therapy was deemed necessary. While the diagnosis of DM was made later, the possibility of refractory IP preceding PM/DM or CADM prompted us to consider the early use of combination immunosuppressive therapy.

It should be noted that the use of immunosuppressants for the treatment of IP does not ensure rapid improvement in patient condition. In a similar case report, a pregnant woman at 16 weeks of gestation had developed IP preceding PM and was treated with a combination of steroid pulse therapy and tacrolimus [11]. Due to that patient's worsening respiratory condition, the pregnancy was terminated in the 21st week of gestation to save the mother. Cyclophosphamide pulse therapy was subsequently added to the treatment regimen, and the patient began to show signs of improvement. Cases of IP complicated by PM/DM or CADM in pregnant women are extremely rare. Therefore, it remains unclear if the use of combination immunosuppressive therapy (including cyclophosphamide) would produce quick therapeutic effects in cases without termination of pregnancy.

Cardiac involvement has been reported in patients with DM, and the incidence has reached as high as 45.7% [12]. Moreover, interstitial pneumonia has been reported as one of the major predictive factors of cardiac dysfunction in patients with DM [12]. Left ventricular diastolic dysfunction is an early feature of cardiac involvement in patients with PM/DM [13], and cardiac involvement is a common cause of death [14]. This case has not clinically revealed cardiac dysfunction, but diastolic dysfunction might have potentially progressed because of elevation of NT-pro BNP, slight dilatation of the left ventricle, and alveolar syndrome with air bronchogram on the CT chest. HFNC might have suitably applied positive end expiratory pressure [15]. HFNC oxygen therapy was seamlessly provided without interruption throughout the patient's treatment in the intensive care unit, the operating theater, and the general ward and during transfers between these units. As the pregnancy had progressed to the point where the baby could be treated in the neonatal intensive care unit after delivery, the nonuse of intubation allowed the patient to be quickly transitioned from the cesarean section to immunosuppressive therapy. This way, we were able to save both the mother and the child.

4. Conclusions

This case report describes the successful use of HFNC oxygen therapy for respiratory management in a pregnant patient who developed rapidly progressive IP complicated by DM. Both the mother and the child were saved. It is necessary to quickly treat such cases with a combination of steroid pulse

therapy and immunosuppressants. HFNC oxygen therapy is a useful respiratory management method that negates the need for intubation and allows for greater freedom of treatment and patient comfort.

References

[1] Y. Horio, T. Takihara, K. Niimi et al., "High-flow nasal cannula oxygen therapy for acute exacerbation of interstitial pneumonia: A case series," *Respiratory Investigation*, vol. 54, no. 2, pp. 125–129, 2016.

[2] H. Y. Lee, C. K. Rhee, and J. W. Lee, "Feasibility of high-flow nasal cannula oxygen therapy for acute respiratory failure in patients with hematologic malignancies: A retrospective single-center study," *Journal of Critical Care*, vol. 30, no. 4, pp. 773–777, 2015.

[3] J. P. Frat, A. W. Thille, A. Mercat et al., "High-flowoxygen-through nasal cannula inacutehypoxemicrespiratory failure," *New England Journal of Medicine*, vol. 372, no. 23, pp. 2185–2196, 2015.

[4] B. A. Rosenzweig, S. Rotmensch, S. P. Binette, and M. Phillippe, "Primary idiopathic polymyositis and dermatomyositis complicating pregnancy: diagnosis and management," *Obstetrical & Gynecological Survey*, vol. 44, no. 3, pp. 162–170, 1989.

[5] Y. Nawata, K. Kurasawa, K. Takabayashi et al., "Corticosteroid resistant interstitial pneumonitis in dermatomyositis/polymyositis: Prediction and treatment with cyclosporine," *The Journal of Rheumatology*, vol. 26, no. 7, pp. 1527–1533, 1999.

[6] M. Fathi and I. E. Lundberg, "Interstitial lung disease in polymyositis and dermatomyositis," *Current Opinion in Rheumatology*, vol. 17, no. 6, pp. 701–706, 2005.

[7] K. Tanimoto, K. Nakano, S. Kano et al., "Classification criteria for polymyositis and Dermatomyositis," *The Journal of Rheumatology*, vol. 22, no. 4, pp. 668–674, 1995.

[8] J. R. Masclans, P. Pérez-Terán, and O. Roca, "The role of high flow oxygen therapy in acute respiratory failure," *Medicina Intensiva*, vol. 39, no. 8, pp. 505–515, 2015.

[9] P. Gerami, J. M. Schope, L. McDonald, H. W. Walling, and R. D. Sontheimer, "A systematic review of adult-onset clinically amyopathic dermatomyositis (dermatomyositis siné myositis): a missing link within the spectrum of the idiopathic inflammatory myopathies," *Journal of the American Academy of Dermatology*, vol. 54, no. 4, pp. 597–613, 2006.

[10] R. D. Sontheimer and S. Miyagawa, "Potentially fatal interstitial lung disease can occur in clinically amyopathic dermatomyositis," *Journal of the American Academy of Dermatology*, vol. 48, no. 5, pp. 797-798, 2003.

[11] R. Okad, Y.-S. Miyabe, S. Kasai et al., "Successful treatment of interstitial pneumonia and pneumomediastinum associated with polymyositis during pregnancy with a combination of cyclophosphamide and tacrolimus: A case report," *Japanese Journal of Clinical Immunology*, vol. 33, no. 3, pp. 142–148, 2010.

[12] C. Zuo, X. D. Wei, Y. L. Ye et al., "Risk factors associated with cardiac involvement in patients with dermatomyositis/polymyositis," *Sichuan DaXueXueBao YiXue Ban*, vol. 44, no. 5, pp. 801–804, 2013.

[13] Z. Lu, Q. Wei, Z. Ning, Z. Qian-Zi, S. Xiao-Ming, and W. Guo-Chun, "Left ventricular diastolic dysfunction - early cardiac impairment in patients with polymyositis/dermatomyositis: a tissue doppler imaging study," *The Journal of Rheumatology*, vol. 40, no. 9, pp. 1572–1577, 2013.

[14] Z. Lu, W. Guo-Chun, M. Li, and Z. Ning, "Cardiac involvement in adult polymyositis or dermatomyositis: a systematic review," *Clinical Cardiology*, vol. 35, no. 11, pp. 686–691, 2012.

[15] A. Corley, L. R. Caruana, A. G. Barnett, O. Tronstad, and J. F. Fraser, "Oxygen delivery through high-flow nasal cannulae increase end-expiratory lung volume and reduce respiratory rate in post-cardiac surgical patients," *British Journal of Anaesthesia*, vol. 107, no. 6, pp. 998–1004, 2011.

36

A Rare Case of Persistent Lactic Acidosis in the ICU: Glycogenic Hepatopathy and Mauriac Syndrome

Kirsten S. Deemer[1] and George F. Alvarez[2]

[1]Department of Critical Care Medicine, South Health Campus ICU, 4448 Front Street SE, Calgary, AB, Canada T3M 1M4
[2]Department of Critical Care Medicine, University of Calgary, AB, Canada

Correspondence should be addressed to Kirsten S. Deemer; kirsten.deemer@ahs.ca

Academic Editor: Gerhard Pichler

Mauriac syndrome is a rare disorder that can present with the single feature of glycogenic hepatopathy in children and adults with poorly controlled diabetes mellitus. An often underrecognized finding of glycogenic hepatopathy is lactic acidosis and hyperlactatemia. Primary treatment of glycogenic hepatopathy is improved long-term blood glucose control. Resolution of symptoms and hepatomegaly will occur with improvement in hemoglobin A1C. We present here a case of a young adult female presenting to the intensive care unit with Mauriac syndrome. This case demonstrates *exacerbation* of lactic acidosis in a patient with glycogenic hepatopathy treated for diabetic ketoacidosis with high dose insulin and dextrose.

1. Introduction

Lactic acidosis is a common finding in critically ill patients admitted to the intensive care unit (ICU) and it is associated with increased mortality [1, 2]. An anion gap and pH of less than 7.35 are not required for a definition of lactic acidosis as additional causes for anion gap and metabolic alkalosis often exist [3]. Seventy percent of lactate metabolism to glucose takes place in the liver via gluconeogenesis. Anaerobic glycolysis generates pyruvate, NADA, and H+, which is converted into lactate. When lactate production rises and exceeds that of consumption, hyperlactatemia and lactic acidosis result [3].

The most common cause of lactic acidosis in the ICU is type A. Currently there is debate among researchers surrounding the pathogenesis of some forms of type A lactic acidosis and whether it is attributed to tissue hypoxia and anaerobic glycolysis or simply an adrenergic response during stress and increased aerobic glycolysis [4]. Nevertheless, it is often found in disease states such as cardiogenic and hypovolemic shock, sepsis, trauma, and severe hypoxemia [1, 3].

Type B lactic acidosis is less commonly seen in critically ill patients and occurs without evidence of tissue hypoperfusion or shock [3, 5]. Several etiologies of type B lactic acidosis have been described, such as drug metabolites, toxins, congenital enzyme deficiencies, grand Mal seizures, liver failure, hematologic malignancies, renal disease, ethanol intoxication, thiamine deficiency, and diabetes mellitus (DM) [1–3, 5].

The correlation between DM and lactic acidosis is previously described in diabetic ketoacidosis (DKA); however, it can also be seen in clinically well patients with diabetes and glycogenic hepatopathy [6]. This paper will describe a case of persistent lactic acidosis in a young adult female with poorly controlled diabetes and hepatomegaly.

2. Case Presentation

An 18-year-old female with a history of type 1 DM diagnosed at the age of 6 presented to the ER with complaints of nausea, vomiting, and diarrhea. Her blood glucose was 22 mmol/L with an anion gap of 25 and lactate of 2.1 mmol/L. Urine tested positive for ketones. She complained of three days of upper respiratory tract infection symptoms and stated that she had high blood sugars for days but did not take enough insulin and omitted a dose with her last meal. She had two

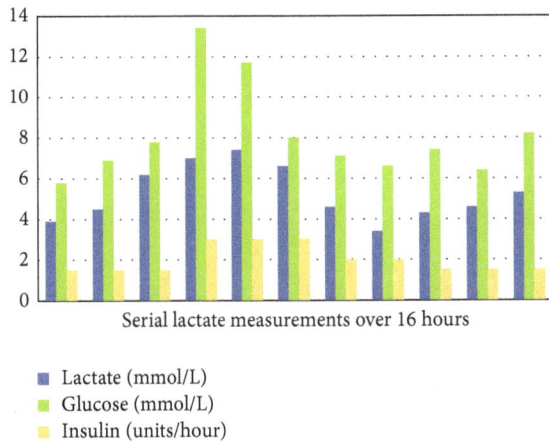

FIGURE 1: Persistent lactic acidosis with dextrose and insulin therapy in an 18-year-old female patient with hepatomegaly.

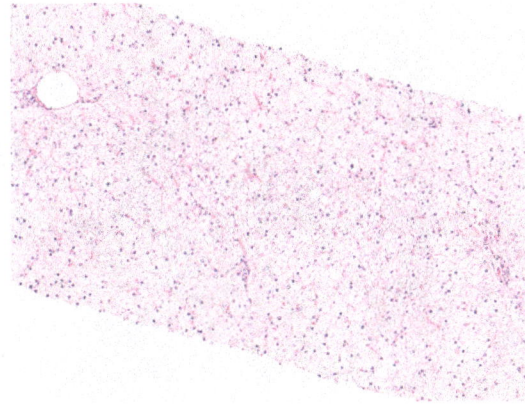

FIGURE 2: Liver Biopsy. Diffusely pale and swollen hepatocytes with numerous glycogenated nuclei. There is no architectural distortion, significant inflammation, or large droplet steatosis.

prior admissions to hospital with DKA and was noted to have chronically suboptimal glucose control (hemoglobin A1C 11.3%). The patient was afebrile and blood and urine cultures were negative for bacteria.

After one day in hospital with insulin and dextrose infusions, the anion gap closed and the patient was converted to subcutaneous insulin. However, the following day, plasma lactate levels were noted to be 3.9 mmol/L with an elevated anion gap. Insulin and dextrose infusions were restarted due to concerns of recurrent DKA. Due to persistent lactic acidosis and labor-intensive DKA management, the patient was moved to the ICU.

Upon examination, the patient looked well. She was hemodynamically stable and afebrile and had no respiratory distress. She had no signs or symptoms of shock. Abdomen on palpation was soft, nondistended, and nontender. Liver was palpated at 8 cm below the costal margin with no palpable splenomegaly. Blood glucose was 5.8 mmol/L with an insulin infusion at 3 units/hour and 5% dextrose infusion at 100 mL/hour. Serum total bilirubin was 2 umol/L, ALT 36 U/L, alkaline phosphate was 120 U/L, and lipase was 12 U/L. Abdominal ultrasound revealed a liver span of 27 cm with hepatosteatosis and mild splenomegaly.

Serial measurements of arterial blood gases revealed persistent lactic acidosis and anion gap despite insulin and dextrose infusions (Figure 1).

The patient was transitioned from insulin infusion to subcutaneous insulin the following day. Her blood sugars stabilized in the range of 6–9 mmol/L and her last measured lactate was 5.3 mmol/L. She was discharged home with an endocrinologist referral for a suspected diagnosis of glycogenic hepatopathy and Mauriac syndrome.

Subsequently, the patient underwent a chronic liver disease screen. Alpha-1 antitrypsin, ceruloplasmin, iron studies, viral hepatitis, celiac and immunological testing were normal. A FibroScan showed no evidence of hepatic fibrosis. After discharge, an abdominal ultrasound again revealed hepatomegaly with liver span of 24 cm. Mitochondrial disorder and respiratory chain defects were ruled out. A liver biopsy revealed numerous hepatocytes with glycogenated nuclei, abundant cytoplasmic and nuclear glycogen deposits, and no large droplet steatosis (Figure 2). Periodic Acid-Schiff (PAS) stain was positive for glycogen accumulation (Figure 3(a)), which was abolished with diastase pretreatment (Figure 3(b)). Therefore, a diagnosis of Mauriac syndrome was given with the only manifestation being that of glycogenic hepatopathy with lactic acidosis. The patient was referred to a diabetes management clinic for further optimization of blood glucose. Lactate level six months following discharge was 4.9 mmol/L.

3. Discussion

First described in 1930, Mauriac syndrome is typically diagnosed in young patients with poorly controlled type 1 DM with growth retardation, delayed puberty, cushingoid features, hypercholesterolemia, and hepatomegaly [7, 8]. However, the single presenting feature of Mauriac syndrome can be glycogenic hepatopathy in both adults and children [6].

Glycogenic hepatopathy is an underrecognized and uncommon complication of poorly controlled DM type 1 manifested by hepatomegaly, abdominal pain, nausea and vomiting, elevated serum transaminases, and elevated plasma lactate levels [9, 10].

3.1. Pathophysiology of Glycogenic Hepatopathy. Glucose is transported into hepatocytes without the aid of insulin. In Mauriac syndrome, hepatic glycogen deposition is achieved during hyperglycemia. Large amounts of insulin drive glycogen synthesis and decrease gluconeogenesis and glycogenolysis. Further insulin administration and hyperglycemia facilitate further glycogen synthesis, which creates congested hepatocytes resulting in storage overload [10, 11].

Subsequent episodes of DKA and hyperglycemia only compound the problem. Inherent in the treatment of DKA are high amounts of insulin and dextrose, which promotes

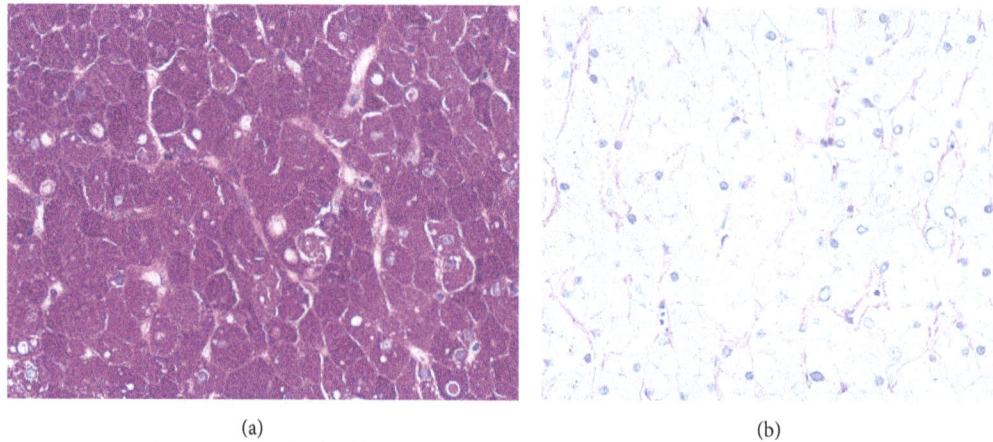

(a)   (b)

FIGURE 3: (a) Liver Biopsy. Periodic Acid-Schiff stain-positive for glycogen accumulation. (b) Glycogen abolishes after pretreatment with diastase.

glycogen synthesis within hepatocytes. The resultant manifestation is hepatomegaly and sometimes elevated transaminases but preserved synthetic liver function in patients with poor glucose control and a history of DKA admissions [8, 10].

A poorly recognized consequence of glycogenic hepatopathy is lactic acidosis. Fitzpatrick et al. described half of all pediatric study participants with hepatopathy of Mauriac syndrome having elevated lactate levels despite no signs of illness or DKA [7]. Elevation of lactate in chronic liver diseases, such as cirrhosis, may be partially due to accelerated glycolysis in the splanchnic region [12]. However, the mechanism of hyperlactatemia in Mauriac syndrome and type B lactic acidosis is poorly understood [5]. A reduction in gluconeogenesis in the liver may raise lactate levels in the body. Therefore, lactic acidosis in Mauriac syndrome could be explained by reduced gluconeogenesis and lack of conversion of pyruvate to glucose [12].

Given that large amounts of insulin and glucose are required for the development of glycogenic hepatopathy, this would explain the persistent and worsening lactic acidosis in our patient with typical DKA treatment of dextrose and insulin infusions [10]. In patients with poorly controlled diabetes, initial treatment of hyperglycemia with insulin has been shown to cause transient elevation of liver enzymes [13].

3.2. Diagnosis and Treatment. Diagnosis of glycogenic hepatopathy involves ruling out infectious disease, oncologic, autoimmune, metabolic (glycogen storage disease) or, more commonly in diabetic patients, nonalcoholic fatty liver disease [10]. Imaging includes abdominal ultrasonography; however, ultrasound does not differentiate fatty liver from glycogen overload [8, 11, 13]. Liver biopsy is the gold standard in diagnosing glycogenic hepatopathy and reveals marked glycogen accumulation within hepatocytes leading to enlarged, pale cells [8, 10]. Mild large droplet steatosis may be present [9].

Treatment of Mauriac syndrome and glycogenic hepatopathy involves improved blood glucose management [11, 13]. Resolution of symptoms, normalizing of liver enzymes

and resolved hepatomegaly, has been demonstrated with only minor improvements to hemoglobin A1C levels [11].

4. Conclusion

Mauriac syndrome is a rare complication of poorly controlled DM and may present with lactic acidosis. This case demonstrates lactic acidosis exacerbated by high dose insulin and dextrose therapy. Further research is required to explain the pathophysiology of lactic acidosis in glycogenic hepatopathy.

Competing Interests

The authors declare no competing interests.

Acknowledgments

The authors acknowledge Lanie Galman, M.D. anatomic pathologist, Calgary Laboratory Services, and clinical assistant professor, Pathology and Laboratory Medicine, University of Calgary, and Kari Taylor R.N., MN Department of Critical Care Medicine, South Health Campus, Calgary, AB, Canada.

References

[1] S. Nandwani, M. Saluja, M. Vats, and Y. Mehta, "Lactic acidosis in critically ill patients," *People's Journal of Scientific Research*, vol. 3, no. 1, pp. 43–47, 2010.

[2] A. J. Reddy, S. W. Lam, S. R. Bauer, and J. A. Guzman, "Lactic acidosis: clinical implications and management strategies," *Cleveland Clinic Journal of Medicine*, vol. 82, no. 9, pp. 615–624, 2015.

[3] J. A. Kraut and N. E. Madias, "Lactic acidosis," *The New England Journal of Medicine*, vol. 371, no. 24, pp. 2309–2319, 2014.

[4] P. Marik and R. Bellomo, "Lactate clearance as a target of therapy in sepsis: a flawed paradigm," *OA Critical Care*, vol. 1, no. 1, article 3, 2013.

[5] M. Chen, T. Y. Kim, and A. M. Pessegueiro, "Elevated lactate levels in a non-critically ill patient," *The Journal of the American Medical Association*, vol. 313, no. 8, pp. 849–850, 2015.

[6] M. C. G. J. Brouwers, J. C. Ham, E. Wisse et al., "Elevated lactate levels in patients with poorly regulated type 1 diabetes and glycogenic hepatopathy: a new feature of mauriac syndrome," *Diabetes Care*, vol. 38, no. 2, pp. e11–e12, 2015.

[7] E. Fitzpatrick, C. Cotoi, A. Quaglia, S. Sakellariou, M. E. Ford-Adams, and N. Hadzic, "Hepatopathy of Mauriac syndrome: a retrospective review from a tertiary liver centre," *Archives of Disease in Childhood*, vol. 99, no. 4, pp. 354–357, 2014.

[8] M. Torbenson, Y.-Y. Chen, E. Brunt et al., "Glycogenic hepatopathy: an underrecognized hepatic complication of diabetes mellitus," *The American Journal of Surgical Pathology*, vol. 30, no. 4, pp. 508–513, 2006.

[9] S. Messeri, L. Messerini, F. Vizzutti, G. Laffi, and F. Marra, "Glycogenic hepatopathy associated with type 1 diabetes mellitus as a cause of recurrent liver damage," *Annals of Hepatology*, vol. 11, no. 4, pp. 554–558, 2012.

[10] S. Giordano, A. Martocchia, L. Toussan et al., "Diagnosis of hepatic glycogenosis in poorly controlled type 1 diabetes mellitus," *World Journal of Diabetes*, vol. 5, no. 6, pp. 882–888, 2014.

[11] N. Parmar, M. Atiq, L. Austin, R. A. Miller, T. Smyrk, and K. Ahmed, "Glycogenic hepatopathy: thinking outside the box," *Case Reports in Gastroenterology*, vol. 9, no. 2, pp. 221–226, 2015.

[12] J. B. Jeppesen, C. Mortensen, F. Bendtsen, and S. Møller, "Lactate metabolism in chronic liver disease," *Scandinavian Journal of Clinical and Laboratory Investigation*, vol. 73, no. 4, pp. 293–299, 2013.

[13] R. Kant, H. B. Loper, V. Verma, R. Malek, C. B. Drachenberg, and K. M. Munir, "Glycogenic hepatopathy with persistent hepatomegaly in a patient with uncontrolled type 1 diabetes," *Journal of Endocrinology and Metabolism*, vol. 5, no. 1-2, pp. 189–191, 2015.

37

Beta Lactamase Producing *Clostridium perfringens* Bacteremia in an Elderly Man with Acute Pancreatitis

Rashmi Mishra,[1] **Nupur Sinha,**[2] **and Richard Duncalf**[1]

[1]*Division of Pulmonary and Critical Care Medicine, Bronx Lebanon Hospital Center, 1650 Grand Concourse, Bronx, NY 10457, USA*
[2]*Division of Pulmonary and Critical Care, Community Hospital of the Monterey Peninsula, 23625 Pacific Grove-Carmel Highway, Monterey, CA 93942, USA*

Correspondence should be addressed to Rashmi Mishra; rashmi_mishra1987@yahoo.com

Academic Editor: Zsolt Molnar

Clostridium perfringens bacteremia is associated with adverse outcomes. Known risk factors include chronic kidney disease, malignancy, diabetes mellitus, and gastrointestinal disease. We present a 74-year-old man admitted with confusion, vomiting, and abdominal pain. Exam revealed tachycardia, hypotension, lethargy, distended abdomen, and cold extremities. He required intubation and aggressive resuscitation for septic shock. Laboratory data showed leukocytosis, metabolic acidosis, acute kidney injury, and elevated lipase. CT scan of abdomen revealed acute pancreatitis and small bowel ileus. He was started on vancomycin and piperacillin-tazobactam. Initial blood cultures were positive for *C. perfringens* on day five. Metronidazole and clindamycin were added to the regimen. Repeat CT (day 7) revealed pancreatic necrosis. The patient developed profound circulatory shock requiring multiple vasopressors, renal failure requiring dialysis, and bacteremia with vancomycin-resistant enterococci. Hemodynamic instability precluded surgical intervention and he succumbed to multiorgan failure. Interestingly, our isolate was beta lactamase producing. We review the epidemiology, risk factors, presentation, and management of *C. perfringens* bacteremia. This case indicates a need for high clinical suspicion for clostridial sepsis and that extended spectrum beta lactam antibiotic coverage may be inadequate and should be supplemented with use of clindamycin or metronidazole if culture is positive, until sensitivities are known.

1. Introduction

Clostridium species are Gram-positive, spore-forming, obligate anaerobic bacilli. Malignancies, renal insufficiency, and other chronic illnesses have been associated with *Clostridium perfringens* (*C. perfringens*) bacteremia [1]. This entity is associated with adverse outcomes, especially if not clinically suspected early in the course of disease [1]. We present a rare case of resistant *C. perfringens* bacteremia associated with acute pancreatitis. The purpose of this case report is to alert physicians to suspect *C. perfringens* bacteremia in elderly patients presenting with abdominal symptoms and sepsis. Additionally, providers should be aware that although rare, *C. perfringens* can produce beta lactamase which can complicate antibiotic management.

2. Case Presentation

A 74-year-old man was brought to our emergency room with altered mental status, abdominal pain, and multiple episodes of vomiting and diarrhea for one day. Review of systems was negative for any other systemic complaints including fever. His medical history was significant for hypertension. He had no prior history of diabetes or surgery and had no pertinent family history. Personal history included prior alcohol use for fifty years with a reported intake of approximately 3-4 beers daily.

On physical exam, he was tachycardic, hypotensive, and obtunded with cold extremities. His abdomen was tense and distended with sluggish bowel sounds. He was emergently intubated and aggressive resuscitation initiated for presumptive septic shock.

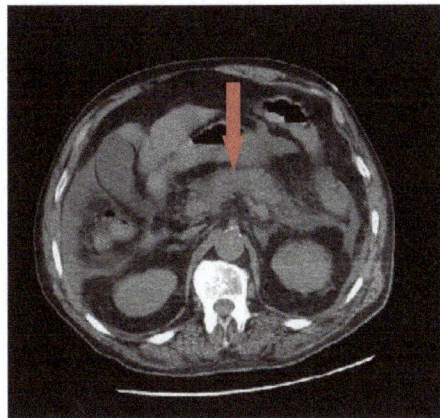

FIGURE 1: Axial cut of abdomen on day 1: arrow showing mildly edematous pancreas, with moderate peripancreatic infiltrative changes secondary to moderate acute pancreatitis.

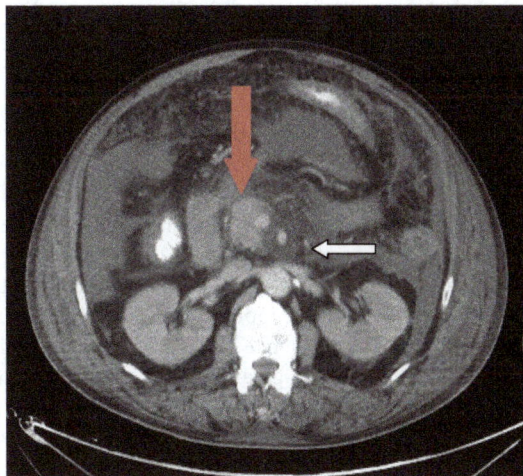

FIGURE 2: Axial cut of abdomen on day 7: red arrow pointing at a partially loculated fluid within the body of the pancreas. The white arrow shows an area of focal necrosis within the body of the pancreas.

Laboratory parameters revealed leukocytosis (12 × $10^3/\mu$L), anion gap metabolic acidosis (pH 7.10 with anion gap of 31), acute kidney injury (creatinine level 2.6 mg/dL), elevated lipase (1088 U/L), and mildly elevated transaminases (aspartate aminotransferase level 95 IU/L, alanine aminotransferase level 256 IU/L, and alkaline phosphatase level 195 IU/L). Mean corpuscular volume (MCV) was 98 fL and there was no evidence of hemolysis. Of note, his HbA1c was 8.4% suggesting undiagnosed diabetes mellitus. Urine toxicology screen was negative and serum ethanol level was less than 10 mg/dL. Computerized tomography (CT) scan of the abdomen (Figure 1) revealed moderate peripancreatic infiltrative changes and dilated loops of small bowel consistent with moderate acute pancreatitis and small bowel ileus.

A blood culture drawn on admission was reported to be positive for C. perfringens on day five. Metronidazole and clindamycin were then added to the existing regimen of vancomycin and piperacillin-tazobactam. Subsequent antibiotic sensitivity testing of the C. perfringens isolate revealed beta lactamase positivity; hence clindamycin was continued to treat the C. perfringens bacteremia. Metronidazole was also continued for suspected colitis. Stool studies including Clostridium difficile toxin and cultures were negative. The patient continued to require vasopressor support despite appropriate antibiotics and continued aggressive medical therapy, with worsening renal failure requiring hemodialysis.

A contrast enhanced CT of the abdomen on day seven revealed extensive acute pancreatitis with a new focus of likely necrotic pancreatitis in the pancreatic body with an associated 8.2 cm fluid collection consistent with a developing pseudocyst (Figure 2). Bilateral pleural effusions were also demonstrated. The patient's tenuous hemodynamic status precluded surgery. CT guided percutaneous aspiration of the pseudocyst fluid as well as pleural fluid was performed by interventional radiology. Cultures from these samples were subsequently negative. The remainder of the patient's hospital course was complicated by vancomycin-resistant enterococcus bacteremia and continued septic shock with worsening multiorgan failure and death.

3. Discussion

Advanced age increases the risk of clostridial infection independent of comorbidities which could be explained by age-related increase of clostridial species in the normal intestinal flora [2]. C. perfringens is frequently isolated from the biliary tree and gastrointestinal tract [2–4]. C. perfringens bacteremia has been reported after colonoscopy and gynecologic procedures [5, 6], and in association with choledocholithiasis in the absence of gallbladder stones and with normal common bile duct diameter [7].

Five subtypes of C. perfringens (A to E) exist and can produce as many as 12 different toxins. The 4 principal toxins of C. perfringens are alpha, beta, epsilon, and iota [8–10]. Alpha toxin can cause gas gangrene [11] as well as hemolysis and platelet destruction [12–14]. C. perfringens bacteremia has been associated with intravascular hemolysis and death [9, 10, 15, 16]. Low MCV and hemolysed samples in a patient with fever should alert the clinician to the possibility of clostridial infection. Beta toxin is associated with necrotic enteritis [17]. Epsilon toxin is known to cause fatal enterotoxemia in sheep and other animals [18]. When injected intradermally, iota toxin causes an increase in capillary permeability and intradermal necrosis in guinea-pigs. Larger doses injected intravenously are lethal in animals [18].

C. perfringens bacteremia, especially with a penicillinase producing strain, is a rare clinical entity. Epidemiological studies examining Clostridium bacteremia have been conducted in Taiwan, Japan, Canada, and the United States.

A study from northern Taiwan [1] demonstrated an overall annual incidence of C. perfringens bacteremia of 0.97 per 100,000 population. Elderly patients with comorbid illnesses, especially renal insufficiency or malignancy, were at increased risk. The 30-day and attributed mortalities were 26.9% and 8.6%, respectively. Nosocomial acquired C. perfringens infection was a significant predictor of 30-day mortality.

Most *C. perfringens* blood isolates were susceptible to the antibiotics tested. Resistance was observed in only seven out of ninety-three isolates, primarily to penicillin and clindamycin.

A review of all blood cultures drawn in a Japanese tertiary center from 2001 to 2009 demonstrated only 18 patients with *C. perfringens* bacteremia. Overall 30-day mortality was 27%. Septic shock at initial presentation was significantly associated with mortality [19]. A population-based surveillance of clostridial bacteremia among all residents of the Calgary Health Region (population 1.2 million) during 2000–2006 revealed a prevalence of clostridial bacteremia at 1.8/100,000 per year. Older age and multiple comorbidities, most importantly malignancy and Crohn's disease, were risk factors for acquiring *Clostridium* bacteremia. *C. perfringens* was the most common species isolated [2].

Review of blood cultures drawn in a rural hospital in Wisconsin from 1990 to 1997 yielded *Clostridium* infection in 0.12% with *C. perfringens* again, being the most common isolate (21.7%) [20].

Several studies have identified other conditions associated with the pathogenicity of *Clostridium* species and have demonstrated that failure to institute early, appropriate antimicrobial therapy may be associated with a poor outcome [2, 21, 22].

In another Taiwanese study, a review of 73 patients with clostridial bacteremia in an 11-year period identified diabetes mellitus and liver cirrhosis as the most common underlying comorbidities. Etiological species identified were *C. perfringens* (77%), *Clostridium bifermentans* (9%), and *Clostridium septicum* (4%). *Clostridium* bacteremia in patients with underlying liver cirrhosis and septic shock on initial presentation were poor prognostic factors [21].

The significance of positive blood culture for *Clostridium* was also studied in Israel. They found that growth of *Clostridium* species in blood cultures, even in the absence of one of the histotoxic syndromes, is often of clinical significance. Patients with *Clostridium* bacteremia were older, had a higher frequency of gastrointestinal disease, especially colorectal tumors, were more frequently associated with polymicrobial bacteremia, and had a higher mortality rate [22].

Our patient had several known risk factors for clostridial infection and subsequent mortality. He was older, apparently diabetic, had gastrointestinal disease, and presented in shock. However, none of the histotoxic syndromes associated with *Clostridium* infection were readily apparent. Although *C. perfringens* bacteremia was not initially suspected in our patient, he was treated with appropriate antibiotics.

Our isolate was reported to be beta lactamase producing. Based on the susceptibility report (see Table 1), our patient appeared to have a penicillinase producing organism as opposed to being a cephalosporinase producer.

The patient was initiated on piperacillin-tazobactam and vancomycin, both of which could be expected to have efficacy towards our isolate. Nevertheless, our patient deteriorated, requiring the addition of metronidazole and clindamycin. It is conceivable that penicillinase *C. perfringens* in vitro may predict cephalosporinase activity in vivo. Beta lactam resistance has been well studied in many pathogenic bacteria. In vitro

TABLE 1

Antibiotic	Interpretation	MIC mcg/mL
Ampicillin/sulbactam	S	<1
Cefotaxime	S	4
Cefoxitin	S	<2
Ceftizoxime	S	<2
Chloramphenicol	S	4
Clindamycin	S	<0.5
Metronidazole	S	<0.5
Penicillin	R	
Piperacillin	S	<4
Tetracycline	S	<0.5

susceptibility does not necessarily produce in vivo activity of an apparently appropriate antibiotic [23]. Unfortunately, we could not find any specific studies of this phenomenon related to *C. perfringens*. Early studies have demonstrated in vitro susceptibility of *C. perfringens* strains to vancomycin [24]. However a more recent study has shown that vancomycin is not bactericidal against *C. perfringens* [25].

4. Conclusion

Although rare, given the significant mortality of *C. perfringens* bacteremia, clinicians should be aware of the risk factors and presentation associated with this pathogen. We recommend immediate initiation of additional antibiotic coverage, for example, clindamycin or metronidazole, as soon as *C. perfringens* is isolated in culture, pending sensitivity. Data regarding clinical outcomes in beta lactamase producing Clostridia are scarce and may warrant further subgroup analysis. Furthermore, more microbiologic studies are required exploring in vitro and in vivo susceptibility patterns.

Abbreviations

C. perfringens: *Clostridium perfringens*
CT: Computerized tomography
MCV: Mean corpuscular volume.

References

[1] C.-C. Yang, P.-C. Hsu, H.-J. Chang, C.-W. Cheng, and M.-H. Lee, "Clinical significance and outcomes of *Clostridium perfringens* bacteremia—a 10-year experience at a tertiary care hospital," *International Journal of Infectious Diseases*, vol. 17, no. 11, pp. e955–e960, 2013.

[2] J. Leal, D. B. Gregson, T. Ross, D. L. Church, and K. B. Laupland, "Epidemiology of *Clostridium* species bacteremia in Calgary, Canada, 2000–2006," *Journal of Infection*, vol. 57, no. 3, pp. 198–203, 2008.

[3] G. Hill, S. Osterhous, and H. Willet, "Histotoxic clostridia," in *Zinsser Microbiology*, W. Joklik, H. Willet, and D. Amos, Eds., pp. 697–706, Appleton-Century-Crofts, Norwalk, Conn, USA, 1984.

[4] S. Gorbach, "Clostridium perfringens and other clostridia," in *Infectious Diseases*, S. Gorbach, J. Bartlett, and N. Blacklow, Eds., W.B. Saunders, Philadelphia, Pa, USA, 1998.

[5] A. N. Kunz, D. Riera, and P. Hickey, "Case of *Clostridium perfringens* bacteremia after routine colonoscopy and polypectomy," *Anaerobe*, vol. 15, no. 5, pp. 195–196, 2009.

[6] S. Halawa, A. Kassab, and R. Fox, "*Clostridium perfringens* infection following endometrial ablation," *Journal of Obstetrics & Gynaecology*, vol. 28, no. 3, p. 360, 2008.

[7] A. Atia, T. Raiyani, P. Patel, R. Patton, and M. Young, "Clostridium perfringens bacteremia caused by choledocholithiasis in the absence of gallbladder stones," *World Journal of Gastroenterology*, vol. 18, no. 39, pp. 5632–5634, 2012.

[8] C. M. Miller, S. Florman, L. Kim-Schluger et al., "Fulminant and fatal gas gangrene of the stomach in a healthy live liver donor," *Liver Transplantation*, vol. 10, no. 10, pp. 1315–1319, 2004.

[9] W. Hübl, B. Mostbeck, H. Hartleb, H. Pointner, K. Kofler, and P. M. Bayer, "Investigation of the pathogenesis of massive hemolysis in a case of *Clostridium perfringens* septicemia," *Annals of Hematology*, vol. 67, no. 3, pp. 145–147, 1993.

[10] A. Merino, A. Pereira, and P. Castro, "Massive intravascular haemolysis during *Clostridium perfrigens* sepsis of hepatic origin," *European Journal of Haematology*, vol. 84, no. 3, pp. 278–279, 2010.

[11] J. Sakurai, M. Nagahama, and M. Oda, "*Clostridium perfringens* alpha-toxin: characterization and mode of action," *Journal of Biochemistry*, vol. 136, no. 5, pp. 569–574, 2004.

[12] G. C. Diaz, T. Boyer, and J. F. Renz, "Survival of *Clostridium perfringens* sepsis in a liver transplant recipient," *Liver Transplantation*, vol. 15, no. 11, pp. 1469–1472, 2009.

[13] B. Eigenberger, I. Königsrainer, H. Kendziorra, and R. Riessen, "Fulminant liver failure due to *Clostridium perfringens* sepsis 9 years after liver transplantation," *Transplant International*, vol. 19, no. 2, pp. 172–173, 2006.

[14] D. L. Stevens and A. E. Bryant, "The role of clostridial toxins in the pathogenesis of gas gangrene," *Clinical Infectious Diseases*, vol. 35, supplement 1, pp. S93–S100, 2002.

[15] G. Rajendran, P. Bothma, and A. Brodbeck, "Intravascular haemolysis and septicaemia due to *Clostridium perfringens* liver abscess," *Anaesthesia and Intensive Care*, vol. 38, no. 5, pp. 942–945, 2010.

[16] S. D. Boyd, B. C. Mobley, D. P. Regula, and D. A. Arber, "Features of hemolysis due to *Clostridium perfringens* infection," *International Journal of Laboratory Hematology*, vol. 31, no. 3, pp. 364–367, 2009.

[17] M. R. Popoff and P. Bouvet, "Clostridial toxins," *Future Microbiology*, vol. 4, no. 8, pp. 1021–1064, 2009.

[18] J. L. McDonel, "*Clostridium perfringens* toxins (type A, B, C, D, E)," *Pharmacology and Therapeutics*, vol. 10, no. 3, pp. 617–655, 1980.

[19] H. Fujita, S. Nishimura, S. Kurosawa, I. Akiya, F. Nakamura-Uchiyama, and K. Ohnishi, "Clinical and epidemiological features of *Clostridium perfringens* bacteremia: a review of 18 cases over 8 year-period in a tertiary care center in metropolitan Tokyo area in Japan," *Internal Medicine*, vol. 49, no. 22, pp. 2433–2437, 2010.

[20] P. M. Rechner, W. A. Agger, K. Mruz, and T. H. Cogbill, "Clinical features of clostridial bacteremia: a review from a rural area," *Clinical Infectious Diseases*, vol. 33, no. 3, pp. 349–353, 2001.

[21] Y.-M. Chen, H.-C. Lee, C.-M. Chang, Y.-C. Chuang, and W.-C. Ko, "Clostridium bacteremia: emphasis on the poor prognosis in cirrhotic patients," *Journal of Microbiology, Immunology and Infection*, vol. 34, no. 2, pp. 113–118, 2001.

[22] B. Benjamin, M. Kan, D. Schwartz, and Y. Siegman-Igra, "The possible significance of *Clostridium* spp. in blood cultures," *Clinical Microbiology and Infection*, vol. 12, no. 10, pp. 1006–1012, 2006.

[23] D. M. Livermore, "Beta-lactamases in laboratory and clinical resistance," *Clinical Microbiology Reviews*, vol. 8, no. 4, pp. 557–584, 1995.

[24] F. L. Sapico, Y. Y. Kwok, V. L. Sutter, and S. M. Finegold, "Standardized antimicrobial disc susceptibility testing of anaerobic bacteria: in vitro susceptibility of *Clostridium perfringens* to nine antibiotics," *Antimicrobial Agents and Chemotherapy*, vol. 2, no. 4, pp. 320–325, 1972.

[25] K. L. Tyrrell, D. M. Citron, Y. A. Warren, H. T. Fernandez, C. V. Merriam, and E. J. C. Goldstein, "In vitro activities of daptomycin, vancomycin, and penicillin against *Clostridium difficile*, *C. perfringens*, *Finegoldia magna*, and *Propionibacterium acnes*," *Antimicrobial Agents and Chemotherapy*, vol. 50, no. 8, pp. 2728–2731, 2006.

38

Compartment Syndrome as a Result of Systemic Capillary Leak Syndrome

Kwadwo Kyeremanteng,[1,2] **Gianni D'Egidio,**[1,2] **Cynthia Wan,**[3]
Alan Baxter,[1,4] **and Hans Rosenberg**[1,5]

[1]*The Ottawa Hospital, Ottawa, ON, Canada*
[2]*Division of Critical Care, Department of Medicine, The University of Ottawa, Ottawa, ON, Canada*
[3]*School of Psychology, The University of Ottawa, Ottawa, ON, Canada*
[4]*Department of Anesthesiology, The University of Ottawa, Ottawa, ON, Canada*
[5]*Department of Emergency Medicine, The University of Ottawa, Ottawa, ON, Canada*

Correspondence should be addressed to Kwadwo Kyeremanteng; kkyeremanteng@toh.ca

Academic Editor: Martin Albert

Objective. To describe a single case of Systemic Capillary Leak Syndrome (SCLS) with a rare complication of compartment syndrome. *Patient.* Our patient is a 57-year-old male, referred to our hospital due to polycythemia (hemoglobin (Hgb) of 220 g/L), hypotension, acute renal failure, and bilateral calf pain. *Measurements and Main Results.* The patient required bilateral forearm, thigh, and calf fasciotomies during his ICU stay and continuous renal replacement therapy was instituted following onset of acute renal failure and oliguria. Ongoing hemodynamic (Norepinephrine and Milrinone infusion) and respiratory (ventilator) support in the ICU was provided until resolution of intravascular fluid extravasation. *Conclusions.* SCLS is an extremely rare disorder characterized by unexplained episodic capillary hyperpermeability, which causes shift of volume and protein from the intravascular space to the interstitial space. Patients present with significant hypotension, hemoconcentration, hypovolemia, and oliguria. Severe edema results from leakage of fluid and proteins into tissue. The most important part of treatment is maintaining stable hemodynamics, ruling out other causes of shock and diligent monitoring for complications. Awareness of the clinical syndrome with the rare complication of compartment syndrome may help guide investigations and diagnoses of these critically ill patients.

1. Introduction

Systemic Capillary Leak Syndrome (SCLS, Clarkson Syndrome) was first described by Clarkson et al. in 1960 [1]. SCLS is an extremely rare disorder characterized by unexplained episodic capillary hyperpermeability, which causes shift of volume and protein from the intravascular space to the interstitial space. Patients present with significant hypotension, hemoconcentration, hypovolemia, and oliguria. Severe edema results from leakage of fluid and proteins into tissue. The etiology of SCLS is not known. The most frequent association between patients is an IgG monoclonal gammopathy. There have been approximately 100 reported cases since 2007. Most patients were previously healthy and

middle-aged, and both sexes appear equally represented [2–4]. A familial component has not been identified [5].

2. Case Report

Our patient is a 57-year-old male, referred to our hospital from a neighboring community hospital due to polycythemia (hemoglobin (Hgb) of 220 g/L), hypotension, and bilateral calf pain. His past medical history was significant for gastroesophageal reflux disease and hypertension. In the 5 weeks prior to presentation, he had begun an exercise program, which included running on a treadmill, and over the last week he complained of progressive bilateral leg swelling and pain.

TABLE 1: Laboratory assessments, patient results, and the expected range of analyses.

Laboratory analyses	Results	Normal range
White blood cells (WBC)	27.3×10^9/L	3.0–10.5
Hemoglobin (Hgb)	210 g/L	130–170
Platelets (PLAT)	296×10^9/L	125–400
International normalized ratio (INR)	1.3	0.9–1.2
Partial thromboplastin time (PTT)	47 s	22–33
Sodium (Na)	135 mmol/L	136–144
Potassium (K)	4.7 mmol/L	3.6–5.1
Chloride (Cl)	113 mmol/L	101–111
Carbon dioxide (CO2)	14 mmol/L	22–32
Glucose random	10.3 mmol/L	3.8–11.0
Urea	10 mmol/L	2.9–7.1
Creatinine	135 mmol/L	62–106
Albumin	26 g/L	35–48
Lactate	2.7 mmol/L	0.5–2.2
CK	1353 U/L	20–215
Blood gas		
Source	Arterial	
Blood pH	7.14	
Blood pCO2	36 mm Hg	
Blood pO2	162 mm Hg	
Bicarbonate	12 mmol/L	
O2 saturation (calculated)	99 (% O2SAT)	
O2 saturation (measured)	99 (% O2SAT)	
% oxyhemoglobin (FO2Hb)	97%	
Base excess	−15.8 mmol/L	

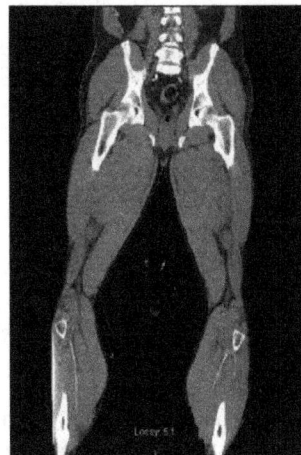

FIGURE 1: CT angiogram of the lower limbs showing marked narrowing of the distal vessels (arterial and venous) but no occlusive pathology.

Additionally, he experienced significant nausea and weakness over that same time. In the two days prior to presentation, the bilateral calf pain and swelling rapidly progressed resulting in the "worst pain of his life." The remaining review of systems was unremarkable.

On presentation to our Emergency Department, the patient was alert and oriented, his vital signs were initially stable including blood pressure of 150/99 (blood pressure in community hospital noted to be 68/40 before receiving 2 L bolus of normal saline), and his physical exam was unremarkable except for bilateral swollen calves, described as "rock hard" and tender to palpation. There was also limited range of motion at his ankle, with severe pain on plantar and dorsiflexion. At this point, compartment syndrome was suspected and the Orthopedics team was consulted. This diagnosis was confirmed by compartment pressure measurements of 110 mmHg and the patient was booked for emergent bilateral fasciotomies.

His initial blood work showed Hgb of 210 g/L, WBC of 27.3×10^9/L, albumin of 26 g/L, and creatinine of 135 umol/L (see Table 1). Due to his elevated Hgb, phlebotomy of 600 cc was performed prior to his operation. Throughout the operation, the patient's blood pressure was unstable despite significant crystalloid fluids administered (3 L of normal saline) requiring institution of vasopressor support.

Following his bilateral fasciotomies, the patient remained hypotensive and difficult to wean from the ventilator, resulting in his admission to the intensive care unit.

His initial resuscitation included administration of 6 liters of crystalloid over the first 12 hours with further boluses of albumin 5% for a total of 2.5 L, continued vasopressor support (Norepinephrine titrated to MAP > 65), broad spectrum antibiotic coverage (Pip-Tazo 3.375 g q6 h), and parenteral steroids (Solucortef 100 mg IV q8 hr) while working up the cause of his ongoing shock. Measures of our patient's Cardiac Index (CI) using the CardioQ™ esophageal device showed significant decline in cardiac function with CIs of 0.9–1.6 L/min during his initial presentation, prompting initiation of a Milrinone infusion. An urgent CT angiogram of the lower limbs was performed which showed marked narrowing of the distal vessels (arterial and venous) but no occlusive pathology (Figure 1).

Due to oliguria, increasing creatinine, CK (initially 1353 U/L and rising to 11590 U/L by postoperative day one), and positive urine myoglobin, the patient was thought to be in acute renal failure secondary to relative intravascular hypovolemia and rhabdomyolysis. For this reason, continuous renal replacement therapy was started and continued for three days.

Continuing intravascular fluid extravasation on postoperative days one and two necessitated performance of bilateral fasciotomies of the thighs and forearms. Continued ventilator support was required for eleven days related to his gross edema. He had mild pulmonary edema, moderate bilateral effusions, and mild ascites. On further work up, the patient was found to be JAK-2 mutation negative, with normal C3 and C4 complement levels, and serum immunofixation showed a monoclonal IgG band.

Given the initial presentation of hemoconcentration, hypoalbuminemia, and hypotension, with the concomitant presence of the monoclonal IgG band, a diagnosis of Systemic Capillary Leak Syndrome (Clarkson Syndrome) was made.

Our patient eventually stabilized, allowing for admission to the Orthopedic service, followed by a discharge home with minimal sequelae other than a persisting bilateral median and ulnar nerve neuropathies. Hemoglobin and albumin were 93 g/L and 23 g/L, respectively.

3. Discussion

3.1. Clinical Features. SCLS typically presents in three phases: a prodromal, an extravasation, and a recovery phase [4, 5]. In prodromal phase, the patient presents with signs typical of a viral illness such as lethargy, fever, nausea, and vomiting. During the extravasation phase, the patient shows signs of increased capillary permeability, such as significant generalized edema and hypotension. The edema can be profound, manifesting as pleural effusions, pericardial effusions, and rarely cerebral, epiglottic, and macular edema [2]. In the most severe cases, tissue edema can lead to compartment syndrome requiring fasciotomies; however, this is a rare complication. Moreover, tissue edema can also lead to rhabdomyolysis, and hypotension may be considerable.

Despite being edematous, the patient may require several liters of fluid and vasoactive agents to maintain adequate blood pressure. Acute renal failure can also occur secondary to hypovolemic shock. The recovery phase of SCLS is associated with the mobilization of extravascular fluid. This point is when the patient is at high risk of developing pulmonary edema.

3.2. Lab Features. High hemoglobin and hematocrit are present in almost all cases. Serum protein and albumin are also low. Elevated CK secondary to rhabdomyolysis is also seen. A monoclonal protein is present on serum electrophoresis in most cases. One review stated that there was no monoclonal protein detected in only 10 cases [2].

3.3. Pathophysiology. The pathophysiology of SCLS has not been established. Imaging with radio labelled albumin and dye has shown increased capillary permeability which can result in loss of up to 70% of total intravascular volume [5]. Polycythemia takes place because the RBCs are too large to permeate through the capillaries and often the degree of polycythemia reflects the severity of illness. Unfortunately, these episodes can reoccur spontaneously. It has been hypothesized that higher levels of circulating factors associated with capillary permeability such as coagulation factors, bradykinin generation, complement, serotonin, prostaglandins, and histamine levels would be associated with SCLS. These factors do not appear to be altered in patients with SCLS [4, 6]. Some medications (gemcitabine, retinoids, sirolimus, and interferon-α) are among the rare drug-induced causes of SCLS.

3.4. Differential Diagnosis. It is essential to rule out other forms a shock, that is, distributive (sepsis/anaphylaxis/pancreatitis), cardiogenic, obstructive, and other forms of hypovolemia (bleeding, etc.). Although edemas may not be present in these cases, it is important to rule them out because lack of recognition can be fatal. Other rare conditions such as Cl-esterase deficiency and systemic mastocytosis can present like SCLS. As in our case, SCLS can be mistaken as polycythemia vera, possibly resulting in phlebotomies which can worsen the patient's shock. An important differentiating factor is that polycythemia vera is not associated with hypotension.

3.5. Treatment. The most important part of treatment is maintaining stable hemodynamics. Due to the severe loss of intravascular volume, aggressive fluid resuscitation is often necessary. There does not appear to be any benefit whether crystalloids or colloids are used [7]. We favoured the use of colloids for volume expansion in the hope that the fluid would remain intravascularly for longer. In our case, there was difficult balance between maintaining adequate volume expansion and increasing edema causing worsening compartment syndrome. Fortunately compartment syndrome requiring fasciotomy is rare. During the recovery phase when the patient begins mobilizing fluid, diuretics may be considered to prevent pulmonary edema (assuming stable renal function). There is no proven therapy to prevent future occurrences. Multiple therapies including theophylline and terbutaline, steroids, IVIG, and plasmapheresis have not shown clear benefit.

In terms of prognosis, the progression to multiple myeloma appears rarely [8]. The average of recurrences is about three [2]. Regrettably, 5-year mortality of SCLS has been as high as 76% [9]; but in the most recent reviews [2, 4], in cases between 1990 and 2006, mortality rates were between 25 and 30%. Differences in mortality rate appear to be strongly impacted by the treatment administered to the patients. In a recent series of case studies, Gousseff et al. [10] reported that five years after diagnosis, survival was 85% in 23 patients who had received prophylactic treatment whereas the survival rate plummeted to 20% for five patients who had not. Increasing awareness of SCLS may account for the decreased mortality rates.

Disclosure

This work was performed at the Ottawa Hospital, Ottawa, Ontario, Canada.

Competing Interests

The authors declare that they have no competing interests.

References

[1] B. Clarkson, D. Thompson, M. Horwith, and E. H. Luckey, "Cyclical edema and shock due to increased capillary permeability," *The American Journal of Medicine*, vol. 29, no. 2, pp. 193–216, 1960.

[2] V. Dhir, V. Arya, I. C. Malav, B. S. Suryanarayanan, R. Gupta, and A. B. Dey, "Idiopathic Systemic Capillary Leak Syndrome(SCLS): case report and systematic review of cases reported in the last 16 years," *Internal Medicine Journal*, vol. 46, no. 12, pp. 899–904, 2007.

[3] W. Kai-Feng, P. Hong-Ming, L. Hai-Zhou, S. Li-Rong, and Z. Xi-Yan, "Interleukin-11-induced capillary leak syndrome in primary hepatic carcinoma patients with thrombocytopenia," *BMC Cancer*, vol. 11, article 204, 2011.

[4] K. M. Druey and P. R. Greipp, "Narrative review: the systemic capillary leak syndrome," *Annals of Internal Medicine*, vol. 153, no. 2, pp. 90–98, 2010.

[5] K. Dams, W. Meersseman, E. Verbeken, and D. C. Knockaert, "A 59-year-old man with shock, polycythemia, and an underlying paraproteinemia," *Chest*, vol. 132, no. 4, pp. 1393–1396, 2007.

[6] J. P. Atkinson, T. A. Waldmann, S. F. Stein et al., "Systemic capillary leak syndrome and monoclonal IgG gammopathy: studies in a sixth patient and a review of the literature," *Medicine*, vol. 56, no. 3, pp. 225–239, 1977.

[7] S. Teelucksingh, P. L. Padfield, and C. R. W. Edwards, "Systemic capillary leak syndrome," *Quarterly Journal of Medicine*, vol. 75, no. 277, pp. 515–524, 1990.

[8] Z. Amoura, T. Papo, J. Ninet et al., "Systemic capillary leak syndrome: report on 13 patients with special focus on course and treatment," *The American Journal of Medicine*, vol. 103, no. 6, pp. 514–519, 1997.

[9] S. Kawabe, T. Saeki, H. Yamazaki, M. Nagai, R. Aoyagi, and S. Miyamura, "Systemic capillary leak syndrome," *Internal Medicine*, vol. 41, no. 3, pp. 211–215, 2002.

[10] M. Gousseff, L. Arnaud, M. Lambert et al., "The systemic capillary leak syndrome: a case series of 28 patients from a European registry," *Annals of Internal Medicine*, vol. 154, no. 7, pp. 464–471, 2011.

39

A Fatal Case of Influenza B Myocarditis with Cardiac Tamponade

Dominick Roto ⓘ,[1] **Michelle L. Malnoske ⓘ,**[2] **Shira Winters,**[3] **and Steve N. Georas**[2]

[1]*Department of Medicine, University of Rochester Medical Center, 601 Elmwood Avenue, Rochester, NY 14642, USA*
[2]*Division of Pulmonary and Critical Care, Department of Medicine, University of Rochester Medical Center,*
601 Elmwood Avenue, Rochester, NY 14642, USA
[3]*Department of Pathology, University of Rochester Medical Center, 601 Elmwood Avenue, Rochester, NY 14642, USA*

Correspondence should be addressed to Dominick Roto; dominick_roto@urmc.rochester.edu

Academic Editor: Kurt Lenz

Background. Influenza B is generally regarded as a less severe counterpart to influenza A, typically causing mild upper respiratory symptoms. Myocardial involvement with influenza B is a rare complication, better described in children than adults. However, when it occurs, it can lead to profound myocarditis with progression to shock requiring aggressive supportive care. *Case Presentation.* We present a case of cardiac tamponade in the setting of influenza B infection in a previously healthy 57-year-old woman, with progression to refractory shock and death. Autopsy revealed myocardial necrosis with infiltration of CD3+ lymphocytes, and little evidence of viral pneumonia. *Conclusions.* Myocarditis is a rare complication of influenza B in adults, and subsequent pericardial effusion with tamponade physiology is a previously unreported event in an otherwise healthy adult without other medical comorbidities. While rare, this is a serious and potentially fatal complication that clinicians should be aware of when evaluating a patient with suspected viral illness who is exhibiting shock physiology.

1. Introduction

Influenza infections are a substantial cause of morbidity and mortality worldwide. Influenza viruses infect respiratory tract epithelial cells, leading to a range of clinical outcomes ranging from mild self-limited infections to severe respiratory failure and death. The factors explaining this wide range in clinical outcomes after influenza infection are under investigation and include both host- and virus-specific factors. Severe pneumonia and respiratory failure after influenza infections are often due to overexuberant immune responses leading to neutrophilic lung inflammation and lung injury (i.e., immunopathology), but why this occurs in some patients and not others is currently not known. It is also not clear why influenza can spread to distant organs and cause tissue damage outside of the lungs.

Although myocardial involvement as a result of influenza infection has been described, this is an uncommon complication. Influenza myocarditis typically presents as a mild self-limited disease, but fulminant shock has been rarely reported [1–3]. Cardiac involvement is also more common and is better described with influenza A infections, and there are only a few case reports of cardiac involvement from influenza B infections in adults [1–4]. We present a case of influenza B infection in a previously healthy 57-year-old woman presenting with cardiac tamponade with rapid progression to refractory shock and death despite aggressive resuscitative measures.

2. Case Presentation

A 57-year-old female without past medical history presented to the Emergency Department (ED) at the end of May with altered mental status, nausea, and vomiting. She had felt unwell for the past week with symptoms of mild cough and intermittent fevers peaking at 39.4° Celsius (C). She had been seen by her primary care physician two days prior and was diagnosed with a urinary tract infection based on a positive urine culture for Enterococcus species. She had not started the antibiotics prior to presentation to the ED.

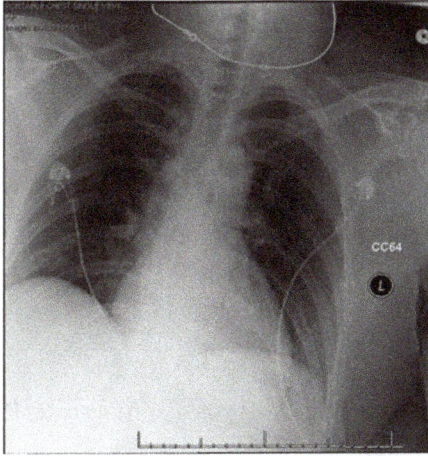

FIGURE 1: Presenting CXR showing no focal infiltrates or other evidence of cardiopulmonary disease.

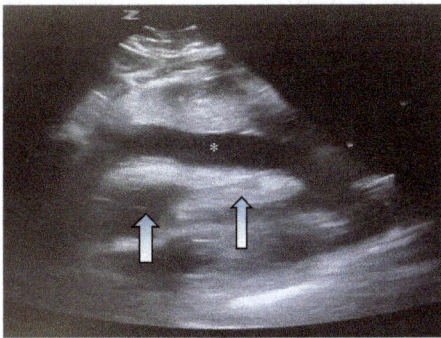

FIGURE 2: Subxiphoid window on bedside echocardiography demonstrating a large pericardial effusion (indicated by the *) associated with right ventricular (RV) and right atrial (RA) collapse (indicated by the arrows).

In the ED, she appeared acutely ill. She was hypotensive (blood pressure 58/41 mmHg by cuff), tachycardic (heart rate 120 beats/minute), and hypothermic (32.4°C). Physical exam revealed dry mucus membranes, clear lung fields, and cold and mottled extremities. Initial blood work demonstrated an arterial blood gas with pH of 7.0, pCO2 32mmHg, pO2 450 mmHg on supplemental oxygen, and arterial lactate 9.6 mmol/L. Chemistries and hepatic function testing showed creatinine of 1.64 mg/dL, glucose 330 mg/dL, alanine transferase 23 U/L, and total bilirubin <0.2mg/dL. Complete blood count was notable for leukocytosis 16,300/uL with 77.4% neutrophils and 16.9% lymphocytes and hemoglobin of 18.6 g/dL. CRP was normal at 2mg/L. Procalcitonin was 0.89 ng/mL. Troponin T was elevated to 0.20 ng/mL which subsequently rose to 0.97 ng/mL on repeat. Urine toxicology screen was negative. Initial chest X-ray (CXR) showed no acute cardiopulmonary disease (Figure 1). Initial ECG demonstrated sinus tachycardia. Three liters of isotonic intravenous fluids were given as bolus infusion, which resulted in transient increases in blood pressure, but systolic blood pressure remained low (<70 mm Hg) despite

fluid resuscitation. A left subclavian triple lumen catheter was inserted, norepinephrine was initiated to maintain mean arterial pressure >60 mmHg, and the patient received cefepime and vancomycin for presumed septic shock.

A bedside cardiac ultrasound was performed which demonstrated a large pericardial effusion with tamponade physiology (Figure 2). The patient was taken to the cardiac catheterization lab for an urgent pericardiocentesis. Prior to the procedure, the patient suffered an asystolic cardiac arrest secondary to pump failure requiring 10 minutes of cardiopulmonary resuscitation. She was intubated and started on mechanical ventilation. The patient underwent pericardiocentes with immediate evacuation of 90ml of serous fluid, and a pericardial drain was subsequently placed to manage any ongoing or residual effusion. After successful pericardiocentesis, the patient also underwent coronary angiography, which revealed angiographically normal coronaries, with no evidence of plaque or obstruction.

The patient was admitted to the Medical Intensive Care Unit. Over the following 24 hours her condition deteriorated with hypotension and a marked metabolic acidosis despite IV fluids, high dose vasopressors, broad-spectrum antibiotics, stress dose steroids, and a bicarbonate drip. Arterial lactate continued to trend up to 16.2mmol/L. Repeat transthoracic echocardiogram 12 hours after the pericardiocentesis revealed only a small anterior pericardial effusion, with normal left and right ventricular ejection fractions. Total pericardial drain output was 150mL over this time. During this time, her respiratory viral panel taken by nasal swab on admission returned positive for influenza B by PCR. Repeat CXR showed bilateral infiltrates concerning for acute respiratory distress syndrome. Oxygenation deteriorated despite high FiO2 and PEEP, and the patient was paralyzed and started on low tidal volume ventilation. Despite maximal supportive care, later that day the patient experienced another asystolic cardiac arrest from persistent hypoxia, respiratory failure, and worsening acidosis for which resuscitative efforts were unsuccessful. All blood cultures remained negative. Urine culture from presentation returned positive for 50,000 colonies of Enterococcus species; however, the urinalysis was not compatible with active infection, showing only 12 white blood cells. Repeat urine culture collected later during the admission remained negative.

Autopsy was performed after consent was obtained from family members. On gross evaluation, the myocardium was grossly firm, dense, and mottled in appearance. Lung histology revealed relatively preserved lung architecture with only focal evidence of lung injury in the left lower lobe, but no widespread evidence of pneumonitis or pneumonia. All cultures from the lung were negative for infection. In contrast the heart was markedly abnormal, with multifocal cardiac cell necrosis and subendocardial septal hemorrhage consistent with myocarditis. The pericardium was normal. Immunohistochemistry revealed extensive infiltration of the myocardium with CD3 positive lymphocytes, and hemoxylin and eosin stain demonstrated hemorrhage and myocyte necrosis (Figure 3). The cause of death was felt to be myocarditis secondary to influenza B infection, given the strongly positive viral PCR.

(a)

(b)

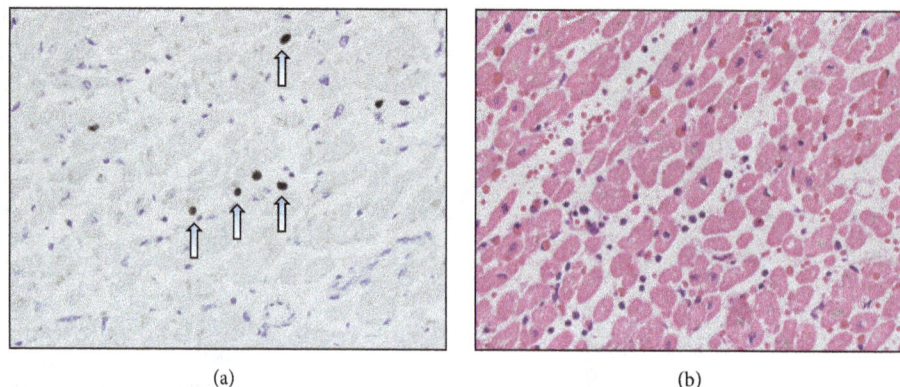

FIGURE 3: (a) Immunohistochemical stain of CD3 lymphocytes in the intraventricular septum (indicated by the arrows), 400x. (b) Hemoxyline and Eosin stain of the intraventricular septum showing hemorrhage and myocyte necrosis, 400x.

3. Discussion and Conclusions

Cardiac complications of influenza infections have been described in the literature as early as the 1900s [4]. These complications are generally more common among those infected with influenza A. While case reports of myocarditis and subsequent shock associated with influenza B have been reported, this presentation is more common in children [3–5]. The data on these complications in adults are limited to a small number of case studies [6–9]. To our knowledge, there have not been any reports of influenza B leading to pericardial effusion and tamponade in adults.

Influenza myocarditis is traditionally defined by a viral prodrome followed by abrupt decline in cardiac function [10]. Spontaneous recovery is the most common outcome, though there have been case reports of abrupt and sudden death, as well as progression to a chronic, dilated cardiomyopathy [10–12]. Diagnosis is generally made by transthoracic echocardiogram in the appropriate clinical context, with findings typically consisting of a globally reduced ejection fraction, though often times the diagnosis is only made postmortem [13]. Histologically, myocarditis is most often associated with patchy infiltrate of the lateral free wall of the left ventricle and consists primarily of macrophages. The right ventricle is typically spared [13].

This case exhibits numerous uncommon features when comparing it to current literature for influenza-associated myocarditis. While the initial clinical presentation was consistent with a viral prodrome leading to septic shock, the development of cardiogenic shock secondary to cardiac tamponade has not been previously described. In general, infection makes up a small percentage of large volume pericardial effusions, with influenza B not being regarded as a common causative agent [14]. Moreover, infection without concurrent pericarditis is very poorly reported in the literature. In this case, there was no evidence of pericarditis on postmortem evaluation. In terms of clinical course, the patient deviated from previous described cases quite drastically in terms of physiologic presentation. While initially presenting in cardiogenic shock, the subsequent transthoracic echocardiograms showed normal cardiac function as determined by ejection fraction. Although all cultures obtained from this patient both pre- and postmortem were negative for infectious etiology, at the time of death she exhibited septic shock type physiology. Previously reported cases of influenza myocarditis generally maintain cardiogenic shock physiology, at times requiring mechanical cardiac support such as an intra-aortic balloon pump or extracorporeal membrane oxygenation (ECMO) [15]. Additionally, previously reported cases typically are self-limited, unlike the fatal course in our patient.

Treatment for influenza-induced myocarditis remains supportive. It is not known if the patient received an influenza vaccine for the season. She was not treated with antiviral therapy given her late presentation. Why exactly this patient developed such a fulminant and fatal course is not known. We suggest that clinicians remain alert for unusual complications of influenza infection for patients presenting with shock physiology, including pericardial tamponade and myocarditis.

Abbreviations

ED: Emergency Department
C: Celsius
mmHg: Millimeters of mercury
EF: Ejection fraction
CXR: Chest X-ray.

Acknowledgments

We would like to thank the medical team that cared for the patient and for the family for providing consent to autopsy. The authors are employed by the University of Rochester Medical Center. No external funding was used in the preparation of this case report.

References

[1] K. Kumar, M. Guirgis, S. Zieroth et al., "Influenza Myocarditis and Myositis: Case Presentation and Review of the Literature," *Canadian Journal of Cardiology*, vol. 27, no. 4, pp. 514–522, 2011.

[2] Z. R. Estabragh and M. A. Mamas, "The cardiovascular manifestations of influenza: A systematic review," *International Journal of Cardiology*, vol. 167, no. 6, pp. 2397–2403, 2013.

[3] H. Frank, C. Wittekind, U. G. Liebert et al., "Lethal influenza B myocarditis in a child and review of the literature for pediatric age groups," *Infection*, vol. 38, no. 3, pp. 231–235, 2010.

[4] D. G. Jaimovich, A. Kumar, C. L. Shabino, and R. Formoli, "Influenza B virus infection associated with non-bacterial septic shock-like illness," *Infection*, vol. 25, no. 3, pp. 311–315, 1992.

[5] R. D. Craver, K. Sorrells, and R. Gohd, "Myocarditis with influenza B infection," *The Pediatric Infectious Disease Journal*, vol. 16, no. 6, pp. 629-630, 1997.

[6] C. D. Paddock, L. Liu, A. M. Denison et al., "Myocardial injury and bacterial pneumonia contribute to the pathogenesis of fatal influenza B virus infection," *The Journal of Infectious Diseases*, vol. 205, no. 6, pp. 895–905, 2012.

[7] M. Taremi, A. Amoroso, H. L. Nace, and B. L. Gilliam, "Influenza B-induced refractory cardiogenic shock: A case report," *BMC Infectious Diseases*, vol. 13, no. 1, 2013.

[8] C. G. Ray, T. B. Icenogle, L. L. Minnich, J. G. Copeland, and T. M. Grogan, "The Use Of Intravenous Ribavirin To Treat Influenza Virus-Associated Acute Myocarditis," *The Journal of Infectious Diseases*, vol. 159, no. 5, pp. 829–836, 1989.

[9] E. N. Silber, "Respiratory viruses and heart disease," *Annals of Internal Medicine*, vol. 48, no. 2, pp. 228–241, 1958.

[10] R. E. McCarthy, J. P. Boehmer, R. H. Hruban et al., "Long-term outcome of fulminant myocarditis as compared with acute (nonfulminant) myocarditis," *The New England Journal of Medicine*, vol. 342, no. 10, pp. 690–695, 2000.

[11] G. M. Felker, J. P. Boehmer, R. H. Hruban et al., "Echocardiographic findings in fulminant and acute myocarditis," *Journal of the American College of Cardiology*, vol. 36, no. 1, pp. 227–232, 2000.

[12] K. P. Theleman, J. J. Kuiper, and W. C. Roberts, "Acute myocarditis (Predominately Lymphocytic) causing sudden death without heart failure," *American Journal of Cardiology*, vol. 88, no. 9, pp. 1078–1083, 2001.

[13] H. Mahrholdt, C. Goedecke, A. Wagner et al., "Cardiovascular magnetic resonance assessment of human myocarditis: a comparison to histology and molecular pathology," *Circulation*, vol. 109, no. 10, pp. 1250–1258, 2004.

[14] J. Sagristà-Sauleda, J. Mercé, G. Permanyer-Miralda, and J. Soler-Soler, "Clinical clues to the causes of large pericardial effusions," *American Journal of Medicine*, vol. 109, no. 2, pp. 95–101, 2000.

[15] S. Kato, S.-I. Morimoto, S. Hiramitsu, M. Nomura, T. Ito, and H. Hishida, "Use of percutaneous cardiopulmonary support of patients with fulminant myocarditis and cardiogenic shock for improving prognosis," *American Journal of Cardiology*, vol. 83, no. 4, pp. 623–625, 1999.

40

A Case of MDMA-Associated Cerebral and Pulmonary Edema Requiring ECMO

A. Thakkar,[1] K. Parekh,[2] K. El Hachem,[3] and E. M. Mohanraj[2]

[1]*Department of Internal Medicine, Mount Sinai St. Luke's-West Hospital, New York, NY, USA*
[2]*Division of Pulmonary, Critical Care & Sleep Medicine, Mount Sinai St. Luke's-West Hospital, New York, NY, USA*
[3]*Division of Nephrology, Mount Sinai St. Luke's-West Hospital, New York, NY, USA*

Correspondence should be addressed to A. Thakkar; astha.thakkar@mountsinai.org

Academic Editor: Kenneth S. Waxman

A 20-year-old female presented with confusion, generalized tonic-clonic seizures, and severe hyponatremia after ingesting 3,4-methylenedioxymethamphetamine (MDMA). Brain computed tomography (CT) demonstrated cerebral edema. Her hospital course was rapidly complicated by respiratory failure and shock requiring intubation and vasopressors. Refractory acute respiratory distress syndrome (ARDS) was diagnosed which was unresponsive to conventional and salvage therapies, requiring initiation of extracorporeal membrane oxygenation (ECMO), leading to normalization of oxygenation parameters. Hyponatremia was corrected and the encephalopathy resolved. The patient was decannulated and extubated after three days. MDMA-induced hyponatremia is hypothesized to result from enhanced serotonergic activity and arginine vasopressin (AVP) release in the brain leading to hyperthermia-induced polydipsia and syndrome of inappropriate antidiuretic hormone (SIADH) secretion. A common but often unrecognized complication of severe hyponatremia is the Ayus-Arieff syndrome where cerebral edema causes neurogenic pulmonary edema via centrally mediated increases in catecholamine release and capillary injury. For our patient, ECMO was required for three days while the hyponatremia was corrected which led to rapid clearing of the cerebral edema and neurogenic pulmonary edema. This case illustrates that, in selecting patients with refractory ARDS from MDMA-associated cerebral and pulmonary edema, ECMO may be a temporizing and life-saving modality of treatment.

1. Introduction

MDMA (3,4-methylenedioxymethamphetamine), a synthetic substance initially patented as an appetite inhibitor or tranquilizer, is now a frequently used recreational drug. Common street names for the drug are *ecstasy* or *molly*. The drug has become popular amongst teenagers and young adults as it is marketed as a "safe" drug without long-term side effects and lack of addiction tendencies. What is not widely advertised is that MDMA has potentially life-threatening acute and chronic effects on several organ systems. There are reports of fatalities associated with MDMA related to hyperpyrexia, rhabdomyolysis, cardiac arrhythmias, hepatic necrosis, cerebrovascular accidents, and drug-related accidents or suicide [1]. We present the case of a young female who ingested MDMA and presented with confusion, severe hyponatremia, seizures, and rapid progression to acute respiratory distress syndrome (ARDS) requiring mechanical ventilation and extracorporeal membrane oxygenation (ECMO).

2. Case

A 20-year-old healthy female presented to the emergency room with confusion, vomiting, and generalized tonic-clonic seizure. She was last seen in her usual state of health 12 hours prior to arrival. Friends reported that she consumed an unknown amount of alcohol and ingested a quarter tablet of MDMA. The patient subsequently became paranoid, attempted to climb up walls, and drank ten bottles of water. She had a witnessed generalized tonic-clonic seizure with frothing at the mouth and recurrent seizure en route the Emergency Department. Both seizures broke spontaneously. Her initial vital signs were notable for a temperature of

TABLE 1: Laboratory values.

Relevant labs	Arterial blood gas		Others
	Pre-ECMO	Post-ECMO	
Serum sodium 112 mmol/L	pH 7.28	pH 7.42	Urine toxicology-positive for amphetamines
Urine sodium 112 mmol/L	pO2 53 mm Hg	pO2 99 mm Hg	Serum hCG < 2.39 mIU/ml
Serum osmolality 239 mmol/L	pCO2 41.6 mm Hg	pCO2 23.0 mm Hg	Serum creatinine kinase 1308 IU/mL
Urine osmolality 439 mmol/L	O2 saturation 82.9%	O2 saturation 100%	Troponin (peak) 0.497 mg/mL
Lactic acid 2.8 mmol/L	A-a gradient 492		
TSH 1.8 IU/ml			

38.0 degrees Celsius, heart rate of 88 beats/minute, blood pressure of 140/70 mm Hg, respiratory rate of 14 per minute, and oxygen saturation of 97% on room air. The patient was obtunded, and pupils were dilated, equal, and reactive to light bilaterally. Mucus membranes were moist. Neck was supple. Lung auscultation demonstrated good air entry with bilateral rhonchi. Cardiovascular examination was normal without any murmurs, rubs, or gallops. Abdominal exam was normal. Neurologic examination was limited but the patient had normal extremity tone, hyporeflexia was noted in biceps, triceps, knees, and ankles bilaterally, clonus was absent, and normal bilateral Babinski reflexes were noted. She received 10 mg of IV lorazepam for additional seizures and was intubated for airway protection. A summary of relevant laboratory findings is mentioned in Table 1. Her initial complete blood count had a white blood cell count of 20,600/μliter, hemoglobin of 12.8 g/dl, and platelet count of 233,000/μliter. Her chemistry panel was as follows: sodium 112 mmol/L, potassium 3.5 mmol/L, chloride 84 mmol/L, bicarbonate 16 mmol/L, blood urea nitrogen of 7 mg/dl, serum creatinine of 0.5 mg/dl, and serum glucose of 117 mg/dl. A liver function panel was normal.

Serum lactic acid was 2.8 and osmolality was 239 mmol/L. Urine chemistries were significant for a urine sodium 112 mmol/L and urine osmolality of 439 mmol/L. The urine electrolytes were checked prior to administration of any hypertonic saline. These electrolyte derangements suggested a state of syndrome of inappropriate antidiuretic hormone (SIADH). She received three doses of 3% hypertonic normal saline without a significant change in her serum sodium. A brain computed tomography (CT) scan showed cerebral edema.

Over the next couple of hours, she had increasing oxygen requirements on the ventilator of up to 100% FiO2 and a positive end-expiratory pressure of 20 mm Hg. The initial chest-radiograph was concerning for multifocal pneumonia; however a repeat chest-radiograph, twelve hours later, revealed diffuse bilateral hazy opacities concerning for acute respiratory distress syndrome (ARDS). Her blood gas analysis showed a pH of 7.28 with PaO2 of 53 mm Hg and an alveolar-arterial oxygen gradient of 492 mm Hg. Her PaO2 : FiO2 ratio was 53 suggesting severe ARDS. At that time, she was paralyzed with cis-atracurium and started on inhaled nitric oxide as salvage therapy. She subsequently developed hemodynamic compromise and was started on norepinephrine, ultimately requiring addition of vasopressin and dopamine

to maintain stable hemodynamics. Finally, venovenous extracorporeal membrane oxygenation (ECMO) was started with immediate resolution of hypoxemia. Hyponatremia was corrected gradually with 3% hypertonic saline that led to resolution of altered mental status and improvement in hypoxemia. She was gradually weaned off of ECMO and extubated within three days.

3. Discussion

MDMA is a synthetic compound, which is usually marketed in the form of pills and is taken orally. The drug is readily bound to tissues and metabolized by CYP2D6 and a few other enzymes. These enzymes have a very high affinity and get saturated at low concentrations of the drug, thereby greatly increasing the concentration of MDMA in brain with small increase in drug dosage [1]. The drug exerts effects on all systems of the body, most pronounced in the central nervous system. There is evidence that MDMA leads to local increase in the concentration of monoamine neurotransmitters (norepinephrine, serotonin, and, to an extent, dopamine) at the axon terminals. MDMA blocks the reuptake of serotonin by blocking the serotonin receptor, thereby increasing the local concentration of serotonin. Serotonin affects the thermostat and leads to increased body temperature coupled with increased activity leading to profuse sweating. This triggers intense thirst and the individual tends to drink lots of water. However, studies have demonstrated that ecstasy also independently increases the amount of arginine vasopressin (AVP) in the brain, leading to a state of SIADH, leading to increased water retention by the kidneys. Combined, these two pathological mechanisms lead to hyponatremia which can lead to cerebral edema and increase the intracranial pressure, which can trigger generalized tonic-clonic seizures and potentially compression of brainstem and cerebellum into the foramen magnum leading to fatal disruption of circulation or respiration. Cardiovascular effects of MDMA are mediated by the norepinephrine surge. Increase in blood pressure is the direct effect, which indirectly leads to major and minor cerebral and retinal hemorrhages. Cardiac arrhythmias have also been reported. Patients who have ecstasy intoxication are often jaundiced. The mechanism of hepatic injury is postulated to be oxidative injury to hepatocytes secondary to excess glutathione consumption by MDMA metabolites. Elevation in liver enzymes is typically seen. Biopsy usually shows nonspecific acute hepatitis. Resolution of hepatic injury occurs within a few days to weeks. The excess activity induced by sympathetic overdrive and hyperpyrexia induced by serotonin leads to rhabdomyolysis which can potentially lead to myoglobinuria and renal failure [1]. Hence, MDMA can lead to multiorgan failure. This has been described in many cases as well [2–4]. Risk of death from MDMA intoxication is very high in these patients given risk of cerebral herniation as well as severe systemic effects as described above. Apart from short-term effects, MDMA also leads to long-term psychiatric and physical effects. Psychiatric disturbances include severe depression, paranoias, memory impairment, and panic attacks. Long-term physical disturbances include bruxism, low sympathetic tone leading to labile blood pressure and heart rates, and neurologic impairment [1].

MDMA-induced hyponatremia has been reported in several cases [3, 5–14]. A complication of severe hyponatremia is Ayus-Arieff syndrome where hyponatremia-induced cerebral edema drives pulmonary edema [14, 15]. The mechanism behind Ayus-Arieff syndrome is postulated as follows: cerebral edema leads to increase in intracranial pressure. This in turn leads to a centrally mediated increase in vascular permeability and catecholamine release causing capillary injury. This effect seems to be most pronounced in the pulmonary vasculature. Pulmonary artery hypertension and plasma leakage through injured capillaries result in pulmonary edema and subsequent acute respiratory distress syndrome (ARDS) [15]. This phenomenon has also been described in marathon runners who develop hyponatremia secondary to dehydration and develop pulmonary edema, frequently requiring mechanical ventilation [14]. Our patient presented with symptomatic hyponatremia from MDMA-induced SIADH and primary polydipsia leading to Ayus-Arieff syndrome and resultant severe ARDS with $PaO_2 : FiO_2$ ratio of 53 refractory to conventional management and salvage therapies. She responded instantaneously to venovenous ECMO, a modality associated with medical and mechanical complications and increased mortality ratios in some patient groups (elderly individuals and patients with underlying hematologic malignancies) [16]. In this patient, it proved instrumental as a bridge therapy [17]. ECMO gave us the opportunity to correct the underlying hyponatremia which helped clear the pulmonary edema and resolution of ARDS and saved our patient's life.

Disclosure

This paper was partly presented as a poster at American Thoracic Society (ATS) International Conference 2016.

References

[1] H. Kalant, "The pharmacology and toxicology of 'ecstasy' (MDMA) and related drugs," *Canadian Medical Association Journal*, vol. 165, no. 7, pp. 917–928, 2001.

[2] T. Vakde, M. Diaz, K. Uday, and R. Duncalf, "Rapidly reversible multiorgan failure after ingestion of "molly" (pure 3,4-methylenedioxymethamphetamine): A case report," *Journal of Medical Case Reports*, vol. 8, no. 1, article no. 204, 2014.

[3] Y.-M. Sue, Y.-L. Lee, and J.-J. Huang, "Acute hyponatremia, seizure, and rhabdomyolysis after ecstasy use," *Journal of Toxicology—Clinical Toxicology*, vol. 40, no. 7, pp. 931-932, 2002.

[4] G. R. Screaton, H. S. Cairns, M. Sarner, M. Singer, A. Thrasher, and S. L. Cohen, "Hyperpyrexia and rhabdomyolysis after MDMA ("ecstasy") abuse," *The Lancet*, vol. 339, no. 8794, pp. 677-678, 1992.

[5] I. Ajaelo, K. Koenig, and E. Snoey, "Severe hyponatremia and inappropriate antidiuretic hormone secretion following ecstasy use," *Academic Emergency Medicine*, vol. 5, no. 8, pp. 839-840, 1998.

[6] S. J. Traub, R. S. Hoffman, and L. S. Nelson, "The "ecstasy" hangover: Hyponatremia due to 3,4-methylenedioxymethamphetamine," *Journal of Urban Health*, vol. 79, no. 4, pp. 549–555, 2002.

[7] A. C. de Braganca, R. L. Moreau, T. de Brito et al., "Ecstasy induces reactive oxygen species, kidney water absorption and rhabdomyolysis in normal rats. Effect of N-acetylcysteine and Allopurinol in oxidative stress and muscle fiber damage," *PLoS ONE*, vol. 12, no. 7, p. e0179199, 2017.

[8] R. Farah and R. Farah, "Ecstasy (3,4-methylenedioxymethamphetamine)-induced inappropriate antidiuretic hormone secretion," *Pediatric Emergency Care*, vol. 24, no. 9, pp. 615–617, 2008.

[9] S. C. Satchell and M. Connaughton, "Inappropriate antidiuretic hormone secretion and extreme rises in serum creatinine kinase following MDMA ingestion," *British Journal of Hospital Medicine*, vol. 51, no. 9, p. 495, 1994.

[10] T. K. Hartung, E. Schofield, A. I. Short, M. J. A. Parr, and J. A. Henry, "Hyponatraemic states following 3,4-methylenedioxymethamphetamine (MDMA, 'ecstasy') ingestion," *QJM: An International Journal of Medicine*, vol. 95, no. 7, pp. 431–437, 2002.

[11] M. Gomez-Balaguer, H. Peña, C. Morillas, and A. Hernández, "Syndrome of Inappropriate Antidiuretic Hormone Secretion and "Designer Drugs" (Ecstasy)," *Journal of Pediatric Endocrinology and Metabolism*, vol. 13, no. 4, 2000.

[12] M. Brvar, G. Kozelj, J. Osredkar, M. Mozina, M. Gricar, and M. Bunc, "Polydipsia as another mechanism of hyponatremia after 'ecstasy' (3,4 methyldioxymethamphetamine) ingestion," *European Journal of Emergency Medicine*, vol. 11, no. 5, pp. 302–304, 2004.

[13] L. Braback and M. Humble, "Young woman dies of water intoxication after taking one tablet of ecstasy. Today's drug panorama calls for increased vigilance in health care," *Läkartidningen*, vol. 98, no. 8, pp. 817–819, 2001.

[14] J. C. Ayus, J. Varon, and A. I. Arieff, "Hyponatremia, cerebral edema, and noncardiogenic pulmonary edema in marathon runners," *Annals of Internal Medicine*, vol. 132, no. 9, pp. 711–714, 2000.

[15] J. C. Ayus and A. I. Arieff, "Pulmonary complications of hyponatremic encephalopathy: noncardiogenic pulmonary edema and hypercapnic respiratory failure," *CHEST*, vol. 107, no. 2, pp. 517–521, 1995.

[16] S. Vaquer, C. de Haro, P. Peruga et al., "Systematic review and meta-analysis of complications and mortality of veno-venous extracorporeal membrane oxygenation for refractory acute respiratory distress syndrome," *Annals of Intensive Care*, vol. 7, p. 51, 2017.

[17] D. Abrams and D. Brodie, "Novel Uses of Extracorporeal Membrane Oxygenation in Adults," *Clinics in Chest Medicine*, vol. 36, no. 3, pp. 373–384, 2015.

41

Recurrence of Postoperative Stress-Induced Cardiomyopathy Resulting from Status Epilepticus

Grant A. Miller, Yousef M. Ahmed, and Nicki S. Tarant

Department of Critical Care Medicine, Naval Medical Center Portsmouth, Portsmouth, VA, USA

Correspondence should be addressed to Grant A. Miller; grant.miller75@gmail.com

Academic Editor: Won S. Park

Introduction. Classically, stress-induced cardiomyopathy (SIC), also known as takotsubo cardiomyopathy, displays the pathognomonic feature of reversible left ventricular apical ballooning without coronary artery stenosis following stressful event(s). Temporary reduction in ejection fraction (EF) resolves spontaneously. Variants of SIC exhibiting mid-ventricular regional wall motion abnormalities have been identified. Recent case series present SIC as a finding in association with sudden unexplained death in epilepsy (SUDEP). This case presents a patient who develops recurrence of nonapical cardiomyopathy secondary to status epilepticus. *Case Report.* Involving a postoperative, postmenopausal woman having two distinct episodes of status epilepticus (SE) preceding two incidents of SIC. Preoperative transthoracic echocardiogram (TTE) confirms the patient's baseline EF of 60% prior to the second event. Postoperatively, SE occurs, and the initial electrocardiogram exhibits T-wave inversions with subsequent elevation of troponin I. Postoperative TTE shows an EF of 30% with mid-ventricular wall akinesia restoring baseline EF rapidly. *Conclusion.* This case identifies the need to understand SIC and its diagnostic criteria, especially when cardiac catheterization is neither indicated nor available. Sudden cardiac death should be considered as a possible complication of refractory status epilepticus. The pathophysiology in SUDEP is currently unknown; yet a correlation between SUDEP and SIC is hypothesized to exist.

1. Introduction

Classically, stress-induced cardiomyopathy (SIC), more commonly known as takotsubo cardiomyopathy, displays the pathognomonic feature of echocardiographic, reversible left ventricular apical ballooning without angiographic coronary artery stenosis occurring after a stressful event [1, 2]. SIC is much more common among females than males, especially in older adults [3]. Typically, the temporary decline in ejection fraction (EF) resolves within a few days to weeks. More recently, variants of SIC that exhibit mid-ventricular regional wall motion abnormalities have been identified [3, 4]. Recent data suggests that SIC may be secondary to status epilepticus (SE) in up to 56% of cases [5]. Additionally, recurrence is associated with sudden unexplained death in epilepsy (SUDEP) in 3% of cases [5]. It is important to note that a study by Belcour et al. reports incidence of SIC in ICU patients admitted with convulsive status epilepticus, but these refractory cases do not represent all cases [5]. Recent case series present SUDEP as a one-time finding in a possible association with neurologic pathologies (i.e., seizures) [6]. In

this case, we are presenting a patient who develops recurrence of nonapical SIC secondary to status epilepticus.

2. Case Presentation

Our patient is a 49-year-old female with medical history significant for hypertension, refractory status epilepticus, and recent diagnosis of endometrioid endometrial carcinoma initially admitted to our institution for elective total abdominal hysterectomy and bilateral salpingoooophorectomy. She required an ICU admission for postoperative generalized tonic-clonic status epilepticus. Of note, she was hospitalized six months priorly for new onset seizure and subsequently identified stress-induced cardiomyopathy. During her previous hospitalization, her SIC resolved 10 days after initial identification of mid-ventricular to apical akinesia, demonstrated by EF of 25% on echocardiogram and minimal increase in troponin T to 0.03 (reference < 0.01). A coronary angiogram did not occur as part of the work-up of cardiomyopathy. Resolution of her episode of SIC was defined by a repeat echocardiogram showing EF of 60% without identifiable

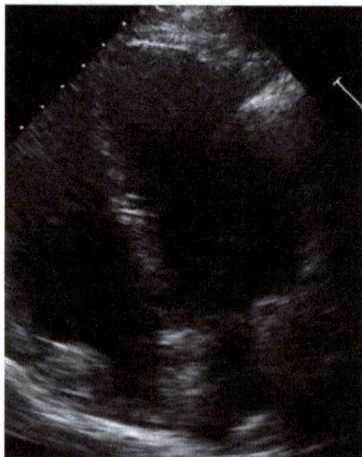

FIGURE 1: Preoperative TTE, end diastole (preop pics).

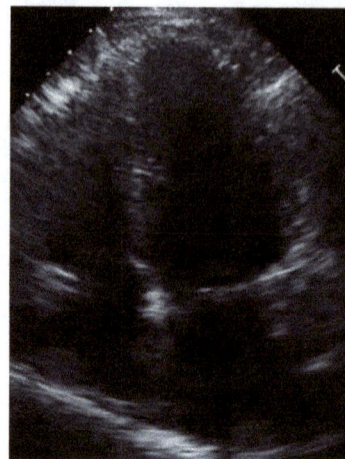

FIGURE 3: Preoperative TTE, end systole (preop pics).

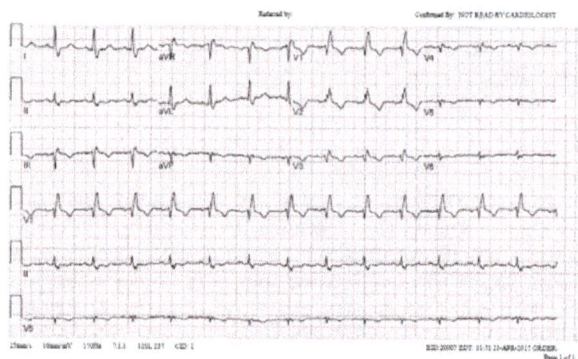

FIGURE 2: Preoperative/4 months after prior takotsubo cardiomy-opathy (preop pics).

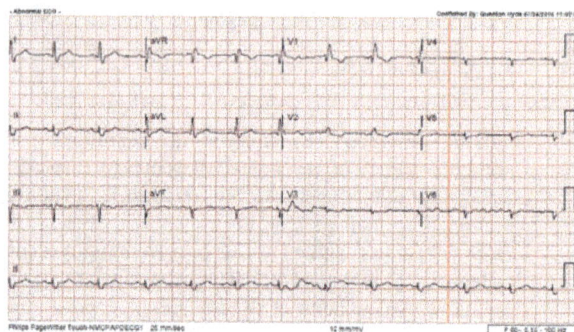

FIGURE 4: Immediately after seizure (postop pics).

wall motion abnormality (Figure 1, preoperative TTE, end diastole). After the first hospitalization, she had a follow-up nuclear stress test with EF of 72% without wall motion abnormality and electrocardiogram (ECG) with normal sinus rhythm (NSR) and right bundle branch block (RBBB) (Figure 2, preoperative/4 months after initial SIC).

Six months following her initial hospital discharge, a preoperative TTE demonstrated an EF of 60–65% without wall motion abnormality and an ECG having NSR and RBBB (Figures 1–3). In the postanesthesia care unit (PACU), though initially stable after surgery, the patient experienced a seizure and developed refractory status epilepticus (RSE) requiring admission to the ICU. Her seizures were described as being generalized tonic-clonic. Following management of her episode of RSE, her ECG demonstrated no ST segment elevation and sinus tachycardia (Figure 4, immediately after seizure). During this period, she was transferred to the ICU and a bedside TTE was performed. Though quality of imaging was limited by tachycardia, inferior and lateral wall akinesia was identified. Troponin I was obtained and elevated at 0.563 initially and after 6 hours at 0.762 (reference < 0.01). A formal TTE was performed the following day, which revealed posterior wall akinesia, septal wall dyskinesia, and

an EF of 15–20% (Figures 5 and 6, mid-ventricular akinesis at end systole and end diastole). Coronary angiogram was initially not performed due to the risk-benefit analysis of continued seizure activity on triple antiepileptic therapy and breakthrough benzodiazepine therapy. Combination of previous history of SIC after seizure, quick resolution of cardiac complications, and conversion to benzodiazepine coma to stop all seizure activity precluded the ability to perform coronary angiogram.

Four days after the initial cardiac event, another formal TTE was obtained which demonstrated no wall motion abnormality and her EF returned to a baseline of 60%, which was consistent with her previous admission (Figures 7 and 8, resolution SIC, end systole and end diastole). Three weeks postoperatively, she was hypertensive and tachycardic after extubation and required labetalol to control catecholamine surge to prevent exacerbation of SIC. Prior to discharge, she was restarted on carvedilol to prevent recurrent cardiomy-opathy, which was prescribed after her previous event. The patients' cardiovascular findings continued to improve after resolution of cardiomyopathy.

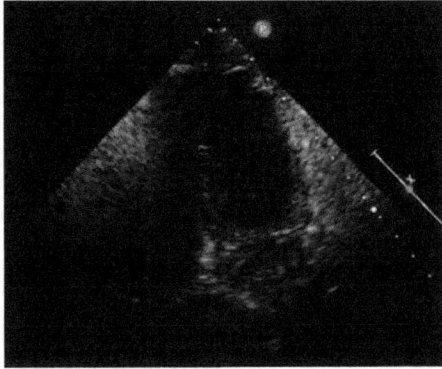

FIGURE 5: Mid-ventricular akinesis, end systole (postop pics).

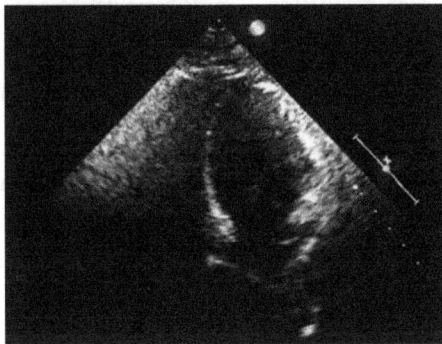

FIGURE 6: Mid-ventricular akinesis, end diastole (postop pics).

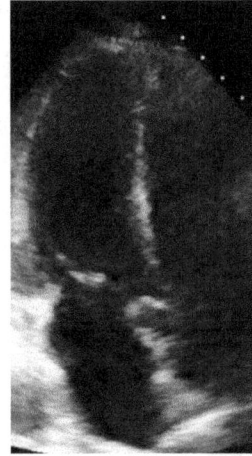

FIGURE 7: Resolution of SIC, end systole (SIC resolution pics).

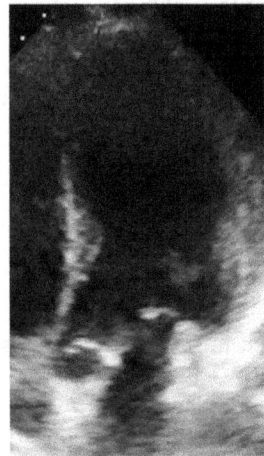

FIGURE 8: Resolution of SIC, end diastole (SIC resolution pics).

3. Discussion

During the management of our patient, close evaluation of ECG changes became necessary due to prolonged QT interval (QTI) effects of antiepileptic medications. Consideration for SIC after seizure warrants checking troponins as undiagnosed SIC may progress to cardiogenic shock and SUDEP [6]. As previously described, SIC may be secondary to surgery and the status may be secondary to cerebral hypoxia or metabolic abnormalities in the setting of surgery [7]. A cardiac catheterization could not be performed due to risks associated with RSE; in addition, other diagnostic information indicates SIC as a likely diagnosis. However, cardiac catheterization is not mandatory in typical SIC. Resolution of cardiac dysfunction ultimately occurred within four days, excluding the need for cardiac catheterization. The decision not to catheterize the coronary arteries was made on clinical risk-benefit analysis of patient safety. Vasospasm and plaque rupture could not be excluded in this case, due to resolution of cardiac complications prior to establishing a seizure-free baseline. However, our patient met all the other criteria for SIC and resolution of cardiac injury occurred within four days, making an infarct unlikely. This patient never requires hemodynamic pressor augmentation, making cardiogenic shock very unlikely.

This raises the question of whether the current guidelines are adequate and necessary for diagnosing this condition. Another important question to consider is how to best delineate subtypes of stress-induced cardiomyopathy. Our patient exhibited no apical ballooning and other case series have shown patients to have either dyskinesia/akinesia in wall motion or mid-ventricular ballooning especially following convulsive seizures [5, 8, 9]. Likewise, the association with varying stressors may involve other pathophysiologic pathways other than catecholamine surge that are not fully understood. Of consideration is the possibility of a neurocardiac pathway, as similar cardiomyopathy findings have been seen in intracranial hemorrhage [3, 4]. Recent case studies have shown an increased risk of SIC after seizure without classic symptoms of acute coronary syndromes (chest discomfort, radiating pain, shortness of breath, or crushing chest pain) [6].

Recent case studies and case series have elucidated the presence of nonapical involved cardiomyopathy associated with various stress precursors [4, 6]. Current subtypes recognized are apical and nonapical regional wall dysfunction, which in some instances may be associated with a subset of precipitating stressors. Recent case studies have involved patients with nonapical ballooning cardiomyopathy following hemorrhagic stroke or seizures in particular [5, 9, 10]. The case presented here involves recurrence of nonapical stress-induced cardiomyopathy following status epilepticus. SIC is observed to have recurrence by up to 11.4% over the first 4 years [9]. Future case series should review the incidence of recurrence of SIC associated with seizures. Additional topics of interest, assessing for recurrence of SIC as associated with type and severity of epileptic activity, and consideration of antiepileptic therapy and serum concentrations prove to increase risk of SIC and recurrence.

The current diagnostic standard for patients suspicious for SIC requires ruling out acute myocardial infarction, acute coronary syndrome, myocarditis, neurogenic pulmonary edema, and nonischemic cardiomyopathy. Therefore, ECG, TTE, cardiac enzymes (especially troponins), and cardiac catheterization should occur in order to rule out other causes [3, 8]. Diagnostic criteria include the following: transient apical or mid-ventricular ballooning with subsequent left ventricle (LV) dyskinesia/akinesia that extends beyond one coronary distribution, the absence of CAD or acute plaque rupture by cardiac catheterization as the source of myocardial dysfunction, new ECG changes such as transient ST segment elevation or diffuse T-wave inversions, and a mild to moderate elevation of troponins. The underlying pathophysiology is believed to be related to catecholamine surge generating a transient stress-induced demand ischemia [3, 4, 8].

Disclosure

The views expressed in this article are those of the authors and do not necessarily reflect the official policy or position of the Department of the Navy, Department of Defense, or the United States Government. The authors are military service members. This work was prepared as part of their official duties. Title 17 U.S.C. 105 provides that "Copyright protection under this title is not available for any work of the United States Government." Title 17 U.S.C. 101 defines a United States Government work as a work prepared by a military service member or employee of the United States Government as part of that person's official duties.

Competing Interests

The authors declare that there is no conflict of interests regarding the publication of this paper.

References

[1] M. Gianni, F. Dentali, A. M. Grandi, G. Sumner, R. Hiralal, and E. Lonn, "Apical ballooning syndrome or takotsubo cardiomyopathy: a systematic review," European Heart Journal, vol. 27, no. 13, pp. 1523–1529, 2006.

[2] T. M. Pilgrim and T. R. Wyss, "Takotsubo cardiomyopathy or transient left ventricular apical ballooning syndrome: a systematic review," International Journal of Cardiology, vol. 124, no. 3, pp. 283–292, 2008.

[3] K. A. Bybee and A. Prasad, "Stress-related cardiomyopathy syndromes," Circulation, vol. 118, no. 4, pp. 397–409, 2008.

[4] Y.-P. Lee, K.-K. Poh, C.-H. Lee et al., "Diverse clinical spectrum of stress-induced cardiomyopathy," International Journal of Cardiology, vol. 133, no. 2, pp. 272–275, 2009.

[5] D. Belcour, J. Jabot, B. Grard et al., "Prevalence and risk factors of stress cardiomyopathy after convulsive status epilepticus in ICU patients," Critical Care Medicine, vol. 43, no. 10, pp. 2164–2170, 2015.

[6] M. Dupuis, K. Van Rijckevorsel, F. Evrard, N. Dubuisson, F. Dupuis, and P. Van Robays, "Takotsubo syndrome (TKS): a possible mechanism of sudden unexplained death in epilepsy (SUDEP)," Seizure, vol. 21, no. 1, pp. 51–54, 2012.

[7] B. Acar, O. Kirbas, S. Unal, Z. Golbasi, and S. Aydogdu, "Reverse Takotsubo cardiomyopathy following intraabdominal surgery," Archives of the Turkish Society of Cardiology, vol. 44, no. 6, pp. 514–516, 2016.

[8] T. A. Boland, V. H. Lee, and T. P. Bleck, "Stress-induced cardiomyopathy," Critical Care Medicine, vol. 43, no. 3, pp. 686–693, 2015.

[9] S. Legriel, F. Bruneel, L. Dalle et al., "Recurrent Takotsubo cardiomyopathy triggered by convulsive status epilepticus," Neurocritical Care, vol. 9, no. 1, pp. 118–121, 2008.

[10] N. Benyounes, M. Obadia, J.-M. Devys, A. Thevenin, and S. Iglesias, "Partial status epilepticus causing a transient left ventricular apical ballooning," Seizure, vol. 20, no. 2, pp. 184–186, 2011.

42

Creutzfeldt-Jakob Disease Presenting as Expressive Aphasia and Nonconvulsive Status Epilepticus

Hafiz B. Mahboob ⓘ,[1,2] **Kazi H. Kaokaf,**[1,2] **and Jeremy M. Gonda**[1,2]

[1]*University of Nevada School of Medicine, Reno, NV, USA*
[2]*Renown Regional Medical Center, Reno, NV, USA*

Correspondence should be addressed to Hafiz B. Mahboob; hmahboob@medicine.nevada.edu

Academic Editor: Petros Kopterides

Creutzfeldt-Jakob disease (CJD), the most common form of human prion diseases, is a fatal condition with a mortality rate reaching 85% within one year of clinical presentation. CJD is characterized by rapidly progressive neurological deterioration in combination with typical electroencephalography (EEG) and magnetic resonance imaging (MRI) findings and positive cerebrospinal spinal fluid (CSF) analysis for 14-3-3 proteins. Unfortunately, CJD can have atypical clinical and radiological presentation in approximately 10% of cases, thus making the diagnosis often challenging. We report a rare clinical presentation of sporadic CJD (sCJD) with combination of both expressive aphasia and nonconvulsive status epilepticus. This patient presented with slurred speech, confusion, myoclonus, headaches, and vertigo and succumbed to his disease within ten weeks of initial onset of his symptoms. He had a normal initial diagnostic workup, but subsequent workup initiated due to persistent clinical deterioration revealed CJD with typical MRI, EEG, and CSF findings. Other causes of rapidly progressive dementia and encephalopathy were ruled out. Though a rare condition, we recommend consideration of CJD on patients with expressive aphasia, progressive unexplained neurocognitive decline, and refractory epileptiform activity seen on EEG. Frequent reimaging (MRI, video EEGs) and CSF examination might help diagnose this fatal condition earlier.

1. Introduction

We report a rare clinical presentation of sporadic CJD (sCJD) with combination of both expressive aphasia and NCSE. Isolated language problems and aphasia have been described in CJD before [1–8]; however, this combination is unique. This patient had an atypical clinical presentation with normal initial workup, but subsequent workup revealed CJD with typical EEG finding of spike-wave complexes (PSWCs) as well as hyperintensities in basal ganglia and cortical ribboning on MRI and positive CSF analysis for 14-3-3 proteins. Due to the extremely high mortality rate and often atypical clinical presentation and/or inconclusive initial workup, a high degree of suspicion and thus repeating workup might aid in early diagnose of this fatal condition.

2. Case Report

A 60-year-old male with a past medical history significant only for benign prostatic hyperplasia presented to our Emergency Department (ED) with chief complaints of gradual onset of progressively worsening speech difficulty (predominantly word finding with stuttering) and confusion (inability to recognize his family members).

His symptoms started four weeks priorly, beginning with constitutional symptoms of headache, fatigue, and vertigo. This slowly led to intermittent confusion, slurred speech, and intermittent spasms of his right upper and lower extremities. His spasms and weakness resulted in a fall from a tractor one week into the course of his symptoms fortunately without significant trauma nor loss of consciousness. His family gave additional potentially relevant information of a recent visit to Mexico where he stayed for four months before returning home. He was asymptomatic upon return to the USA, but symptoms started approximately four weeks later. Interestingly, while in Mexico, he worked in the cattle manure industry which he does locally as well. He was relatively healthy at baseline without any previous surgeries and no family history of diabetes, seizure, dementia, nor neurodegenerative conditions.

He initially visited an urgent care center with these complaints ten days prior to this hospital encounter. At that time, he was found to have a normal neurological examination, brain MRI, and carotid Doppler. He was discharged home with a working diagnosis of transient ischemic attack. His symptoms continued to worsen however, thus motivating him to present to the ED for further evaluation.

Upon arrival to the ED, he complained of photophobia, neck pain, and vertigo but was afebrile. His initial physical examination included vital signs: pulse 85 beats per minute, blood pressure 135/78 mmHg, temperature 98 F, and a respiratory rate of 18 per minute. Initial neurological examination was unremarkable except for persistent word finding difficulty. Initial lab work is summarized in table format (Table 1). A noncontrast head computed tomography (CT) scan was negative for any acute intracranial pathology. Initial CSF analysis was inconclusive for any acute infectious etiology although he had a mildly elevated protein level of 65 mg/dl (Table 2). He was admitted to the neurology unit and diagnosed with a complex migraine and treated with intravenous (IV) ketorolac, sumatriptan, and promethazine. A neurology consult was obtained and an EEG ordered.

Initial EEG on his second hospital day showed focal seizures emanating from the left frontal region (Figure 1(a)) and he was started on oral levetiracetam (loading dose of 1 gram followed by 750 mg PO twice daily thereafter). He started complaining of right upper extremity weakness and on repeat physical exam was found to have diminished deep tendon reflexes of his right upper extremity (RUE) with weakness in pronation and fine motor activity. On hospital day #3, he developed intermittent myoclonic jerking of his RUE with a fine, persistent tremor. At this point intermittent focal seizure activity was thought to be precipitated from his minor head trauma related to his fall. Differential diagnoses, though less likely, included an infectious etiology which was excluded with negative microbiology, a stroke despite a normal MRI, or other common metabolic causes including electrolyte abnormalities, ammonia, toxins, and liver and kidney dysfunction. Medications were also considered which could potentially lower seizure threshold, and tramadol and diphenhydramine were discontinued.

Over the next few days he gradually became drowsier and confused with worsening of his expressive aphasia and development of cerebellar dysfunction on exam. His dose of levetiracetam was increased to 1 gm twice daily. Initial MRI of brain during this hospital encounter was performed which did not show any acute intracranial lesion except mild cerebral and cerebellar substance loss (Figure 2(a)).

His cognition and right upper extremity shaking/tremor rapidly worsened and, on hospital day #4, EEG was significant for persistent focal seizures in left hemisphere despite being on levetiracetam (Figure 1(a)). He was started on lacosamide 200 mg twice daily in addition to the ongoing levetiracetam increased now to 1 gm three times daily. Continuous EEG was started at this point to closer monitor effectiveness of therapies. A repeat MRI brain with contrast on hospital day #5 showed developing cytotoxic edema in the left frontal and

TABLE 1: Laboratory data.

Variable	Value
Microbiology	
CSF	Negative for bacterial growth
	Negative for acid fast bacilli (AFB)
Autoimmune panel serum:	
Microsomal TPO antibody	<0.2 IU/ml
Thyroxine binding globulin	19.3 microgram/ml
Anti-TG Ab	<0.2 IU/ml
HIV 1/2 PCR	None
Lyme	0.07 (Ref: ≤0.99 LIV)
FT Ab	Non-reactive
West Nile Virus (IgM)	None
SSA, 52 (Ro)	1 AU/ml
SSA, 60 (Ro)	1 AU/ml
Sjogren's Ab	0 AU/ml
ANA	None
Cysticercosis Ab, IgG by ELISA	0.0 (Ref: OD ≤ 0.34)
Paraneoplastic antibodies serum:	
ANNA (1–3)	Negative
AGNA-1	Negative
PCA (1-2)	<1 : 240 Negative
PCA-Tr	<1 : 240 Negative
Amphiphysin	<1 : 240 negative
CRMP-% IgG	<1 : 120 Negative
Striational Ab	0.0 nmol/L
P/Q type calcium channel Ab	0.0 nmol/L
	0.0 nmol/L
Ach receptor (muscle binding AB)	0.0 nmol/L
	0.0 nmol/L
Ach receptor (ganglionic neuronal Ab)	0.0 nmol/L
Neuronal (V-G) K+ channel Ab	0.0 nmol/L
Other labs:	
WBC	6.1×10^9/L
Neutrophil	73%
Hemoglobin	15.9 g/dl
Hematocrit	45.3%
Platelets	211×10^9/L
MCV	86 fl
Lymphocyte	30.70%
Eosinophil	1.88%
Polys	62%

TABLE 1: Continued.

Variable	Value
Sodium	136 mEq/L
Potassium	3.5 mEq/L
Chloride	105 mEq/L
Bicarbonate	22 mEq/L
BUN	15 mg/dl
Creatinine	0.79 mg/dl
Anion Gap	9 mEq/L
Vitamin B 12	800 pg/ml
Thyroglobulin	2.0 ng/ml
TSH	4.016 microIU/ml
CRP	0.14 mg/L
AST	22 unit/L
ALT	21 unit/L
ALP	61 unit/L
Calcium	9.6 mg/dl
T-Bili	0.5 mg/dl
Albumin	4.4 g/dl
Total protein	7.5 g/dl

parietal lobe with punctate calcified lesions in right cortex (Figure 2(b)) which was considered likely due to persistent seizure activity. Given the initial CSF result showing elevated proteins (65 mg/dl), ongoing myoclonus, and the newly developed vasogenic edema on MRI, the decision was made by neurology at this point, to start a 3-day course of pulse dose steroids (solumedrol 1 gm IV/daily) for possible autoimmune encephalitis (AE) while awaiting the finalized autoimmune workup [9, 10].

Unfortunately, despite the increasing doses of antiepileptics and the high dose steroids, the patient continued to decline neurologically. Continuous EEG revealed persistent epileptogenic activity with bilateral hemispheric discharges (left > right) (Figure 1(b)). Valproic acid (500 mg orally three times daily) was added to his regimen and lacosamide increased to 200 mg three times daily. His initial CSF (collected on the first hospital day) was sent for oligoclonal bands and infectious encephalopathies which all eventually came back negative (Table 2). Acyclovir was started empirically for possible viral encephalitis but subsequently discontinued two days later when CSF resulted negative.

During the next few days (hospital days nine to eleven) he remained globally aphasic with RUE flaccidity. He would awaken but was unable to follow commands. A repeat MRI showed persistent ribboning in the left hemispheric region (Figure 2(c)) and EEG (Figure 1(c)) showed "diffuse epileptiform discharge suggestive of encephalopathic state with presence of continuous left frontal and sometimes synchronized bifrontal sharps spikes with a more generalized appearance, which was concerning for nonconvulsive status epilepticus." Perampanel was added to his antiseizure regimen at dose of 4 mg twice daily. Efficacy of perampanel has been established as an adjunct treatment for partial-onset seizures with or without secondary generalization and primary generalized tonic-clonic seizures in idiopathic generalized epilepsy as well as for treatment of refractory seizures. This patient was having refractory seizures; therefore, this medication was added [11].

At this point CJD was considered among other possible etiologies such as paraneoplastic encephalitis, meningeal carcinomatous, infectious cerebritis, and primary CNS angiitis given his continued deterioration and refractory status epilepticus. Computed tomography angiogram (CTA) excluded the primary central nervous system (CNS) angiitis. A repeat lumbar puncture was performed with additional CSF tests ordered including Epstein-Barr virus (EBV), acid fast bacilli (AFB), fungal culture, Zika virus, 14-3-3 protein, neurocysticercosis antibodies, and an autoimmune and paraneoplastic panel.

Eventually phenobarbital (16.2 mg twice daily) was started yet he continued to deteriorate remaining aphasic with flaccid paralysis in RUE and lost his ability to protect his airway requiring intubation on hospital day #11. His EEG remained without any significant improvement. On hospital day #13, while awaiting results from his repeat CSF analysis, neurology felt it was prudent to again trial high dose steroids (solumedrol 1 gm IV daily) for potential AE which continued for the next 5 days without obvious efficacy.

He remained in a persistent coma at this point and lost reflexes to even deep painful stimuli while cEEG showed continuous episodic sharp wave from left frontal and synchronized bifrontal discharge was obvious on lowering his sedation (Figure 1(c)). Seizures were refractory to extensive antiseizure medication regimen including keppra 1500 mg twice daily, lacosamide 200 mg three times daily, perampanel 4 mg twice daily, phenobarbital 120 mg twice daily, and valproic acid 1 gm twice daily.

On hospital day #23, his course was complicated by development of ventilator associated pneumonia, for which he was started on vancomycin and cefepime. Cultures from bronchoalveolar lavage were negative.

His neurological condition did not improve with EEG persistently showing frequent generalized epileptiform discharges (Figure 1(d)). Repeat MRI brain (Figure 2(d)) showed extensive and persistent worse cortical ribboning particularly around the left hemisphere, and involving right frontal, and limited involvement of the basal ganglia without any acute infarct on diffusion weighted imaging (DWI) (suggestive of cytotoxic edema from prolonged seizure activity and early CJD). Tissue diagnosis from brain biopsy was discussed but, given hospital policy and limitations, deemed not possible.

On hospital day #26, his CSF finally resulted from the national laboratory positive for 14-3-3 protein, tau protein, and Real-Time Quaking-Induced Conversion (RT-QuIC) proteins, confirming prion disease. Before giving his family the news of the results, and for prognostication purposes, his sedation was held for several hours. On physical exam, he lacked any withdrawal response to painful stimuli but maintained cough and gag reflexes with a minimal, sluggish pupillary reflex. EEG (Figure 1(d)) at that time showed a worsening seizure activity pattern which initially started as focal left frontal lobe diffuse spike-wave complexes but now

TABLE 2: Cerebrospinal fluid analysis.

CSF	Day 1	Day 12
Number of tubes	*2*	*4*
Character/color	*Colorless/clear*	*Colorless/clear*
Volume	*4 ml*	*20 ml*
WBC	*0 cells/unit*	*3 cells/unit*
RBC	*7 cells/unit*	*9 cells/unit*
Lymphocytes	*46%*	*14%*
Mononuclear cells	*54%*	*3%*
Glucose CSF	*63 mg/dl*	*66 mg/dl*
Total protein, CSF	*65 mg/dl*	*28 mg/dl*
IgG CSF	*3.5 mg/dl*	-
Lacrosse-California IgG		<1:1
Lacrosse-California IgM		<1:1
East Equine Virus IgG		<1:1
East Equine Virus IgM		<1:1
St Louis Virus IgG		<1:1
St Louis Virus IgM		<1:1
Western Equine Venezuela Virus IgG		<1:1
Western Equine Venezuela Virus IgM		<1:1
West Nile IgG, CSF		0.03
West Nile IgM, CSF		0.01
Varicella Zoster Virus		
Oligoclonal bands		
VDRL		Non-Reactive
Cocci Ab Ig G		0.1
Cocci Ab Ig M		0.0
Coccidioides AB ID		Not detected
Coccidioidomycosis Ab		<1:2
EBV, DNA quant interpretation		Not detected
EBV, Qnt log		<2.6 units: log
EBV, Quant source		CSF
EBV virus, Copy/m		<390 copy/ml
Encephalitis/meningitis panel on CSF by PCR		
E. *Coli K -1*		Not detected
H. *Influenza*		Not detected
L. *Monocytogenes*		Not detected
N *Meningitides*		Not detected
S. *agalactae*		Not detected
S. *Pyogenes*		Not detected
Cytomegalovirus		
Herpes Simplex Virus (HSV 1 & 2)		
Human herpes Virus-6		
Varicella Zoster Virus		
Cryptococcus Neoformans		

TABLE 2: Continued.

CSF	Day 1	Day 12
Paraneoplastic Panel		
AGNA-1		
Amphiphysin Ab		
ANNA-1		
Reflex Added		Negative <1 : 2
ANNA-2		
CRMP-5		
PCA-1 and 2		
PCA-Tr		
S-100B		3230 ng/L
RT QuIC		POSITIVE
14-3-3 Protein		+++
T- Tau Protein		++ 9094 pg/ml

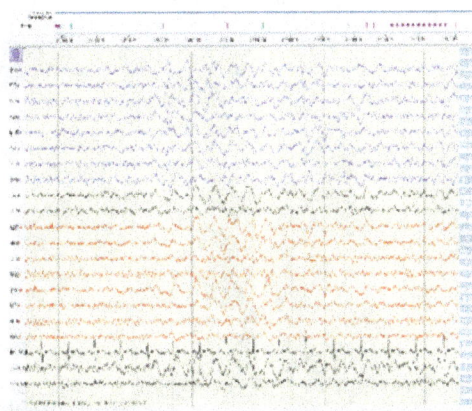

(a) Hospital day one to hospital day four: consistent with focal seizure activity from left hemisphere (frontal)

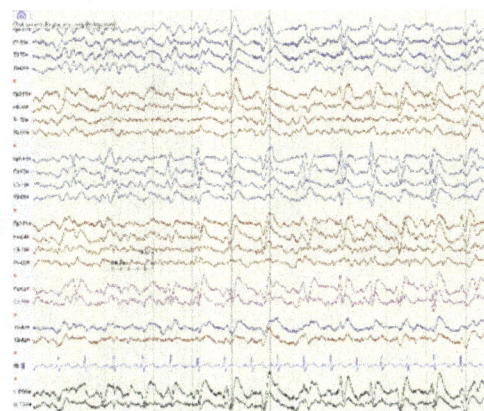

(b) Hospital day eight and day nine: continuous EEG revealed persistent epileptogenic activity with bilateral hemispheric discharges (left > right)

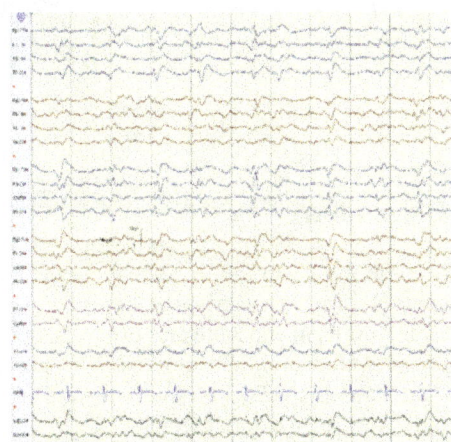

(c) Hospital day fourteen: 24 hours' video EEG showing diffuse epileptiform discharge suggestive of encephalopathic state with presence of continuous left frontal and sometimes synchronized bifrontal sharp spikes with a more generalized appearance suggestive of NCSE

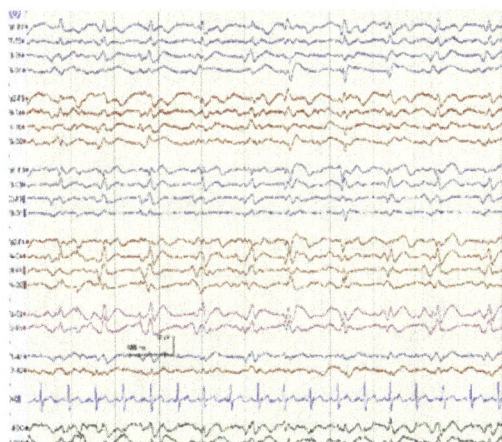

(d) Hospital day twenty-eight: EEG consistent with nonconvulsive status epilepticus (NCSE)

FIGURE 1: *EEG studies.*

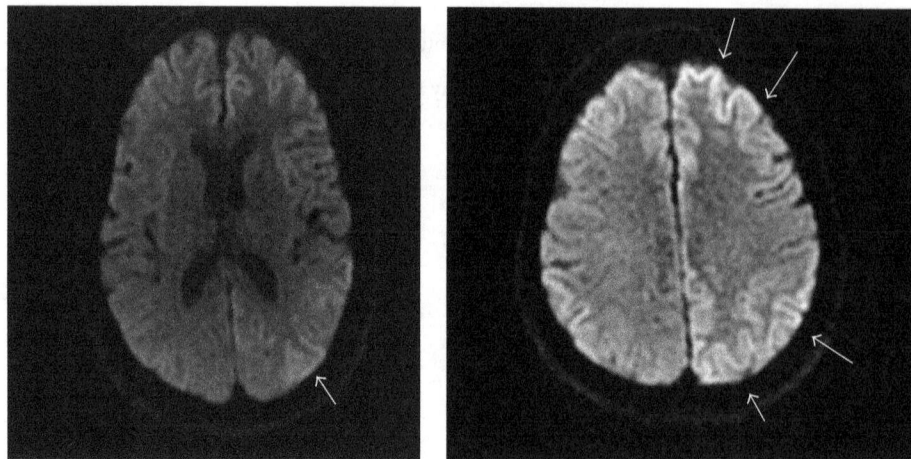

(a) Hospital day two: no evidence of acute pathology except mild diffuse cerebral and cerebellar substance loss on MRI

(b) Hospital day five: DW-MRI showing cortical and gyriform diffusion signal hyperintensity with cortical ribbon edema (cytotoxic edema) in the left frontal and parietal lobes, likely due to persistent seizure activity. Punctate calcification in the right frontal cortex is also visible

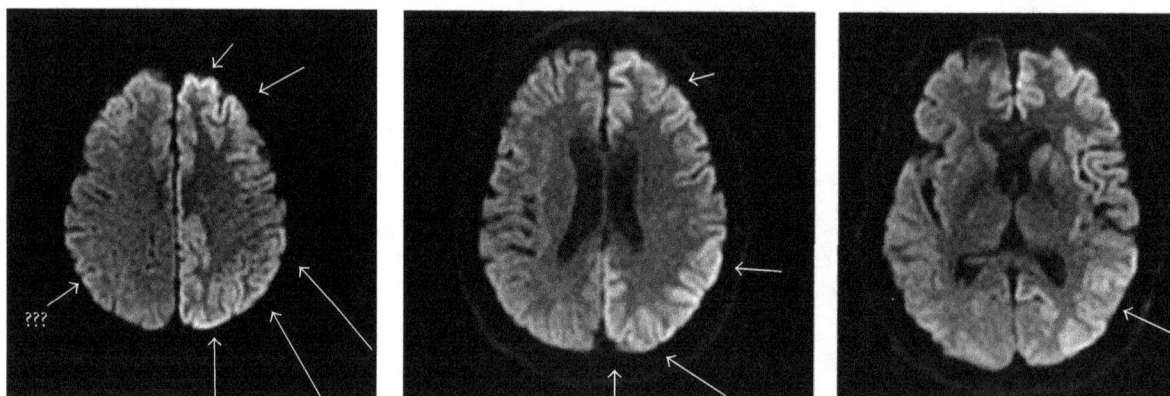

(c) Hospital day nine: persistent cortical ribboning particularly around the left hemisphere with frontal lobe > parietal lobe. There is also involvement of right frontal cortex

(d) Hospital day twenty-three: extensive and persistent worsening of cortical ribboning particularly around the left hemisphere and involving right frontal and limited involvement of the basal ganglia

FIGURE 2: *MRIs.*

had progressed into generalized epileptiform discharges with development of nonconvulsive status epilepticus (NCSE).

A family conference was held discussing the patient's terminal diagnosis and a decision was made to transition the patient to comfort care with compassionate extubation. He died shortly after extubation with family at bedside. The county health department was involved in his case and investigations were performed at the local manure plant to test for potential cow involvement, usually seen in variant (vCJD), which was unremarkable. However, our patient's age of disease onset, typical EEG (PSWC), absent pulvinar sign on MRI as well as lack of past medical/surgical and family history was not consistent with vCJD. Thus, he was diagnosed with probable sCJD. His remains were cremated, and his ashes taken to Mexico by family preventing final genetic testing to be performed.

3. Discussion

CJD is the most commonly seen form of prion diseases in humans [1]. This is a fatal neurodegenerative disease which typically results in subacute and progressive deterioration in cognitive, behavioral, and motor function over a period of weeks to months [12–15]. Typical clinical presentation also includes startle myoclonus, cerebellar, pyramidal, extrapyramidal, behavioral, and visual defects with a characteristic periodic sharp complex on the EEG [16, 17]. Other neurocognitive disorders including Alzheimer's disease, Lewy body dementia, vascular dementia, and frontotemporal dementia tend to have slower course and gradual cognitive decline [18].

Based on its etiology, CJD is divided into sporadic (most common), variant (vCJD), iatrogenic, and familial forms [14, 19]. Genetic analysis of prion protein gene (PRNP) can help to identify different forms of CJD and to subclassify them based on molecular phenotype [20, 21].

Sporadic form is seen in older age and previous diagnosis of psychosis, multiple surgeries, and living in the farm (garden or animal farm) for more than 10 years are associated risk factors [22]. Our patient had worked in a cow manure plant although investigations performed at the local manure plant to test for potential cow involvement were unremarkable. Variant CJD is seen in younger age and represents bovine-to-human transmission. It manifests with early sensory disturbances and psychiatric symptoms rather than cognitive decline [23]. EEG usually do not show PSWCs and a slow wave pattern is predominant [20, 24]. Symmetrical hyperintensity in the pulvinar nuclei of the thalamus termed as "pulvinar" sign is 90% specific for vCJD [25, 26]. Our patient in terms of clinical presentation (age, personal and family history, EEG, and MRI findings) falls under sCJD.

Although the diagnosis may be straightforward in older adults who present with the classic clinical and radiological presentation, the diagnosis becomes challenging if the initial presentation is atypical both clinically and in terms of imaging [27].

CJD have presented with a variety of atypical clinical syndromes including but not limited to amyopathy, deafness, and cataracts [28–30] and often with nonspecific constitutional signs and symptoms such as dizziness [12]. Our patient also did have a work-related fall and difficulty waking but he did not have evidence of amyopathy (absence of fasciculation and areflexia). His right upper extremity weakness was likely related to involvement of left frontal cortex with seizure activity resulting in "postictal" weakness. He did not have an isolated period of constitutional symptoms before cognitive decline as some other patients did [12]. He did not have deafness or cataracts. He did have vertigo, which is hard to differentiate if being of central or of peripheral origin.

CJD is a rare but an important stroke mimic making it challenging to differentiate between the two, as CJD develops mostly in elderly population who usually also have risk factors for stroke [27]. Our patient had no evidence of stroke.

Seizures have been reported in up to 15% of patients with CJD during the disease course [1]. However, seizures are reported as initial manifestation of the CJD disease only in 3% of cases [31]. Status epilepticus is reported in less than 15% of patients of sCJD [14]. Our patient's EEG identified focal seizure activity early during the hospitalization which then progressed to NCSE as patient deteriorated.

Akinetic mutism is a known entity in patients in the final stages of CJD [32]. In contrast to akinetic mutism (again seen in the late stages), patients can have aphasia as a manifestation of CJD [3–8]. Aphasia at disease onset, however, is much less common [2]. This patient is a rare clinical presentation of sporadic CJD (sCJD) with combination of both expressive aphasia and NCSE.

Early recognition of potentially treatable etiologies can minimize the morbidity and mortality. Because of the delayed availability of results for autoimmune and paraneoplastic etiologies on CSF, we empirically used steroids to treat possible underlying autoimmune encephalopathy. Steroids can be empirically given in the setting of an elevated CSF protein (as our case) or personal or family history of an autoimmune disease [10]. However, there is not enough evidence to routinely recommend the use of steroids as a routine treatment in rapidly progressive dementia. We did not use intravenous immunoglobulin (IVIG) or plasmapheresis since we did not have enough evidence to support the diagnosis of AE [11].

CSF analysis for protein 14-3-3 has positive predictive value of 93% to 95% but its sensitivity is low [33]. Other CSF proteins such as tau and neuron-specific enolase are nonspecific general markers of neuronal injury and their utility is questionable due to lack of specificity [15].

The most common EEG finding in CJD is diffuse slowing pattern. However, the characteristic EEG findings for CJD are periodic synchronous bi- or triphasic or mixed sharp wave complexes (PSWCs) which have a specificity for sCJD ranging from 66% to 91% [1, 20, 34, 35]. However, its sensitivity is variable based on genotypes of sCJD [34]. PSWCs are sensitive to disease stage and external stimulation [20]. Lateralized PSWCs are seen during the disease course and represent the prodromal stage of disease onset, which then progresses in bifrontal distribution as disease advances as in our patient [35]. EEG-related spikes are independent of the traditional clinical finding of myoclonic jerking and are usually seen while patient is awake. Sleep deprivation usually exacerbate them, and benzodiazepines can mask the PSWCs [20]. We noticed similar pattern in our patient (Figures 1(c) and 1(d)).

Use of DWI or fluid attenuated inversion recovery (FLAIR) and apparent diffusion coefficient (ADC) modalities have significantly improved the sensitivity and specificity to 96% and 93%, respectively, of MRI for diagnosis of CJD [20, 26]. Hyperintensities in the putamen and head of the caudate nuclei are the most common findings on conventional MRI sequences in patients with CJD [36]. Other typical MRI findings in CJD include hyperintensities with diffusion restriction in the frontal, temporal, occipital, insular, and/or parietal regions referred to as cortical ribboning. Moreover, MRI is helpful to identify any other potential inflammatory, infectious, and toxic-metabolic causes of rapidly progressive dementia which might be mimicking CJD [20, 26]. Our patient had similar extensively worsening cortical ribboning pattern (Figure 2(d)).

MRI pattern may be affected by disease stage. DWI is considered superior during early stages of CJD [26]. Later during the disease course hyperintensity decreases and the only findings may be cortical atrophy [37]. Studies have shown that hyperintensity on DWI and ADC studies correlates with the symptoms and clinical course of the disease. Hyperintensity of basal ganglia on DWI is believed to be associated with a shorter disease duration and higher incidence of myoclonus [20]. Our patient had hyperintensity on basal ganglia and disease course was shorter and he had myoclonus (few weeks). One study reported a potential correlation between hyperintense lesions in the occipital cortex on DWI and shorter time between symptom onset and akinetic mutism [38]. Our patient did not show any occipital lobe lesions and did not develop akinetic mutism.

Definitive diagnosis can be established only with tissue diagnosis from brain biopsy or on autopsy tissue and genetic analysis is required as well. However, getting a biopsy is often not possible (as in our case) because of the concern for appropriate tissue handling and to prevent cross-contamination. Diagnostic yield of brain biopsy is low with traditional sampling methods [20] but newer techniques have shown better diagnostic yield [39]. We did not do biopsy as we have enough evidence from noninvasive work to substantiate the probable diagnosis of CJD. We recommend getting biopsy if it can potentially affect the treatment plan or disease course, and appropriate tissue handling is available.

Currently, there is no definite treatment available for this lethal condition. Antiepileptic drugs are used for myoclonic symptoms along with supportive and palliative care. There is no need to isolate the patient, but careful handling of CSF and brain tissue is strongly recommended.

Our patient had an atypical initial clinical presentation but with progressive changes in his radiological, EEG, and CSF findings becoming more typical and diagnostic for CJD. The progression of his imaging (MRI and EEG) and laboratory (CSF) abnormalities correlated well with his neurological deterioration. This emphasizes that uncommon etiologies must be considered in cases of unexplained and rapid neurological deterioration, especially with altered mentation and/or presence of refractory seizure activity. Close clinical monitoring is prudent and needs to be correlated with neuroimaging and cerebrospinal fluid analysis, which might aid in the early diagnosis of this lethal condition.

4. Conclusion

CJD can often have atypical clinical and radiological presentation. Diffuse epileptiform discharge (NCSE) on EEG in a patient with unexplained rapid cognitive decline and confusion might be a presentation of sCJD [14]. Potential reversible causes of rapidly progressive dementia such as autoimmune, infectious, and toxic-metabolic etiologies must be ruled out before making the final diagnosis of prion disease [12]. Continuous video EEG monitoring is crucial, especially if refractory epileptiform activity is suspected [40]. Due to the fatality of CJD, high degree of suspicion is prudent to initiate subsequent workup in instances of persistent/progressive unexplained neurocognitive decline and atypical clinical presentation and/or inconclusive initial workup.

References

[1] D. Cohen, E. Kutluay, J. Edwards, A. Peltier, and A. Beydoun, "Sporadic Creutzfeldt-Jakob disease presenting with nonconvulsive status epilepticus," *Epilepsy & Behavior*, vol. 5, no. 5, pp. 792–796, 2004.

[2] S. El Tawil, G. Chohan, J. Mackenzie et al., "Isolated language impairment as the primary presentation of sporadic Creutzfeldt

Jakob Disease," *Acta Neurologica Scandinavica*, vol. 135, no. 3, pp. 316–323, 2017.

[3] J.-E. Song, D.-W. Yang, H.-J. Seo et al., "Conduction aphasia as an initial symptom in a patient with Creutzfeldt-Jakob disease," *Journal of Clinical Neuroscience*, vol. 17, no. 10, pp. 1341–1343, 2010.

[4] S. E. McPherson, J. D. Kuratani, J. L. Cummings, J. Shih, P. S. Mischel, and H. V. Vinters, "Creutzfeldt-Jakob disease with mixed transcortical aphasia: Insights into echolalia," *Behavioural Neurology*, vol. 7, no. 3-4, pp. 197–203, 1994.

[5] E. C. Shuttleworth, A. J. Yates, and J. D. Paltan-Ortiz, "Creutzfeldt–Jakob disease presenting as progressive aphasia," *Journal of the National Medical Association*, vol. 77, no. 8, pp. 649-650, 1985.

[6] A. Kirk and L. C. Ang, "Unilateral Creutzfeldt-Jakob disease presenting as rapidly progressive aphasia," *Canadian Journal of Neurological Sciences/Journal Canadien des Sciences Neurologiques*, vol. 21, no. 4, pp. 350–352, 1994.

[7] A. E. Hillis, "Aphasia: Progress in the last quarter of a century," *Neurology*, vol. 69, no. 2, pp. 200–213, 2007.

[8] A. M. Mandell, M. P. Alexander, and S. Carpenter, "Creutzfeldt-jakob disease presenting as isolated aphasia," *Neurology*, vol. 39, no. 1, pp. 55–58, 1989.

[9] F. Zuhorn, A. Hübenthal, A. Rogalewski et al., "Creutzfeldt-Jakob disease mimicking autoimmune encephalitis with CASPR2 antibodies," *BMC Neurology*, vol. 14, no. 1, article no. 227, 2014.

[10] F. Graus, M. J. Titulaer, and R. Balu, "A clinical approach to diagnosis of autoimmune encephalitis," *The Lancet Neurology*, vol. 15, no. 4, pp. 391–404, 2016.

[11] C. Di Bonaventura, A. Labate, M. Maschio, S. Meletti, and E. Russo, "AMPA receptors and perampanel behind selected epilepsies: current evidence and future perspectives," *Expert Opinion on Pharmacotherapy*, vol. 18, no. 16, pp. 1751–1764, 2017.

[12] M. D. Geschwind, H. Shu, A. Haman, J. J. Sejvar, and B. L. Miller, "Rapidly progressive dementia," *Annals of Neurology*, vol. 64, no. 1, pp. 97–108, 2008.

[13] E. Gozke, N. Erdal, and M. Unal, "Creutzfeldt-Jacob Disease:a case report," *Cases Journal*, vol. 1, no. 1, article 146, 2008.

[14] P. S. Espinosa, M. K. Bensalem-Owen, and D. B. Fee, "Sporadic Creutzfeldt-Jakob disease presenting as nonconvulsive status epilepticus case report and review of the literature," *Clinical Neurology and Neurosurgery*, vol. 112, no. 6, pp. 537–540, 2010.

[15] M. H. Rosenbloom and A. Atri, "The evaluation of rapidly progressive dementia," *The Neurologist*, vol. 17, no. 2, pp. 67–74, 2011.

[16] C. C. Weihl and R. P. Roos, "Creutzfeldt-Jakob disease, new variant Creutzfeldt-Jakob disease, and bovine spongiform encephalopathy," *Neurologic Clinics*, vol. 17, no. 4, pp. 835–859, 1999.

[17] R. Roods, D. C. Gajdusek, and C. J. Gibbs, "The clinical characteristics of transmissible creutzfeldt-jakob disease," *Brain*, vol. 96, no. 1, pp. 1–20, 1973.

[18] P. Roohani, M. K. Saha, and M. Rosenbloom, "Creutzfeldt-Jakob disease in the hospital setting: a case report and review," *Minnesota Medicine*, vol. 96, no. 5, pp. 46–49, 2013.

[19] A. Ladogana, M. Puopolo, E. A. Croes et al., "Mortality from Creutzfeldt-Jakob disease and related disorders in Europe, Australia, and Canada," *Neurology*, vol. 64, no. 9, pp. 1586–1591, 2005.

[20] M. Manix, P. Kalakoti, M. Henry et al., "Creutzfeldt-Jakob disease: updated diagnostic criteria, treatment algorithm, and the utility of brain biopsy," *Neurosurgical Focus*, vol. 39, no. 5, article E2, 2015.

[21] P. Parchi, A. Giese, S. Capellari et al., "Classification of sporadic Creutzfeldt-Jakob disease based on molecular and phenotypic analysis of 300 subjects," *Annals of Neurology*, vol. 46, no. 2, pp. 224–233, 1999.

[22] D. P. W. M. Wientjens, Z. Davanipour, A. Hofman et al., "Risk factors for Creutzfeldt-Jakob disease: A reanalysis of case-control studies," *Neurology*, vol. 46, no. 5, pp. 1287–1291, 1996.

[23] C. A. Heath, S. A. Cooper, K. Murray et al., "Diagnosing variant Creutzfeldt - Jakob disease: A retrospective analysis of the first 150 cases in the UK," *Journal of Neurology, Neurosurgery & Psychiatry*, vol. 82, no. 6, pp. 646–651, 2011.

[24] S. Binelli, P. Agazzi, G. Giaccone et al., "Periodic electroencephalogram complexes in a patient with variant Creutzfeldt-Jakob disease," *Annals of Neurology*, vol. 59, no. 2, pp. 423–427, 2006.

[25] R. G. Will, M. Zeidler, G. E. Stewart et al., "Diagnosis of new variant Creutzfeldt-Jakob disease," *Annals of Neurology*, vol. 47, no. 5, pp. 575–582, 2000.

[26] P. Vitali, E. MacCagnano, E. Caverzasi et al., "Diffusion-weighted MRI hyperintensity patterns differentiate CJD from other rapid dementias," *Neurology*, vol. 76, no. 20, pp. 1711–1719, 2011.

[27] D. K. Sharma, M. Boggild, A. W. Van Heuven, and R. P. White, "Creutzfeldt-Jakob disease presenting as stroke: a case report and systematic literature review," *The Neurologist*, vol. 22, no. 2, pp. 48–53, 2017.

[28] P. K. Panegyres, E. Armari, and R. Shelly, "A patient with Creutzfeldt-Jakob disease presenting with amyotrophy: a case report," *Journal of Medical Case Reports*, vol. 7, article 218, 2013.

[29] R. Salazar, M. Cerghet, and V. Ramachandran, "Bilateral hearing loss heralding sporadic Creutzfeldt-Jakob disease: A case report and literature review," *Otology & Neurotology*, vol. 35, no. 8, pp. 1327–1329, 2014.

[30] M. A. Leitritz, B. Leo-Kottler, M. Batra, K. Ostertag, K. U. Bartz-Schmidt, and M. S. Spitzer, "Cataract as 'initial symptom' of Creutzfeld-Jacob disease," *Acta Ophthalmologica*, vol. 90, no. 6, pp. e489–e490, 2012.

[31] R. V. Gibbons, R. C. Holman, E. D. Belay, and L. B. Schonberger, "Creutzfeldt-Jakob disease in the United States: 1979–1998," *Journal of the American Medical Association*, vol. 284, no. 18, pp. 2322-2323, 2000.

[32] A. Otto, I. Zerr, M. Lantsch, K. Weidehaas, C. Riedemann, and S. Poser, "Akinetic mutism as a classification criterion for the diagnosis of Creutzfeldt-Jakob disease," *Journal of Neurology, Neurosurgery & Psychiatry*, vol. 64, no. 4, pp. 524–528, 1998.

[33] M. D. Geschwind, J. Martindale, D. Miller et al., "Challenging the clinical utility of the 14-3-3 protein for the diagnosis of sporadic Creutzfeldt-Jakob disease," *JAMA Neurology*, vol. 60, no. 6, pp. 813–816, 2003.

[34] I. Zerr, W. J. Schulz-Schaeffer, A. Giese et al., "Current clinical diagnosis in Creutzfeldt-Jakob disease: Identification of uncommon variants," *Annals of Neurology*, vol. 48, no. 3, pp. 323–329, 2000.

[35] H. G. Wieser, K. Schindler, and D. Zumsteg, "EEG in Creutzfeldt-Jakob disease," *Clinical Neurophysiology*, vol. 117, no. 5, pp. 935–951, 2006.

[36] D. A. Collie, R. J. Sellar, M. Zeidler, A. C. F. Colchester, R. Knight, and R. G. Will, "MRI of Creutzfeldt-Jakob disease: Imaging features and recommended MRI protocol," *Clinical Radiology*, vol. 56, no. 9, pp. 726–739, 2001.

[37] L. Letourneau-Guillon, R. Wada, and W. Kucharczyk, "Imaging of prion diseases," *Journal of Magnetic Resonance Imaging*, vol. 35, no. 5, pp. 998–1012, 2012.

[38] T. Gao, J.-H. Lyu, J.-T. Zhang et al., "Diffusion-weighted MRI findings and clinical correlations in sporadic Creutzfeldt–Jakob disease," *Journal of Neurology*, vol. 262, no. 6, pp. 1440–1446, 2015.

[39] J. M. Schott, L. Reiniger, M. Thom et al., "Brain biopsy in dementia: Clinical indications and diagnostic approach," *Acta Neuropathologica*, vol. 120, no. 3, pp. 327–341, 2010.

[40] D. Friedman, J. Claassen, and L. J. Hirsch, "Continuous electroencephalogram monitoring in the intensive care unit," *Anesthesia & Analgesia*, vol. 109, no. 2, pp. 506–523, 2009.

43

Severe Rhabdomyolysis due to Presumed Drug Interactions between Atorvastatin with Amlodipine and Ticagrelor

Iouri Banakh,[1] Kavi Haji,[2,3] Ross Kung,[2] Sachin Gupta,[2,3] and Ravindranath Tiruvoipati[2,3]

[1]Department of Pharmacy, Frankston Hospital, Peninsula Health, Frankston, VIC 3199, Australia
[2]Department of Intensive Care Medicine, Frankston Hospital, Peninsula Health, Frankston, VIC 3199, Australia
[3]School of Public Health, Faculty of Medicine, Nursing and Health Sciences, Monash University, Clayton, VIC 3800, Australia

Correspondence should be addressed to Iouri Banakh; ibanakh@phcn.vic.gov.au

Academic Editor: Kurt Lenz

Atorvastatin and ticagrelor combination is a widely accepted therapy for secondary prevention of ischaemic heart disease. However, rhabdomyolysis is a well-known rare side effect of statins which should be considered when treatments are combined with cytochrome P450 3A4 enzyme inhibitors. We report a case of atorvastatin and ticagrelor associated severe rhabdomyolysis that progressed to multiorgan failure requiring renal replacement therapy, inotropes, intubation, and mechanical ventilation. Despite withdrawal of the precipitating cause and the supportive measures including renal replacement therapy, creatinine kinase increased due to ongoing rhabdomyolysis rapidly progressing to upper and lower limbs weakness. A muscle biopsy was performed to exclude myositis which confirmed extensive myonecrosis, consistent with statin associated rhabdomyolysis. After a prolonged ventilatory course in the intensive care unit, patient's condition improved with recovery from renal and liver dysfunction. The patient slowly regained her upper and lower limb function; she was successfully weaned off the ventilator and was discharged for rehabilitation. To our knowledge, this is a second case of statin associated rhabdomyolysis due to interaction between atorvastatin and ticagrelor. However, our case differed in that the patient was also on amlodipine, which is considered to be a weak cytochrome P450 3A4 inhibitor and may have further potentiated myotoxicity.

1. Introduction

Statins are a widely used class of drugs that has an established benefit in patients with ischaemic heart disease (IHD) at the highest tolerated doses [1–3]. Statin associated rhabdomyolysis (SAR), although rare, is a well-recognized life threatening adverse effect [4]. "Rhabdomyolysis is a severe form of muscle damage associated with very high creatinine kinase (CK) levels, with myoglobinaemia and/or myoglobinuria with a concomitantly increased risk of renal failure" [4]. The rise of CK during rhabdomyolysis that is associated with lipid lowering therapy is usually more than 10 times upper limit of normal [5]. The risk of SAR is increased with increased statin potency, increased statin blood concentration, age greater than 75 years, female gender, and low body mass index [4]. This is potentiated by patient characteristics, preexisting comorbidities such as hepatic, renal, metabolic, or neuromuscular diseases, and drug interactions [4].

The incidence of SAR is rare, estimated at 1 per 100,000 per year, but the risk may be increased when statins are combined with Cytochrome P450 3A4 (CYP3A4) enzyme inhibitors [4]. Here we present a case report of an elderly patient with a diagnosis of SAR due to presumed cardiovascular drug interactions with several intrinsic factors for the adverse event.

2. Case Presentation

A 74-year-old Maltese female was transferred to our hospital from a rural emergency department following an unwitnessed collapse preceded by several days of generalized weakness. Her significant past medical history included ST elevated myocardial infarction, hypertension, depression, osteoarthritis requiring a total hip replacement, and osteoporosis. Her weight was stable at 51 kg with a body mass index of 22.5. She was a nonsmoker and she consumed on average

TABLE 1: Changes in haematological and biochemical parameters during the course of the disease.

Parameter	Day 1	Day 6	Day 7	Day 8	Day 11	Day 13	Day 69
Haemoglobin (115–165 g/L)	119	77	104	82	95	88	91
Platelets (150–450)	251	113	170	136	23	29	404
INR (<1.3)	1.8	1.7	1.7	2	1.8	1.8	1.3
APTT (26–36 seconds)	53	41	39	49	40	107	28
Urea (3–10 mmol/L)	18.4	8.7	12.8	11.2	12	9.1	11
Creatinine (40–80 micromol/L)	480	143	173	93	75	48	88
Estimated GFR (>60 mL/min/1.73 m^2)	7	31	25	52	68	90	55
Total bilirubin (<15 micromol/L)	53	108	157	156	167	163	10
ALT (0–30 units/L)	746	1094	1605	1537	1228	1346	30
AST (<35 units/L)	1153	1736	2591	2020	1219	890	46
GGT (<35 units/L)	527	348	399	387	234	224	134
ALP (30–115 units/L)	260	232	293	325	248	208	104
pH (7.38–7.43)	7.34	7.46	7.46	7.5	7.42	7.5	7.43
Bicarbonate (20–24 mmol/L)	11	23	15	21	22	24	34
Base excess (−3.3–1.2 mmol/L)	13.2	0.3	7.2	1.1	1.2	1.8	8.6
Lactate (0.5–2.0 mmol/L)	1.5	3.3	7.4	4.2	4.1	2.9	1.4

APTT: activated partial thromboplastin time, INR: International Normalised Ratio, and GFR: Glomerular Filtration Rate.

one unit of alcohol per day. Her admission medications included amlodipine, atorvastatin, ticagrelor, metoprolol, aspirin, amitriptyline, perindopril, and weekly risedronate. She had been treated with a combination product of amlodipine and atorvastatin for several years. Two and a half months prior to her admission, she was diagnosed with ST elevation myocardial infarction, which was medically managed due to unsuccessful percutaneous coronary intervention to reopen a blocked artery. Her management included an increased dose of amlodipine/atorvastatin combination from 5/20 mg to 5/80 mg and antiplatelet therapy of low-dose aspirin in addition to ticagrelor 90 mg twice a day as per treatment guidelines.

In the rural emergency department, the patient was hypotensive and had minimum urine output. She received fluid resuscitation of 4 litres and was commenced on noradrenaline infusion at 10 micrograms per minute. The initial diagnosis was septic shock and acute kidney injury with a creatinine level of 404 μmol/L and urea of 17 mmol/L. She had mild neutrophilia. The chest X-ray and computed tomography of the brain and the cervical spine were reported as unremarkable. She was then transferred to our intensive care unit (ICU) due to lack of ICU services at the referring hospital.

Upon admission to ICU, the patient appeared confused, but cooperative. She was moving her 4 limbs. Her heart rate, blood pressure, respiratory rate, and temperature were 86 beats per minute, 102/42 mmHg, 15 breaths per minute, and 35.7°C, respectively, while receiving 10 micrograms per minute of noradrenaline. She was well oxygenated on 2 litres per minute of oxygen. She was tender on her right lumber region, while the rest of the physical examination was unremarkable. The liver function was significantly deranged, with alteration in the coagulation profile and worsening renal function (Table 1).

The computed tomography and the ultrasound of the abdomen revealed a calculus thickened gall bladder with pericholecystic fluid and free fluid in the abdomen. The diagnosis of acute cholecystitis that resulted in multiorgan failure was affirmed. On subsequent assessment however, the abdominal symptoms and signs had dissipated, and surgery was no longer indicated. Continuous venovenous haemodialysis and filtration (CVVHDF) was commenced due to worsening metabolic acidosis and acute anuric renal failure.

On day 2, the patient developed worsening muscle pain and progressive weakness in the upper and lower limbs with diminished tendon reflexes. The creatinine kinase (CK) was profoundly elevated approaching 100000 U/L (Figure 1) and there was a progressive deterioration in the liver function (Table 1). On further microbiological, biochemical, and serological assessment, sepsis, haemolysis, vasculitis, thyroid disorders, and paracetamol toxicity were excluded. A provisional diagnosis of autoimmune myositis or SAR was suggested. On day 7 magnetic resonance imaging (MRI) of the musculoskeletal system revealed features consistent with upper and lower limbs proximal myositis. MRI targeted muscle biopsy was also performed. CK was persistently elevated with worsening liver function; disseminated intravascular coagulation developed leading to epistaxis, upper gastrointestinal bleeding, and subcutaneous haemorrhage. She continued to have moderate neutrophilia, modest increase in the C-reactive protein.

The disseminated intravascular coagulopathy was treated with platelets and clotting factors replacement and with Vitamin K. A presumed diagnosis of autoimmune myositis was made. Further deterioration in the patient state, while waiting for the biopsy results, prompted treatment with 1 gram of intravenous methylprednisolone daily for 3 consecutive days for the potential autoimmune aetiology of her presentation. The patient was more fatigued, becoming drowsy and hypoxic and requiring endotracheal intubation and ventilation. The muscle biopsy revealed extensive myonecrosis of similar

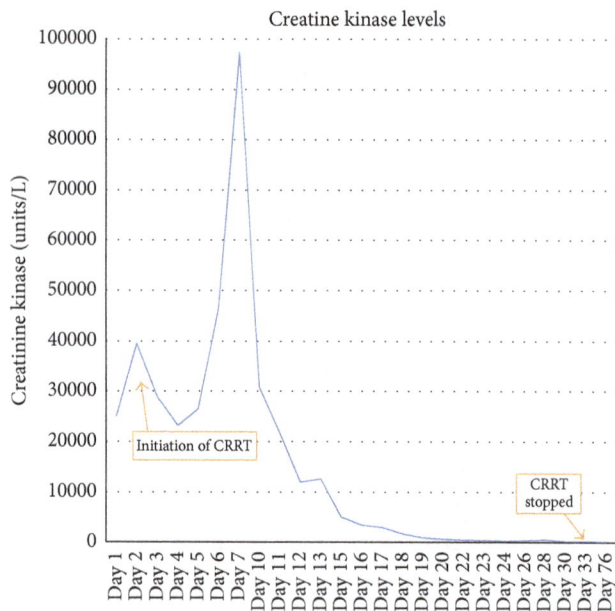

FIGURE 1: Changes in creatinine kinase levels during the course of patient stay.

age and scant regeneration, consistent with toxin induced necrotising myositis.

Her condition gradually improved and CK levels gradually returned to within the normal range (Figure 1). Due to profound weakness, she was rendered difficult to be weaned off mechanical ventilation and subsequently received percutaneous tracheostomy. The renal and liver function gradually improved and CVVHDF was discontinued. The renal biopsy confirmed acute tubular necrosis with extensive myoglobin-related cast formation. She was gradually weaned off the ventilator and the tracheostomy tube was removed in the ICU. She was mechanically ventilated for a total of 1041 hours and she stayed in ICU for 69 days. She was discharged to the medical ward and subsequently discharged to a rehabilitation centre.

3. Discussion

Our case highlights a serious drug induced myotoxicity from high dose atorvastatin, two and a half months after instituting ticagrelor and continuing with amlodipine. A coprescribed statin and a P2Y12 inhibitor are standard therapy for secondary prevention of IHD. However, possibilities of drug interactions in this patient were overlooked. To our knowledge this is the second case of SAR due to an interaction between atorvastatin and ticagrelor [6]. Kido et al. [6] reported a case of similar interaction that led to rhabdomyolysis as the adverse event, though their patient was over a decade younger and was obese. Notably, our patient was also receiving amlodipine, a calcium channel blocker, which may have further contributed to SAR [7]. The patient presented in this case report had no other known causes or predisposing factors for rhabdomyolysis such as trauma, ischaemia, or metabolic disorders [5]. However, rarer

causes of rhabdomyolysis such as mitochondrial disorders or inherited gene mutations were not investigated as the there was a clear drug-related precipitating factor identified early into patient's presentation, as well as the muscle biopsy supporting the diagnosis with a picture consistent with toxin related muscle necrosis [5].

Ticagrelor is an oral antiplatelet agent that binds reversibly to P2Y12 receptors. Ticagrelor differs from clopidogrel, in that it has a faster onset of action, higher platelet inhibition, and a higher morbidity reduction [8]. Dose adjustment is not required to prevent bleeding excluding severe hepatic impairment irrespective of age, gender, ethnicity, or renal impairment [9]. There is a minor increase in the myotoxic effect of atorvastatin when combined with ticagrelor, with area under concentration (AUC) curve 1.4-fold increase, while simvastatin AUC is increased 2-3-fold [10]. Ticagrelor is a known weak inhibitor of the CYP3A enzymes and P-glycoprotein, with the risk of drug interactions with other drugs affected by these pathways considered to be low [9, 11]. The latest American Heart Association (AHA) recommendation from 2016 for using the atorvastatin and ticagrelor is that the "combination is reasonable" [10]. While others have suggested that the interaction between ticagrelor and statins metabolised via CYP3A4 may have provided an added benefit in the primary ticagrelor registration study [12], the interaction may have clinical implications from a safety point of view also [6]. Coadministration of ticagrelor with a high dose of atorvastatin 80 mg had led to a clinically significant rise in statin concentration in our patient's case. Although this is considered a minor risk in young healthy volunteers [9], such a combination with a large dose of atorvastatin was sufficient to cause extensive rhabdomyolysis in our patient. Further, the latest guideline from the AHA has classified ticagrelor as low risk drug interaction for myotoxicity when coadministered with atorvastatin and has recommended that no dose alteration is required [10].

Our patient was also exposed to another drug that may have contributed to the increased risk of rhabdomyolysis. Amlodipine is a dihydropyridine calcium channel blocker that is frequently used for hypertension and angina management [13]. It is frequently combined and sold as a combination product with atorvastatin (Caduet®). In healthy volunteers this product has been found to be safe. One study showed no change in the maximum concentration of atorvastatin from the combination, with the AUC for atorvastatin increasing by 18% [13]. Amlodipine is a weak inhibitor of both CYP3A4 and CYP3A5 enzymes [13, 14] and may effectively not only contribute to a higher atorvastatin AUC, but also increase exposure to ticagrelor and its active metabolite. This boost to ticagrelor levels may in turn add to higher atorvastatin AUC contribution due to a greater extent of enzyme inhibition.

4. Conclusion

This case illustrates that when high doses of atorvastatin are coadministered with ticagrelor, as secondary prevention for IHD, the combination may pose a risk for serious myotoxicity. Moreover, multiple therapies with CYP3A inhibitors, which in this case were ticagrelor and amlodipine, may further increase the risk of statin associated rhabdomyolysis. Further, awareness of statin myotoxic risks should always be raised in susceptible patients; close monitoring and dose alteration are recommended when multiple CYP3A inhibitors are administered.

Authors' Contributions

Iouri Banakh and Kavi Haji have equally contributed to writing of this case report.

References

[1] D. P. Chew, I. A. Scott, L. Cullen, J. K. French, T. G. Briffa, P. A. Tideman et al., "National Heart Foundation of Australia & Cardiac Society of Australia and New Zealand: Australian clinical guidelines for the management of acute coronary syndromes 2016," *Heart Lung and Circulation*, vol. 25, no. 9, pp. 895–951, 2016.

[2] M. Roffi, C. Patrono, and J.-P. Collet, "2015 ESC Guidelines for the management of acute coronary syndromes in patients presenting without persistent ST-segment elevation: task force for the management of acute coronary syndromes in patients presenting without persistent ST-segment Elevation of the European Society of Cardiology (ESC)," *European Heart Journal*, vol. 37, no. 3, pp. 267–315, 2016.

[3] E. A. Amsterdam, N. K. Wenger, R. G. Brindis, D. E. Casey Jr., T. G. Ganiats, D. R. Holmes Jr. et al., "2014 AHA/ACC guideline for the management of patients with non-st-elevation acute coronary syndromes: a report of the American college of cardiology/American heart association task force on practice guidelines," *Journal of American College of Cardiology*, vol. 64, no. 24, pp. e139–228, 2014.

[4] E. S. Stroes, P. D. Thompson, A. Corsini et al., "Statin-associated muscle symptoms: impact on statin therapy—European Atherosclerosis Society Consensus Panel Statement on Assessment, Aetiology and Management," *European Heart Journal*, vol. 36, no. 17, pp. 1012–1022, 2015.

[5] L. O. Chavez, M. Leon, S. Einav, and J. Varon, "Beyond muscle destruction: a systematic review of rhabdomyolysis for clinical practice," *Critical Care*, vol. 20, no. 1, article no. 135, 2016.

[6] K. Kido, M. B. Wheeler, A. Seratnahaei, A. Bailey, and J. A. Bain, "Rhabdomyolysis precipitated by possible interaction of ticagrelor with high-dose atorvastatin," *Journal of the American Pharmacists Association*, vol. 55, no. 3, pp. 320–323, 2015.

[7] N. De Schryver, X. Wittebole, P. Van den Bergh, V. Haufroid, E. Goffin, and P. Hantson, "Severe rhabdomyolysis associated with simvastatin and role of ciprofloxacin and amlodipine coadministration," *Case Reports in Nephrology*, vol. 2015, Article ID 761393, 4 pages, 2015.

[8] L. Wallentin, R. C. Becker, A. Budaj et al., "Ticagrelor versus clopidogrel in patients with acute coronary syndromes," *The New England Journal of Medicine*, vol. 361, no. 11, pp. 1045–1057, 2009.

[9] R. Teng, "Ticagrelor: pharmacokinetic, pharmacodynamic and pharmacogenetic profile: an update," *Clinical Pharmacokinetics*, vol. 54, no. 11, pp. 1125–1138, 2015.

[10] B. S. Wiggins, J. J. Saseen, R. L. Page et al., "Recommendations for management of clinically significant drug-drug interactions with statins and select agents used in patients with cardiovascular disease: a Scientific Statement from the American Heart Association," *Circulation*, vol. 134, no. 21, pp. e468–e495, 2016.

[11] R. Teng, P. D. Mitchell, and K. A. Butler, "Pharmacokinetic interaction studies of co-administration of ticagrelor and atorvastatin or simvastatin in healthy volunteers," *European Journal of Clinical Pharmacology*, vol. 69, no. 3, pp. 477–487, 2013.

[12] J. J. DiNicolantonio and V. L. Serebruany, "Exploring the ticagrelor-statin interplay in the PLATO trial," *Cardiology*, vol. 124, no. 2, pp. 105–107, 2013.

[13] Y.-T. Zhou, L.-S. Yu, S. Zeng, Y.-W. Huang, H.-M. Xu, and Q. Zhou, "Pharmacokinetic drug-drug interactions between 1,4-dihydropyridine calcium channel blockers and statins: factors determining interaction strength and relevant clinical risk management," *Therapeutics and Clinical Risk Management*, vol. 10, no. 1, pp. 17–26, 2014.

[14] Y.-C. Wang, T.-C. Hsieh, C.-L. Chou, J.-L. Wu, and T.-C. Fang, "Risks of adverse events following coprescription of statins and calcium channel blockers: A nationwide population-based study," *Medicine*, vol. 95, no. 2, Article ID e2487, 2016.

44

Icatibant for Angiotensin-Converting Enzyme Inhibitor-Induced Angioedema in Intubated Patients: Case Series and Literature Review

Erin K. Yeung [ID],[1,2] **Haritha Saikumar,**[3] **Jose Castaneda-Nerio,**[3]
Sandra G. Adams [ID],[3,4] **and Mark Wong** [ID][1,2]

[1]*Department of Pharmacy Services, South Texas Veterans Health Care System, 7400 Merton Minter, San Antonio, TX 78229, USA*
[2]*Pharmacotherapy Education & Research Center, The University of Texas Health San Antonio, 7703 Floyd Curl Dr.,*
MSC 6220, San Antonio, TX 78229-3900, USA
[3]*Medicine Service, Pulmonary/Critical Care Division, South Texas Veterans Health Care System, 7400 Merton Minter (111E),*
San Antonio, TX 78229, USA
[4]*Department of Medicine, Pulmonary/Critical Care Division, The University of Texas Health San Antonio,*
7703 Floyd Curl Dr., MSC 7885, San Antonio, TX 78229-3900, USA

Correspondence should be addressed to Erin K. Yeung; erinkyeung@gmail.com

Academic Editor: Natale Daniele Brunetti

Purpose. A case series of icatibant use in intubated patients with angiotensin-converting enzyme inhibitor- (ACEI-) induced angioedema is presented along with a relevant literature review and recommendations for utilization. *Summary.* Three intubated patients admitted to the intensive care unit for ACEI-induced angioedema were treated with icatibant. A literature search identified one controlled study and four case reports describing the use of icatibant in intubated ACEI-induced angioedema patients. *Conclusion.* Icatibant administration in intubated patients may be beneficial in decreasing time to extubation and length of intensive care unit stay. In the three cases described, icatibant administration did not appear to elicit a response in intubated patients, which has been described in previous case reports. For clinicians considering icatibant in the treatment of ACEI-induced angioedema, earlier administration upon arrival to the ED or immediately upon arriving to the intensive care unit is strongly advised. The suggested benefit of icatibant in intubated ACEI-induced angioedema patients should be verified by randomized clinical trials and cost-benefit analyses should be performed at individual institutions.

1. Introduction

ACEI-induced angioedema accounts for approximately one-third of angioedema cases treated in emergency departments (ED) [1]. It is estimated to occur in approximately 0.68% of patients who take an FDA-approved ACEI [2]. Factors contributing to higher risk for ACEI-induced angioedema include: African ancestry; age > 65 years; female gender; history of smoking; heart failure; treatment with statins, aspirin, or sirolimus; and history of drug rashes, seasonal allergies, or previous angioedema [1].

Icatibant is a bradykinin 2 (B2) receptor antagonist that was FDA-approved in 2011 for the treatment of hereditary angioedema [3]. Due to ACEI-induced bradykinin

degradation inhibition and subsequently increased B1/B2 activation, icatibant has also been used as an off-label medication for the treatment of ACE-induced angioedema [2]. Evidence on off-label icatibant usage for ACEI-induced angioedema includes case reports, observational studies, and three randomized, controlled trials [2, 4, 5]. In 2015, Baş et al. treated 13 Caucasian adults presenting to the ED for ACEI-induced angioedema of the upper aerodigestive tract with icatibant and found a significantly shorter time to complete resolution of ACEI-induced angioedema compared to combination glucocorticoid plus antihistamine (prednisolone plus clemastine) therapy within 10 hours of symptom onset. The median time to onset of symptom relief was also significantly shorter with icatibant than with standard therapy (2 hours

TABLE 1: Summary of patient cases.

Patients, n	Case 1	Case 2	Case 3
Characteristics			
Gender	Female	Male	Male
Age, years	60	52	62
Ethnicity	African American	African American	Caucasian
Duration of ACEI therapy, months	81	36	48
Symptoms	Difficulty breathing and swallowing, shortness of breath, coughing	Chest pain, difficulty swallowing and talking, shortness of breath, sensations of "throat closing," swelling of tongue, mouth, and eyes	Macroglossia, muffled voice, shortness of breath
Clinical course			
Symptom onset to ED presentation	1 week	4 hours	5 hours
ED presentation to intubation, mins	20	"Minutes later"	Immediately
ED presentation to icatibant, hrs	12	11	11
Icatibant administration	After intubation	After intubation	After intubation
Icatibant to first symptom resolution, hrs	20	22	11
Hospital day of extubation	Day 4	Day 5	Day 3
ED presentation to discharge	Day 7	Day 6	Day 5

versus 11.7 hours). None of the patients required intubation/tracheostomy. Only one patient in the placebo group experienced no improvement after six hours of initial therapy and required rescue icatibant with prednisolone intervention [4]. Therefore, the authors concluded that icatibant can be used in patients with ACEI-induced angioedema within 10 hours of symptom onset to prevent respiratory intervention (intubation or tracheostomy). On the contrary, Straka et al. treated 13 patients (including Caucasian and African American) with ACEI-induced angioedema within six hours of presentation with icatibant and did not find any difference in the time to symptom resolution compared to placebo. One patient treated with icatibant could not complete the visual analog scale used to measure resolution of symptoms due to intubation and was subsequently excluded from the final analysis [5]. Similarly, a randomized, controlled, double-blind trial by Sinert et al. did not find a difference in time to meeting discharge criteria or time to onset of symptom relief between icatibant and placebo treatment for ACEI-induced angioedema in 121 patients [6].

While evidence exists to suggest significantly faster resolution of ACEI-induced angioedema with icatibant treatment, nearly all patients analyzed in randomized, controlled trials were not intubated [4–6]. Therefore, the efficacy and utility of icatibant in intubated ACEI-induced angioedema patients remain unclear. It may be hypothesized that icatibant administration in an intubated patient may decrease time to extubation and intensive care unit length of stay compared to alternative interventions.

The aim of this article is to share real-life clinical experience of three cases in which patients received icatibant after respiratory intervention, such as intubation and tracheostomy, as a result of ACEI-induced angioedema. In addition, a review of available literature describing other clinical experiences with icatibant utilization in intubated patients is discussed.

2. Methods

A literature review using articles published through April 2017 from PubMed and MEDLINE databases was conducted using the search terms *icatibant, angiotensin-converting enzyme induced angioedema*, and *intubation*. Search results were limited to English-language studies conducted on humans. Studies, case reports, and case series describing patients who received icatibant after receiving respiratory interventions were included.

3. Case Reports

The three patient cases include one female and two male patients who were intubated due to respiratory distress or failure from ACEI-induced angioedema. Their clinical course leading up to icatibant administration and response thereafter is described (Table 1).

3.1. Case 1. A 60-year-old African American female with hypertension presented to the ED with a chief complaint of sudden difficulty in breathing and swallowing after experiencing shortness of breath and coughing for one week. The patient had been on lisinopril therapy for 6 years and 9 months, with a recent increase in dose to 40 mg only two months prior to ED presentation. Home medications also included amlodipine 10 mg daily. The patient was given diphenhydramine en route to the ED and treated with epinephrine nebulization, dexamethasone 10 mg IV, famotidine 20 mg IV, and epinephrine 0.5 mg IM injection upon arrival. Approximately 20 minutes after ED arrival, the patient deteriorated with respiratory failure and required intubation due to severe macroglossia and lip swelling with facial fullness. Her lungs were clear to auscultation. The patient subsequently received two units of fresh frozen plasma (FFP), IV ranitidine, diphenhydramine, and methylprednisolone without improvement. The decision was then made to administer icatibant. Icatibant 30 mg was administered subcutaneously approximately 12 hours after presenting to the ED. Subjective improvement in lip, throat, and tongue edema was not noted until approximately 20 hours after icatibant administration. Steroid therapy was weaned over several days before a laryngoscopy was performed on fourth day of hospitalization. The laryngoscopy showed marked improvement in airway edema and the patient was then successfully extubated. The patient was subsequently downgraded from the intensive care unit on day 5 and discharged from the hospital on seventh day of hospitalization.

3.2. Case 2.

A 52-year-old African American male with a history of hypertension presented to the ED with complaints of chest pain, difficulty in swallowing and talking, shortness of breath, sensations of "throat closing," and swelling of the tongue, mouth, and eyes. Per patient report, the swelling had started approximately four hours prior to ED arrival. Upon chart review, the patient was found to have also presented to the ED two days earlier with similar symptoms of lip swelling. During that ED presentation, the patient was treated with a prednisone burst before being sent home with amoxicillin. The patient was noted to have been on lisinopril for hypertension for nearly 3 years, but patient instructions to discontinue lisinopril were not found in the electronic medical record. Upon the subsequent presentation to the ED, the patient was noted to have labored breathing and massive macroglossia without visualization of the uvula on physical exam. He was immediately treated with IM epinephrine, IV diphenhydramine, dexamethasone, and famotidine. Minutes later, the patient became unresponsive and required cardiopulmonary resuscitation. The patient was successfully intubated after multiple attempts due to a difficult airway. Two units of FFP were subsequently administered and the patient continued treatment on IV methylprednisolone, diphenhydramine, famotidine, and albuterol/ipratropium nebulization. Icatibant 30 mg was administered subcutaneously approximately 11 hours after ED presentation and 15 hours after symptom onset. Subjective improvement of lip and eye swelling was noted within 22 hours after icatibant administration. The patient was extubated and downgraded from the intensive care unit on fifth day and discharged on sixth day of hospitalization.

3.3. Case 3.

A 62-year-old Caucasian male with a history of hypertension presented to the ED with progressive macroglossia and muffled voice which began approximately five hours earlier. Initially, the patient denied shortness of breath but began to develop dyspnea upon arriving to the ED, particularly while supine. Per patient recall, he had experienced a similar episode several years ago and was told that he had an unknown medication allergy. The patient had been on lisinopril for hypertension management for four years. Home medications also included amlodipine 10 mg daily. Upon arrival, the patient was treated with IM epinephrine, IV dexamethasone, diphenhydramine, and famotidine. He was subsequently taken to the operating room, where a

laryngoscopy revealed evidence of significant compromised airway with posterior supraglottic edema, trace edema of the epiglottis, prominent base of tongue mucosa, and uvula hydrops. An awake fiberoptic nasal intubation was then performed. After intubation, the patient continued treatment on methylprednisolone 80 mg IV. The patient then received one subcutaneous dose of icatibant 30 mg approximately 11 hours after ED presentation and 16 hours after symptom onset. Subjective improvement of tongue and submandibular soft tissue swelling was noted approximately 11 hours after icatibant administration. A cuff leak test was attempted one day after icatibant administration to no avail. On third day of hospitalization, a cuff leak was present and the patient was successfully extubated. The patient was then downgraded from the intensive care unit on fourth day and discharged on fifth day of hospitalization.

4. Discussion and Literature Review

No randomized controlled trials have specifically evaluated the utility of icatibant in patients that required respiratory intervention (intubation or tracheostomy) prior to icatibant administration (Table 2). The randomized controlled trial by Straka et al. included three intubated patients treated with icatibant and one intubated patient treated with placebo; there was no statistical difference in the number of intubated patients between groups ($p = 0.32$) [5]. One of the icatibant-treated intubated patients was excluded from final analysis due to sedation and subsequent inability to participate in a visual analog scale. The authors did not specify whether intubation occurred before or after the assigned intervention. Time to extubation was also not described. Overall results found no difference in the time to symptom resolution compared to placebo (Kaplan-Meier curve, $p = 0.192$) [5].

Several other case series and reports have described the use of icatibant in intubated patients for ACEI-induced angioedema. In a case series by Javaud et al. in 2015, one of 62 patients treated with icatibant for ACEI-induced angioedema required immediate tracheal intubation upon presentation to the ED [7]. The age, gender, and ethnicity of this individual and angioedema severity were not specified. The patient was intubated before icatibant injection and successfully extubated on second day after complete resolution of edema [7]. Another case series by Fok et al. in 2015 described four of 13 patients treated with icatibant after requiring intubation upon presenting to the ED with ACEI-induced angioedema [10]. Three of these patients were determined to have type 2 angioedema (angioedema of the floor of the mouth, palate, or oropharynx), while the remaining patient had type 3 angioedema (angioedema of the hypopharynx or larynx). One of the patients with type 2 angioedema received icatibant one hour prior to intubation, while the two other patients received icatibant at the time of intubation. The patient with type 3 angioedema received the dose of icatibant 72 hours after ED presentation per recommendations by immunology consult. Two of the patients were aged >60 years and three of the patients were female, but the ethnicities of each patient were not specified. The duration of ACEI therapy ranged from one day to 20 years. Three of the four patients were

TABLE 2: Review of previously published cases of icatibant utilization in intubated patients.

	Straka et al. [5]	Javaud et al. [7]	Charmillon et al. [8]	Illing et al. [9]
Study type	Randomized controlled trial	Prospective observation study	Case report	Case report
Patients, n	3	1	1	1
Characteristics				
Gender	--	--	Female	Male
Age, years	--	--	65	62
Ethnicity	--	--	Caucasian	--
Duration of ACEI therapy, months	--	--	--	60
Symptoms	--	--	Tongue/facial swelling/severe dyspnea	Drooling/tongue swelling
Clinical course				
Symptom onset to ED presentation	--	--	--	--
ED presentation to intubation, mins	--	--	--	--
ED presentation to icatibant	--	--	--	--
Icatibant administration	--	After intubation	After intubation	Before intubation
Icatibant to first symptom resolution, hrs	--	--	1	"Slow resolution over 48 hours"
Hospital day/time to extubation from icatibant	--	Day 2	Day 3	48 hours
ED presentation to discharge	--	--	Day 3	"A few days later" after extubation
Conclusion	No difference in number of intubated patients between groups or time to symptom resolution compared to placebo	Icatibant use for ACEI-induced angioedema elicits faster symptom relief than placebo	Icatibant recommended for bradykinin mediated angioedema	Icatibant does not always provide rapid and complete resolution of symptoms caused by angioedema

	Fok et al. [10]			
Study type	Case series			
Patients, n	4			
Characteristics				
Gender	Female	Male	Female	Female
Age, years	75	49	40	62
Ethnicity	--	--	--	--
Duration of ACEI therapy	20 years	1 day	2 days	4 years
Symptoms	Lip/tongue swelling	Drooping/facial swelling	Sore throat/drooling	Tongue swelling/hoarse voice
Clinical course				
Symptom onset to ED presentation, hrs	1	24	6	2
ED presentation to intubation, hrs	2	2	1	14
ED presentation to icatibant, hrs	72	2	2	14
Icatibant administration	After intubation	At time of intubation	Before intubation	At time of intubation
Icatibant to first symptom resolution, hrs	7	3	3	2
Hospital day/time to extubation from icatibant, hrs				
ED presentation to discharge		Within 24 hours for 3 out of 4 patients		
Conclusions	Icatibant is effective for adrenaline-unresponsive acute upper airway angioedema involving the larynx or oropharynx			

successfully extubated within 24 hours of treatment, but these patients were not specified. Median time to first symptom resolution after treatment for these four patients was three hours (range: two to seven hours) [10]. A case report by Charmillon et al. in 2014 described a 65-year-old woman presenting with severe dyspnea, facial edema, and macroglossia without urticaria or pruritus [8]. Her medication history included quinapril and everolimus. After failure of tracheal intubation, a tracheostomy was performed followed by subcutaneous administration of icatibant 30 mg. Nearly a total regression of angioedema was observed in one hour. On third day of hospitalization, the patient was decannulated and discharged from the intensive care unit [8]. In 2012, Illing et al. also described a 62-year-old male presenting with sudden onset airway compromise, drooling, and macroglossia [9]. His medication history included fosinopril for five years. The patient was treated with hydrocortisone and chlorphenamine and epinephrine with no clinical improvement. Icatibant 30 mg was subsequently administered subcutaneously, but drooling and inability to speak persisted, while upper airway edema progressed. The patient was then intubated and transferred to the intensive care unit. He remained intubated and ventilated for 48 hours. The authors did not appreciate any immediate benefit from icatibant administration, describing "slow resolution of angioedema over 48 hours" before achieving extubation [9].

Overall, the majority of previous case series and case reports suggest a benefit with icatibant administration in intubated patients presenting with ACEI-induced angioedema, but this benefit has not been compared against any patient controls [7–10]. Insufficient details by Straka et al. limit any inferences from patients included in a randomized controlled trial [5]. The majority of reports described noticeable improvement of symptoms when icatibant was administered at the time of intubation or shortly afterwards, with nearly complete regression reported as early as one hour in severe angioedema [8]. Additionally, all reports described extubation within 48 hours or decannulation by 72 hours [7–10].

In the three cases described by this report, however, icatibant was administered after intubation and past the recommended 10 hours from symptoms onset by Bas et al. [4]. Time to icatibant administration ranged from 11 to 12 hours after presenting to the ED and from 15 hours to one week after symptom onset. This delayed administration of icatibant may explain the discrepancies observed between responses in these patients compared to patients previously described in the literature. In this case series, onset of improvement ranged from 11 to 22 hours compared to an onset of improvement and resolution as early as one hour described in previous case reports [8]. Time to extubation ranged from three to five days compared to the one to three days that have been previously reported [10]. Patients of this case series were also hospitalized for at least two to four days longer than patients previously described in the literature [8, 9]. Therefore, delayed administration of icatibant outside the recommended 10 hours from symptom onset presents a large limitation of this case series. Furthermore, the recommended 10-hour administration window was

determined in the setting of intubation prevention, limiting its applicability in the postintubation setting [4]. The utility of icatibant in intubated patients for improving symptom resolution, reducing time to extubation, and shortening hospitalization remains unclear, but timely administration of icatibant appears essential for improved patient outcomes. These improved outcomes may also manifest as decreased patient morbidity and increased cost savings, but in the United States, this is limited by the cost of icatibant. As of November 2017, the listed average wholesale price of one dose of icatibant 30 mg/3 mL subcutaneous injection in the United States is approximately $12,400 [11]. Considering data that estimates the 2013 median cost of medical intensive care unit hospitalization at approximately $9,000, evidence-based practice and institution specific cost-benefit analyses seem prudent for delivering optimal patient care [12].

5. Conclusion

Icatibant administration in intubated patients may be beneficial in decreasing time to extubation and length of intensive care unit stay. In the three cases described, delayed icatibant administration did not appear to elicit a response in intubated patients, which has been described in previous case reports. For clinicians considering icatibant in the treatment of ACEI-induced angioedema, earlier administration upon arrival to the ED or immediately upon arriving to the intensive care unit is strongly advised. The suggested benefit of icatibant in intubated ACEI-induced angioedema patients should be verified by randomized clinical trials and cost-benefit analyses should be performed at individual institutions.

References

[1] S. Bezalel, K. Mahlab-Guri, I. Asher, B. Werner, and Z. M. Sthoeger, "Angiotensin-converting enzyme inhibitor-induced angioedema," American Journal of Medicine, vol. 128, no. 2, pp. 120–125, 2015.

[2] M. J. Scalese and T. S. Reinaker, "Pharmacologic management of angioedema induced by angiotensin-converting enzyme inhibitors," American Journal of Health-System Pharmacy, vol. 73, no. 12, pp. 873–879, 2016.

[3] Firazyr (Icatibant) Product Information, Shire Orphan Therapies, Inc., Lexington, MA, USA, 2013.

[4] M. Baş, J. Greve, K. Stelter et al., "A randomized trial of icatibant in ACE-inhibitor–induced angioedema," The New England Journal of Medicine, vol. 372, no. 5, pp. 418–425, 2015.

[5] B. T. Straka, C. E. Ramirez, J. B. Byrd et al., "Effect of bradykinin receptor antagonism on ACE inhibitor-associated angioedema," The Journal of Allergy and Clinical Immunology, vol. 140, no. 1, pp. 242–248.e2, 2017.

[6] R. Sinert, P. Levy, J. A. Bernstein et al., "Randomized Trial of Icatibant for Angiotensin-Converting Enzyme Inhibitor–Induced Upper Airway Angioedema," Journal of Allergy and

Clinical Immunology: In Practice, vol. 5, no. 5, pp. 1402–1409.e3, 2017.

[7] N. Javaud, J. Achamlal, P.-G. Reuter et al., "Angioedema Related to Angiotensin-Converting Enzyme Inhibitors: Attack Severity, Treatment, and Hospital Admission in a Prospective Multicenter Study," *Medicine (Baltimore)*, vol. 94, no. 45, article e1939, 2015.

[8] A. Charmillon, J. Deibener, P. Kaminsky, and G. Louis, "Angioedema induced by angiotensin converting enzyme inhibitors, potentiated by m-TOR inhibitors: Successful treatment with icatibant," *Intensive Care Medicine*, vol. 40, no. 6, pp. 893-894, 2014.

[9] E. J. Illing, S. Kelly, J. C. Hobson, and S. Charters, "Icatibant and ACE inhibitor angioedema," *BMJ Case Reports*, vol. 2012, 2012.

[10] J. S. Fok, C. H. Katelaris, A. F. Brown, and W. B. Smith, "Icatibant in angiotensin-converting enzyme (ACE) inhibitor-associated angioedema," *Internal Medicine Journal*, vol. 45, no. 8, pp. 821–827, 2015.

[11] Lexicomp Online®, *Pediatric & Neonatal Lexi-Drugs®*, Lexi-Comp, Inc., Hudson, OH, USA, 2016.

[12] H. B. Gershengorn, A. Garland, and M. N. Gong, "Patterns of daily costs differ for medical and surgical intensive care unit patients," *Annals of the American Thoracic Society*, vol. 12, no. 12, pp. 1831–1836, 2015.

45

Hemodynamic Transesophageal Echocardiography-Guided Venous-Arterial Extracorporeal Membrane Oxygenation Support in a Case of Giant Cell Myocarditis

Juan G. Ripoll,[1] **Robert A. Ratzlaff,**[1,2] **David M. Menke,**[3] **Maria C. Olave,**[3]
Joseph J. Maleszewski,[4] **and José L. Díaz-Gómez**[1,2,5]

[1]*Department of Critical Care Medicine, Mayo Clinic, 4500 San Pablo Road, Jacksonville, FL, USA*
[2]*Department of Anesthesiology, Mayo Clinic, 4500 San Pablo Road, Jacksonville, FL, USA*
[3]*Department of Pathology, Mayo Clinic, 4500 San Pablo Road, Jacksonville, FL, USA*
[4]*Division of Anatomic Pathology, Mayo Clinic, 200 First St SW, Rochester, MN, USA*
[5]*Department of Neurosurgery, Mayo Clinic, 4500 San Pablo Road, Jacksonville, FL, USA*

Correspondence should be addressed to José L. Díaz-Gómez; diazgomez.jose@mayo.edu

Academic Editor: Chiara Lazzeri

Giant cell myocarditis (GCM) is a rare and commonly fatal form of fulminant myocarditis. During the acute phase, while immunosuppressive therapy is initiated, venoarterial extracorporeal membrane oxygenation (VA-ECMO) support is commonly used as a bridge to heart transplantation or recovery. Until recently, conventional transesophageal echocardiography and transthoracic echocardiography were the tools available for hemodynamic assessment of patients on this form of mechanical circulatory support. Nevertheless, both techniques have their limitations. We present a case of a 54-year-old man diagnosed with GCM requiring VA-ECMO support that was monitored under a novel miniaturized transesophageal echocardiography (hTEE) probe recently approved for 72 hours of continuous hemodynamic monitoring. Our case highlights the value of this novel, flexible, and disposable device for hemodynamic monitoring, accurate therapy guidance, and potential VA-ECMO weaning process of patients with this form of severe myocarditis.

1. Introduction

Giant cell myocarditis (GCM) is a rare clinical condition characterized by rapid compromise of cardiac systolic function, ultimately leading to severe cardiogenic shock. It has a grave prognosis with a rate of death or heart transplantation of 70% at 1 year. Recently, venoarterial extracorporeal membrane oxygenation (VA-ECMO) has been used as a bridge to cardiac transplantation or recovery [1, 2]. Although no current guidelines are available for an optimal monitoring device for patients under extracorporeal membrane oxygenation (ECMO) support, conventional transesophageal echocardiography (TEE) or transthoracic echocardiography (TTE) is commonly used for this purpose [3]. Nevertheless, both techniques have limitations [4, 5]. We present a case of fulminant

GCM under VA-ECMO support monitored with a novel, miniaturized, flexible, and disposable hemodynamic transesophageal echocardiography (hTEE) probe that allows for 72 hours of continuous hemodynamic monitoring.

2. Case Presentation

A 54-year-old man with a history of psoriatic arthritis, migraines, osteoarthritis, and hyperlipidemia presented to a primary care facility with complaints of sudden generalized weakness and dizziness. The initial assessment was remarkable for elevated serial troponins and ST elevation in the inferior echocardiogram leads (V2, V3, and aVF). He was transferred to a tertiary care hospital for further management of his cardiac condition.

Upon arrival, he underwent a cardiac catheterization that revealed clear coronary arteries. A subsequent echocardiography displayed a left ventricular ejection fraction of 30%. Despite proper management, the patient experienced a third-degree atrioventricular block requiring the implantation of a dual chamber pacemaker without defibrillator capabilities. After full hemodynamic recovering, the patient was discharged and returned to his daily activities.

Three days later, he was readmitted to the same tertiary care hospital after experiencing 2 syncopal episodes, chest discomfort, and blurry vision. Further clinical studies demonstrated no additional cardiac abnormalities, and a computed tomography scan with angiography of the head, neck, and chest was unremarkable. Autoimmune and infectious diseases tests (including Lyme disease) and a lumbar puncture test were also negative.

The night he was discharged, the patient experienced progressively worsening dyspnea and another syncopal episode. He was readmitted tachycardic (heart rate > 120 bpm), normotensive (blood pressure 110/60 mmHg), tachypneic (respiratory rate > 20 rpm), and diaphoretic, with elevated troponin I levels (10.7 ng/mL) and a positive D-dimer. A second cardiac catheterization was performed in addition to an extensive diagnostic workup for pulmonary embolism. Both diagnostic tests were negative, and the patient's hemodynamics started to deteriorate. He was initiated on vasopressor therapy (dobutamine) but developed rapid ventricular tachycardia requiring antiarrhythmic medication (amiodarone). Once the cardiac rhythm was controlled, he underwent an intra-aortic balloon pump insertion and was transferred to our institution for possible ECMO support.

The initial evaluation was notable for mixed cardiogenic and vasodilatory shock with associated acute kidney injury, metabolic acidosis, acute liver failure, coagulopathy, and acute anemia (Table 1). TTE revealed severe left ventricular systolic dysfunction with an estimated left ventricular ejection fraction of 25% and a concomitant severe right ventricular dysfunction. Due to the high clinical suspicion of GCM, an attempt of endomyocardial biopsy (EMB) was performed. However, the procedure was complicated by rapid ventricular tachycardia and inability to obtain endomyocardial samples.

As a result of incessant slow ventricular tachycardia with spikes of rapid ventricular tachycardia, an elective intubation with direct current cardioversion at 200 J was initiated. Following the procedure, stabilization of mean arterial pressure was achieved. High-dose steroids and antithymocyteglobulin were empirically initiated for a likely diagnosis of GCM. No initial immunosuppressive therapy was considered because of the patient's severe multiorgan compromise.

The day after admission, the intra-aortic balloon pump was removed and VA-ECMO (via left femoral artery-left femoral vein) was initiated as a bridge to cardiac transplantation. A successful intraoperative EMB confirmed the diagnosis of GCM.

As the patient's kidney function continued to deteriorate, he was started on continuous venous-venous hemodialysis. Therefore, the selected immunosuppressive therapy was mycophenolate rather than tacrolimus.

TABLE 1: Overview of notable admission laboratory data.

Admission laboratory data	
General chemistry	
Sodium (Na), mEq/L	131
Potassium (K), mEq/L	4.8
Creatinine (mg/dL)	2.6
Lactate (mmol/L)	4.9
Aspartate aminotransferase (AST) (units per liter)	6693
Alanine aminotransferase (ALT) (units per liter)	4040
B-type natriuretic peptide (BNP) (pg/mL)	960
Blood cell count and differential	
Hemoglobin (g/dL)	10.8
Hematocrit (%)	32.6
Neutrophils (absolute number/% neutrophils)	18.760/92.1
Blood gases	
PH arterial	7.425
$PaCO_2$ (mmHg)	22.9
Bicarbonate (mEq/L)	14.7
SaO_2 (%)	97.4
SvO_2 (%)	55.8
Coagulation studies	
aPTT (sec)	42.3
INR	2.0
Prothrombin time (sec)	23

After immunosuppressive therapy was started, the patient developed fever and purulent secretions. Cultures from a bronchoalveolar lavage revealed the presence of Gram-negative bacilli (*Escherichia coli*). Septic shock, likely a result of pneumonia, was considered, and wide-spectrum antibiotics were initiated.

In the setting of this multifactorial shock (cardiogenic, septic), the hemodynamic status of the patient continued to deteriorate. To better characterize the patient's state of shock and to guide inotropic, vasopressor, and fluid therapy, an initial 72-hour continuous hTEE evaluation was performed. Persistent, severe, right ventricular, and moderate left ventricular dysfunctions were shown. Transfusions of blood products and vasopressor therapy adjustment were decided. As tolerated by the patient, hTEE-guided weaning from VA-ECMO was considered (Figure 1(a)).

Four days later, a second hTEE examination was performed (Figure 1(a)) in order for the cardiology, cardiothoracic surgery, and critical care teams to reassess the patient's heart function and make a decision about weaning the patient from VA-ECMO support. Unfortunately, no signs of cardiac function recovery were identified with hTEE after 11 days of VA-ECMO support (Figure 1(b)). Consequently, the patient was unable to tolerate the definitive weaning trial.

Due to his underlying multisystem organ failure, the patient was not deemed a candidate for heart transplantation or for placement of a left ventricular assist device or a biventricular assist device. Thus, the patient's family was consulted,

(a)

(b)

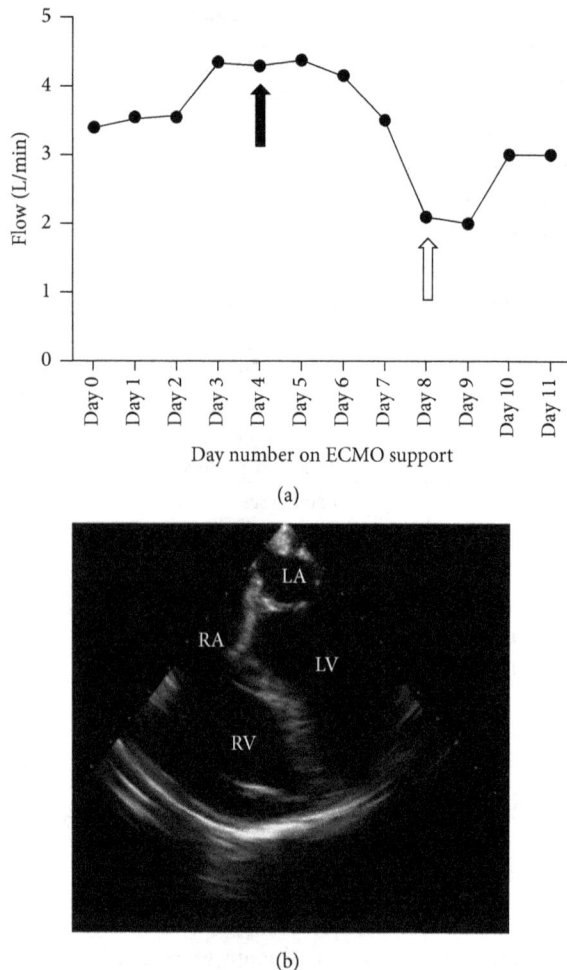

FIGURE 1: hTEE monitoring of VA-ECMO support. hTEE assessments were performed on day 4 (black arrow) and day 8 (white arrow), respectively (a). A mid-esophageal four-chamber view (day 11) revealed persistent biventricular systolic dysfunction despite VA-ECMO support (b).

and compassionate withdrawals of all measures were initiated. Under family consent, a chest autopsy further confirmed the diagnosis of GCM (Figure 2).

3. Discussion

Idiopathic GCM is a rare and fatal form of T-cell mediated inflammatory myocarditis with an estimated incidence between 6.6 and 23.4 cases per 100.000 individuals [6]. It predominantly affects young people with slight male preponderance. Up to 8% of affected patients have concomitant inflammatory bowel disease (ulcerative colitis or Crohn disease) [7]. The most common clinical manifestations of GCM include rapidly progressive heart failure (75%) and incessant ventricular arrhythmias (14%). A syndrome mimicking acute myocardial infarction (6%) and complete heart block (5%) are among the uncommon clinical presentations of the disease. Diagnosis of GCM relies on EMB showing a diffuse multifocal inflammatory infiltrates with associated

myocardial necrosis, presence of multinucleated giant cells, and an absence of sarcoid-like granulomas [7, 8].

Immunosuppressive therapy is a well-established treatment for GCM [9]. On contemporary regimens, two-thirds of patients reached a partial clinical remission characterized by transplant-free survival and reduced risk of severe heart failure [10]. However, there is no data available regarding the maintenance of remission under long-term immunosuppressive therapy. Thus, heart transplantation still remains the definitive treatment for GCM [7, 11].

Acute heart failure is the most common clinical manifestation of GCM. Immunosuppressive agents need time to be effective; meanwhile, cardiovascular support must be assured. Thus, mechanical circulatory devices are valuable alternatives as a bridge both to cardiac transplantation and to myocardial recovery [12–14]. Currently, VA-ECMO is considered a well-known bridging therapy in the setting of fulminant GCM [2, 15]. Although no guidelines are currently available, ECMO monitoring has been commonly performed under TTE or TEE guidance [3]. Nevertheless, several limitations arise with the use of these technologies. On one hand, in the intensive care unit setting, TTE diagnostic performance is considered inferior to TEE due to poorly discernible echocardiographic windows in mechanically ventilated patients [4]. On the other hand, TEE requires highly trained clinicians (cardiac anesthesiologists or cardiologists), the examination is discontinuous in nature, and the need for multiple probe insertions could potentially lead to major injuries such as esophageal trauma and bleeding [4, 5].

To overcome these limitations, a flexible, disposable, and miniaturized hTEE probe has been approved by the Food and Drug Administration. The device can be utilized continuously for up to 72 hours and provides a real-time qualitative and semiquantitative assessment of sudden hemodynamic changes [16]. Simplified insertion and improved tolerance are among the potential benefits for hemodynamically unstable patients requiring mechanical ventilation [17, 18]. In the intensive care unit setting, hTEE provides supplementary information to invasive monitoring [19] and displays good interrater reliability when performed by nonexperienced operators [20]. Thus, hTEE theoretically provides a safer, faster, and more user-friendly assessment of hemodynamic status compared to TTE and continuous TEE.

Only 1 previous study of 21 patients with underlying cardiogenic shock demonstrated the use of hTEE as a monitoring tool for ECMO weaning [21]. To the best of our knowledge, this is the first case reporting the use of an hTEE-guided approach to assess a severe cardiogenic shock in a case of fulminant GCM.

Although our patient ultimately expired as a result of severe multiorgan failure, there are multiple reasons to routinely implement hTEE examination as a monitoring tool in critically ill patients requiring VA-ECMO support. First, this imaging modality allows for 72 hours of continuous monitoring, leading to optimal management of fluid therapy and vasopressor titration. Second, it allows for prompt recognition of sudden cardiac complications emerging from the progressive cardiac damage displayed in disease states, such as GCM. Finally, hTEE provides a real-time assessment of

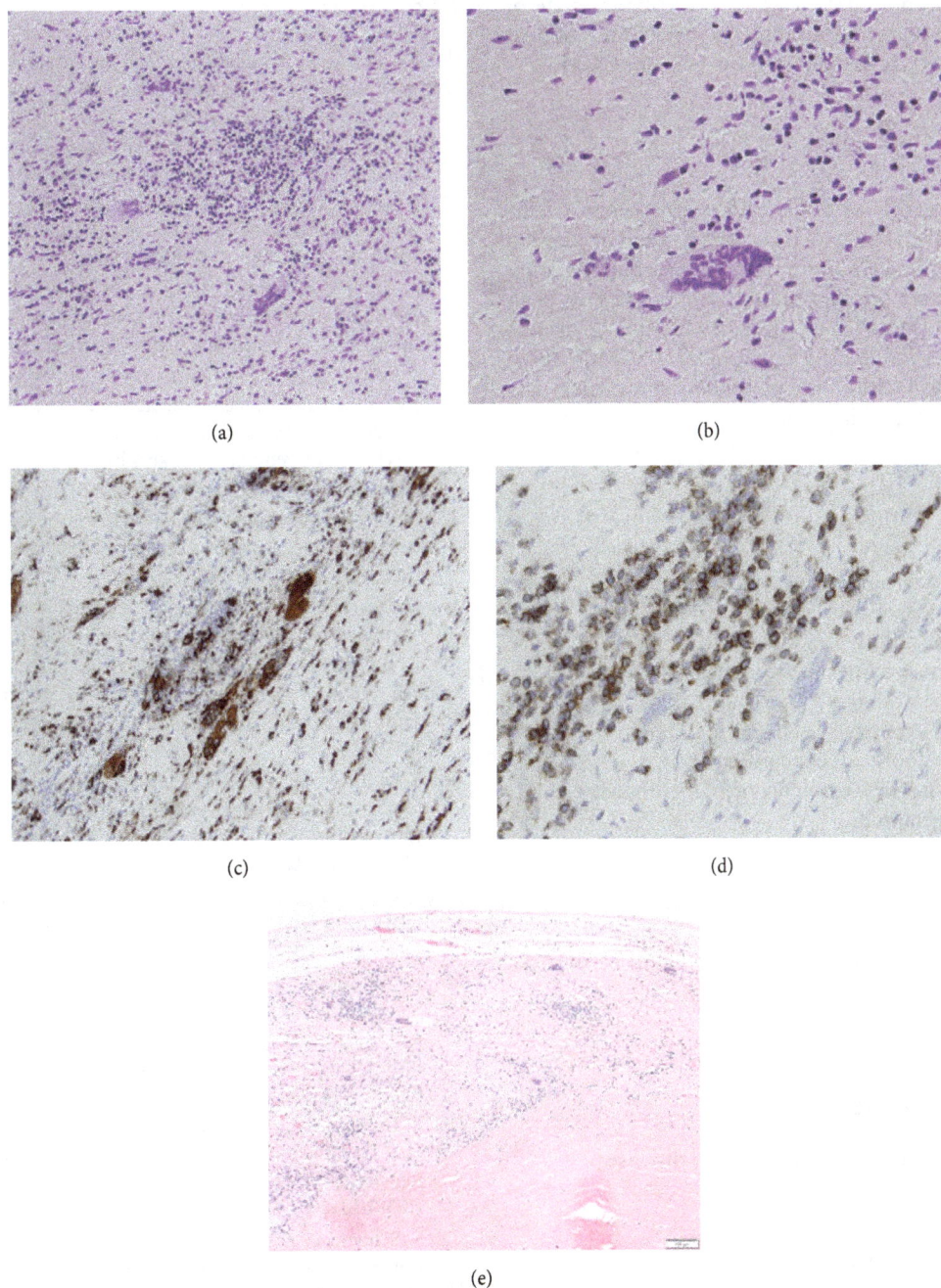

(a)

(b)

(c)

(d)

(e)

FIGURE 2: Histopathology of giant cell myocarditis. (a) Myocardium with prominent lymphohistiocytic infiltrate and well-formed multinucleated giant cells (H&E, original magnification ×200). (b) High power magnification (H&E, original magnification ×400) showing extensive myocardial damage by a dense inflammatory infiltrate. (c) Histiocytic infiltrate (CD68-PGM-1, original magnification ×200). (d) The lymphocytic infiltrate consists primarily of T-lymphocytes (CD3, original magnification ×400). (e) Atrioventricular node involved by giant cell myocarditis (H&E, original magnification, ×100).

cardiac structures, permitting a rapid screening of signs of cardiac recovery in patients under VA-ECMO support and thus favoring the weaning process [21].

In our case, close monitoring of VA-ECMO support with hTEE allowed us to better characterize a complex state of shock (cardiogenic and vasodilatory) [19]. Hence, we have a more appropriate initial resuscitation in the early phase of

our patient's care. Furthermore, we present the usefulness of hTEE for ECMO weaning trial. Although in this case it was utilized for decision-making of withdrawal of life support, it would potentially guide a final decision of ECMO explantation after treatment of severe refractory cardiogenic and septic shock. Although this hTEE management did not lead to better outcome, it can be considered as a valuable tool to a more prompt characterization of complex state of shock since presentation and guiding trials of ECMO support weaning in entities with a high lethality rates like GCM.

4. Conclusion

Our case highlights that an hTEE-guided approach is a valuable alternative for the hemodynamic assessment of patients with GCM under VA-ECMO support. Increased monitoring of mechanical circulatory support in complex states of shock could potentially lead to more accurate clinical decisions, including decision for therapy management, ECMO weaning, and even timely withdrawal of all life-support measures in severely compromised individuals.

Abbreviations

ECMO: Extracorporeal membrane oxygenation
EMB: Endomyocardial biopsy
GCM: Giant cell myocarditis
hTEE: Hemodynamic transesophageal echocardiography
TEE: Transesophageal echocardiography
TTE: Transthoracic echocardiography
VA-ECMO: Venoarterial extracorporeal membrane oxygenation.

Disclosure

Mayo Clinic does not endorse specific products or services included in this paper.

Competing Interests

The authors have no conflict of interests to disclose.

Authors' Contributions

Juan G. Ripoll and Maria C. Olave drafted the paper and performed data collection. Robert A. Ratzlaff, José L. Díaz-Gómez, Joseph J. Maleszewski, and David M. Menke were responsible for patient care and paper revision. All authors read and approved the final paper.

Acknowledgments

The authors would like to thank Victoria L. Clifton, MLIS, ELS, for her assistance with language editing and editorial preparation of this paper.

References

[1] M. A. Acker, "Mechanical circulatory support for patients with acute-fulminant myocarditis," *Annals of Thoracic Surgery*, vol. 71, no. 3, pp. S73–S76, 2001.

[2] A. Le Guyader, F. Rollé, S. Karoutsos, and E. Cornu, "Acute myocarditis supported by extracorporeal membrane oxygenation successfully bridged to transplantation: a giant cell myocarditis," *Interactive Cardiovascular and Thoracic Surgery*, vol. 5, no. 6, pp. 782–784, 2006.

[3] G. Doufle, A. Roscoe, F. Billia, and E. Fan, "Echocardiography for adult patients supported with extracorporeal membrane oxygenation," *Critical Care*, vol. 19, article 326, 2015.

[4] P. Vignon, H. Mentec, S. Terre, H. Gastinne, P. Gueret, and F. Lemaire, "Diagnostic accuracy and therapeutic impact of transthoracic and transesophageal echocardiography in mechanically ventilated patients in the ICU," *Chest*, vol. 106, no. 6, pp. 1829–1834, 1994.

[5] P. Vignon, "Hemodynamic assessment of critically ill patients using echocardiography Doppler," *Current Opinion in Critical Care*, vol. 11, no. 3, pp. 227–234, 2005.

[6] R. Okada and S. Wakafuji, "Myocarditis in autopsy," *Heart and Vessels*, vol. 1, supplement 1, pp. 23–29, 1985.

[7] L. T. Cooper Jr., G. J. Berry, and R. Shabetai, "Idiopathic giant-cell myocarditis—natural history and treatment," *The New England Journal of Medicine*, vol. 336, no. 26, pp. 1860–1866, 1997.

[8] Y. Okura, G. W. Dec, J. M. Hare et al., "A clinical and histopathologic comparison of cardiac sarcoidosis and idiopathic giant cell myocarditis," *Journal of the American College of Cardiology*, vol. 41, no. 2, pp. 322–329, 2003.

[9] J. W. Mason, J. B. O'Connell, A. Herskowitz et al., "A clinical trial of immunosuppressive therapy for myocarditis," *The New England Journal of Medicine*, vol. 333, no. 5, pp. 269–275, 1995.

[10] R. Kandolin, J. Lehtonen, K. Salmenkivi, A. Räisänen-Sokolowski, J. Lommi, and M. Kupari, "Diagnosis, treatment, and outcome of giant-cell myocarditis in the era of combined immunosuppression," *Circulation: Heart Failure*, vol. 6, no. 1, pp. 15–22, 2013.

[11] E. D. Moloney, J. J. Egan, P. Kelly, A. E. Wood, and L. T. Cooper Jr., "Transplantation for myocarditis: a controversy revisited," *Journal of Heart and Lung Transplantation*, vol. 24, no. 8, pp. 1103–1110, 2005.

[12] S. Schenk, L. Arusoglu, M. Morshuis et al., "Triple bridge-to-transplant in a case of giant cell myocarditis complicated by human leukocyte antigen sensitization and heparin-induced thrombocytopenia type II," *Annals of Thoracic Surgery*, vol. 81, no. 3, pp. 1107–1109, 2006.

[13] R. A. Davies, J. P. Veinot, S. Smith, C. Struthers, P. Hendry, and R. Masters, "Giant cell myocarditis: clinical presentation, bridge to transplantation with mechanical circulatory support, and long-term outcome," *Journal of Heart and Lung Transplantation*, vol. 21, no. 6, pp. 674–679, 2002.

[14] D. Marelli, R. Kermani, J. Bresson et al., "Support with the BVS 5000 assist device during treatment of acute giant-cell myocarditis," *Texas Heart Institute Journal*, vol. 30, no. 1, pp. 50–56, 2003.

[15] E. Ammirati, F. Oliva, O. Belli et al., "Giant cell myocarditis successfully treated with antithymocyte globuline and extracor-

poreal membrane oxygenation for 21 days," *Journal of Cardio-vascular Medicine*, 2015.

[16] C. E. Wagner, J. S. Bick, B. H. Webster, J. H. Selby, and J. G. Byrne, "Use of a miniaturized transesophageal echocardiographic probe in the intensive care unit for diagnosis and treatment of a hemodynamically unstable patient after aortic valve replacement," *Journal of Cardiothoracic and Vascular Anesthesia*, vol. 26, no. 1, pp. 95–97, 2012.

[17] A. Vieillard-Baron, M. Slama, P. Mayo et al., "A pilot study on safety and clinical utility of a single-use 72-hour indwelling transesophageal echocardiography probe," *Intensive Care Medicine*, vol. 39, no. 4, pp. 629–635, 2013.

[18] K. T. Spencer, D. Krauss, J. Thurn et al., "Transnasal transesophageal echocardiography," *Journal of the American Society of Echocardiography*, vol. 10, no. 7, pp. 728–737, 1997.

[19] N. Fletcher, M. Geisen, H. Meeran, D. Spray, and M. Cecconi, "Initial clinical experience with a miniaturized transesophageal echocardiography probe in a cardiac intensive care unit," *Journal of Cardiothoracic and Vascular Anesthesia*, vol. 29, no. 3, pp. 582–587, 2015.

[20] L. Cioccari, H.-R. Baur, D. Berger, J. Wiegand, J. Takala, and T. M. Merz, "Hemodynamic assessment of critically ill patients using a miniaturized transesophageal echocardiography probe," *Critical Care*, vol. 17, no. 3, article R121, 2013.

[21] N. C. Cavarocchi, H. T. Pitcher, Q. Yang et al., "Weaning of extracorporeal membrane oxygenation using continuous hemodynamic transesophageal echocardiography," *The Journal of Thoracic and Cardiovascular Surgery*, vol. 146, no. 6, pp. 1474–1479, 2013.

46

Central Pontine Myelinolysis in Pediatric Diabetic Ketoacidosis

Hannah Kinoshita,[1] Leon Grant,[2] Konstantine Xoinis,[3] and Prashant J. Purohit (ID)[3]

[1]University of Hawaii Pediatric Residency Program, USA
[2]Department of Pediatric Neurology, Kapiolani Medical Center for Women & Children, USA
[3]Department of Pediatric Critical Care, Kapiolani Medical Center for Women & Children, USA

Correspondence should be addressed to Prashant J. Purohit; drpurohit22@gmail.com

Academic Editor: Zsolt Molnár

Central pontine myelinolysis (CPM) is rarely reported in pediatric patients with diabetic ketoacidosis (DKA). We report this case of a 16-year-old female with new onset diabetes presenting with DKA, who received aggressive fluid resuscitation and sodium bicarbonate in the emergency department. Later she developed altered mental status concerning for cerebral edema and received hyperosmolar therapy with only transient improvement. Soon she became apneic requiring emergent endotracheal intubation. MRI brain showed cerebral edema, CPM, and subdural hemorrhage. She was extubated on day seven and exhibited mild dysmetria, ataxia, unilateral weakness, and neglect. Upon discharge she was able to ambulate with a walker and speak and eat without difficulty. Although less common than cerebral edema, CPM should be considered in DKA patients with acute neurologic deterioration. Fluid and bicarbonate therapy should be individualized, but larger studies would help guide the management. Although poor outcomes are reported in CPM, favorable outcomes are possible.

1. Introduction

Diabetic ketoacidosis (DKA) is the presenting feature in 10-70% of cases of new onset diabetes in developed countries [1]. One of the most feared complications of DKA, particularly in children, is the development of cerebral edema (CE). The incidence of CE in DKA is approximately 1%; however, when it occurs, it accounts for 57-87% of DKA related mortality and 10-26% of morbidity [2]. Other neurologic complications of DKA include central nervous system infarction, thrombosis, transient grey and white matter changes, and osmotic demyelination [2–8]. The osmotic demyelination syndrome (ODS) consisting of central and extra pontine myelinolysis is a relatively rare complication of DKA. Central pontine myelinolysis (CPM) was originally described as a complication of rapid correction of hyponatremia, particularly in the setting of malnutrition, alcohol abuse, and liver disease [9, 10]. Demyelination is now believed to occur secondary to rapid osmotic shifts from changes in any osmotically active agent including sodium, potassium, glucose, and ammonia [5–8, 11, 12]. To the best of our knowledge, only five other cases of ODS have been reported in association with pediatric DKA [5, 7, 8, 13, 14].

Since these complications are rare and neurological outcomes can be devastating, maintaining a high index of suspicion is important. Some of the suggested risk factors for the development of CE in DKA are young age, severe acidosis, hypocapnia, elevated blood urea nitrogen (BUN), dehydration, aggressive fluid resuscitation, sodium bicarbonate, and bolus/early insulin administration [15–17]. However, no such definite risk factors for the development of CPM have been identified. Here, we present this case of a 16-year-old female with new onset DKA developing features of both CE and CPM.

2. Case Presentation

A previously healthy 16-year-old female visitor from Japan presented to an adult emergency room (ER) with altered mental status and emesis. She was found lying on a bathroom floor in her hotel. There was a history of polyuria and polydipsia for 2 weeks and 8 to 10 kg weight loss during the previous month. Her vital signs upon arrival to the pediatric intensive care unit (PICU) were temperature of 98.1° Fahrenheit, heart rate 110/min, respiratory rate 26/min, blood pressure 140/81 mm of Hg, and 100% oxygen saturations without supplemental oxygen. Her capillary refill time was 4-5 seconds. Her weight was 57 kg. Her Glasgow Coma Scale (GCS) was 13 in the ER, which improved to 15 upon arrival to PICU. Skin rash with infected lesions was noted in her groin. The rest of her physical examination was unremarkable.

Workup in the ER showed hyperglycemia of 472 mg/dL, metabolic acidosis (pH 6.75, pCO2 18.4, pO2 149, HCO3 2.5, base deficit 32.6, anion gap 23.5), ketosis (beta-hydroxybutyrate 11.41), glucosuria, and ketonuria, which were consistent with diabetic ketoacidosis. Her white cell counts were 22.3 k/L, hemoglobin 15.8 g/dL, and hematocrit 47%. The rest of her workup was unremarkable.

The patient received fluid resuscitation with 30 mL/kg of 0.9% normal saline (NS) and 50 mEq of sodium bicarbonate in the ER. Continuous insulin infusion was started at 0.1 unit/kg/hr. After that she was started on intravenous fluids containing 0.45% saline and 75 mEq/L of sodium bicarbonate. This was administered at 150 mL/hr, which was 1.25 times the usual daily maintenance requirement for her weight. A consultation with our PICU was obtained at this stage. No further bicarbonate boluses were given. Her fluids were changed to isotonic fluid with potassium phosphate and potassium chloride and without any bicarbonate. It was administered at the rate of 1.5 times maintenance of daily requirement for weight. She was transferred to the PICU at this stage, where she continued to exhibit severe metabolic acidosis with pH 6.97, pCO2 26.7, HCO3 6.1, and base deficit of 24.5. The DKA management was continued with close monitoring and serial laboratory evaluations.

After few hours of her arrival in the PICU, the patient became disoriented and confused. She was given one time 5 ml/kg of 3% hypertonic saline (HS) due to concern for cerebral edema and she responded well. Four hours later she developed lethargy followed by apnea. She was given additional doses of 3% HS bolus (5 mL/kg) and 0.8 g/kg of 20% mannitol. The hyperosmolar therapy was effective but only transiently; the patient eventually required intubation and mechanical ventilation for recurrent apnea.

CT head obtained at that time showed a thin, right parietal subdural hemorrhage without any evidence of edema or mass effect. Of note, CT scan was obtained after the initiation of hyperosmolar therapy.

Hyperosmolar therapy was continued afterwards with 3% HS and 20% mannitol. It was guided with close monitoring of renal function including serum sodium and serum osmolarity. The doses and other parameters were maintained per standard of care [18, 19].

The patient's serum sodium was 135 upon arrival in the ER and 143 at around 11 hrs before the initiation of hyperosmolar therapy and reached to 160 at 71 hrs when hyperosmolar therapy was discontinued. It was normalized to 143 at 131 hrs of admission. Her osmolarity was 298, 305, 335, and 299 at those timings (sodium in mmol/L and osmolarity in msom/kg). The rate of glucose reduction was < 50 mg/dl/hr.

MRI brain obtained at 60 hrs of admission showed mild edema of the cortex and sulci and diffuse edema of the pons and midbrain with restricted diffusion in the pons consistent with central pontine myelinolysis also known as osmotic

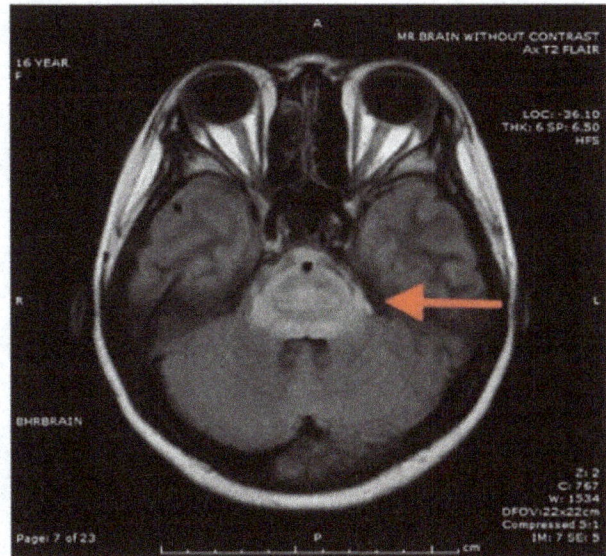

FIGURE 1: T2-FLAIR Axial image showing diffuse pontine edema.

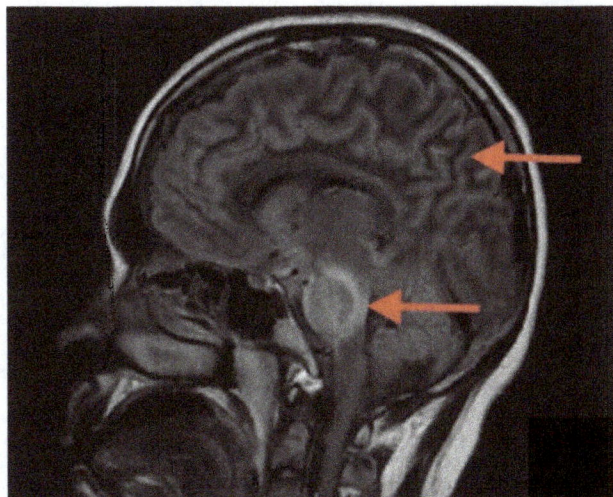

FIGURE 2: T2-FLAIR Sagittal image showing diffuse pontine edema and cerebral edema.

demyelination syndrome. There was no significant change in the subdural hemorrhage (Figures 1–4). MR angiogram showed no evidence of vessel abnormality.

The patient required continued mechanical ventilation and further management in the PICU. She became more responsive on day 5, and her support was gradually weaned until extubation on day 7. At that time she exhibited only mild residual dysmetria, trivial ataxia, mild left sided weakness, and neglect. All deficits subsequently improved.

Her course was complicated by an isolated focal seizure that responded to standard antiepileptic medication. She also developed bilateral upper extremity deep venous thromboses (DVT). Hematology workup showed no underlying hypercoagulability. Thus the DVT was considered as another complication of DKA [20–22].

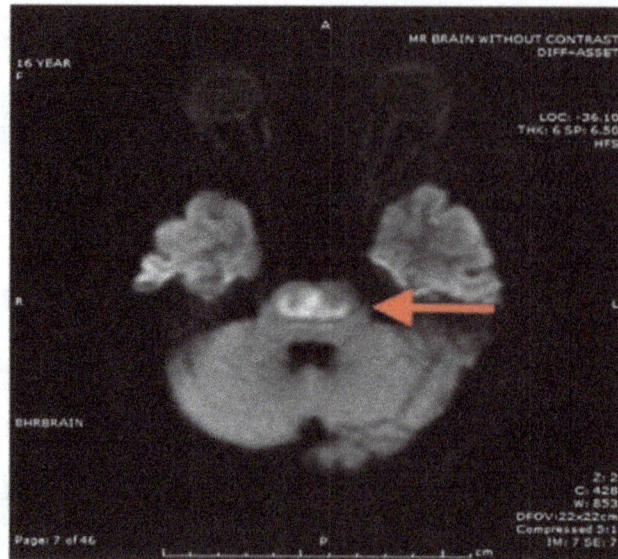

FIGURE 3: Restricted diffusion in pons with relative sparing of corticospinal tract.

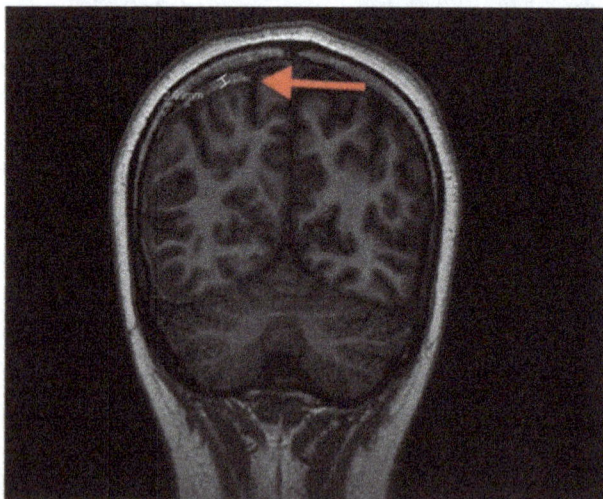

FIGURE 4: FSPGR sequence, coronal image of brain showing right parietal subdural hemorrhage.

Her overall hospital length of stay was 14 days, and by the date of discharge she was able to ambulate with a walker and speak and eat without difficulty.

3. Discussion

This case report portrays two potentially fatal complications of DKA, which are CE and CPM. It is possible that our patient developed these neurologic sequalae due to combination of prolonged cerebral edema and central pontine myelinolysis. It is unclear if our patient developed these complications due to severity of illness, therapies administered, or a combination of these elements.

The major indicators of severity of illness were acidosis (pH of 6.75 on presentation) and the history of 8-10 kg weight loss in one month. Thereafter she was exposed to multiple risk factors including rapid initial rehydration, bicarbonate infusion, and hyperosmolar therapy.

Literature on bicarbonate therapy in the management of diabetic ketoacidosis is diverse. One study supports bicarbonate administration in the adult population for blood pH < 7.20 or in cases of fluid refractory hemodynamic instability [23]. Another adult study found no usefulness of sodium bicarbonate therapy in this population [24]. Pediatric literature is suggestive of increased risk of complications including CE with bicarbonate therapy [2, 3, 15, 17, 25]. The ISPAD [3] recommends use of sodium bicarbonate in case of life threatening hyperkalemia and ESCS [2] in case of profound acidosis affecting action of epinephrine during resuscitation. It is possible that bicarbonate administration contributed to the development of cerebral edema in our case.

There are studies suggesting the association of cerebral edema with aggressive fluid resuscitation in the pediatric DKA patients [16, 26]. Literature also exists which failed to demonstrate this association [27, 28]. The European Society Consensus Statement (ESCS) on DKA and International Society for Pediatric and Adolescent Diabetes (ISPAD) recommend a fluid bolus of 10 to 20 mL/kg over 1-2 hours with repeating if necessary [2, 3]. Our patient received a 30 mL/kg fluid bolus, and it might have contributed to the development of CE. However, further larger studies would be helpful to establish this association.

The usual practice at our institution is to follow the recommendations from ESCS on DKA regarding fluid and bicarbonate administration [2]. However, this patient was initially managed in the ER of another institution.

Hyperosmolar therapy could have contributed to the development of CPM in our case. It is also noteworthy that 3% saline was our first choice of hyperosmolar therapy, which is different from the recommendations from ISPAD and ESCS on DKA. Both these recommendations are based on a retrospective cohort study [29], which actually concluded equipoise on the choice of hyperosmolar agent because of certain limitation of their data. In that study, the mortality was higher in cases treated with HS as a single agent versus mannitol as a single agent. Our patient received combined therapy of HS and mannitol. Among the other reported cases of pediatric ODS, one patient received HS [5], 3 received mannitol [7, 13], and one patient did not receive any hyperosmolar therapy [12]. In the case reported by Sivaswamy et al. [12], there were no wide fluctuations in the sodium level but they noted fluctuations in the osmolarity. While the data are limited in the context of cerebral edema and ODS in the pediatric DKA population, osmotic changes may be responsible for these complications. The available guidelines for the management of cerebral edema in DKA [2, 3] have recommendations on the initiation of the therapy only. The recommendations are lacking on further continuation of the therapy and in the context of rebound ICP and development of SAH and ODS. This would be helpful in cases like ours, where patient was symptomatic for over 5 days with MRI showing cerebral edema on day 3. Hence we extrapolated our management based on the guidelines for TBI population [18, 19]. The rate of rise, the rate of reduction, and the upper limit of sodium and osmolarity were maintained in our case within the guidelines for CE management in cases of TBI. It is plausible that hyperosmolar therapy which increased the level of sodium and the osmolarity significantly contributed to the development of ODS in our patient. However, given the severity of cerebral edema in our patient, it is very likely that it was also a lifesaving intervention. Further larger studies and specific recommendations in terms of serum sodium, osmolarity, and maintenance of hyperosmolar therapy for the CE management in the DKA population will be helpful.

The age group in the other five reported cases of ODS ranged from 18 months to 17 years. The proposed mechanism for the development of ODS varied among the cases but overall included severe acidosis (pH < 7.0), aggressive fluid resuscitation, hyperosmolar therapy, bacteremia with possible meningitis, and wide fluctuations in glucose, sodium, or osmolarity. One patient died and the remaining four survived with full or near full recovery [5, 7, 8, 13, 14].

A larger review of pediatric ODS showed association with a wide array of underlying illnesses including head injury, liver trauma, malignancy, intracranial surgery with or without diabetes insipidus, ornithine transcarbamylase deficiency, acute gastroenteritis, and adrenal insufficiency [5].

The prognosis of CE and ODS varies from full recovery to death. ODS was historically thought to be fatal or to result in severe neurologic deficits including locked-in syndrome. However, in the last 30 years there have been increasing numbers of pediatric cases with complete or near-complete recovery [5, 7, 8, 13, 14, 30]. This shift in outcome is possibly due to improved identification and advancement in medical care.

The etiology of neurologic sequelae in our patient is most likely multifactorial. Despite these severe and rare complications, our patient made near full recovery, which is inspirational.

References

[1] A. Rosenbloom, "Hyperglycemic crises and their complications in children," *Journal of Pediatric Endocrinology and Metabolism*, vol. 20, no. 1, pp. 5–18, 2007.

[2] D. B. Dunger, M. A. Sperling, C. L. Acerini et al., "European society for paediatric endocrinology/lawson wilkins pediatric endocrine society consensus statement on diabetic ketoacidosis in children and adolescents," *Pediatrics*, vol. 113, no. 2, pp. e133–e140, 2004.

[3] J. I. Wolfsdorf, J. Allgrove, M. E. Craig et al., "Diabetic ketoacidosis and hyperglycemic hyperosmolar state," *Pediatric Diabetes*, vol. 15, no. 20, pp. 154–179, 2014.

[4] F. J. Cameron, S. E. Scratch, C. Nadebaum et al., "Neurological consequences of diabetic ketoacidosis at initial presentation of type 1 diabetes in a prospective cohort study of children," *Diabetes Care*, vol. 37, no. 6, pp. 1554–1562, 2014.

[5] P. Gencpinar, H. Tekguc, A. U. Senol, O. Duman, and O. Dursun, "Extrapontine myelinolysis in an 18-month-old boy with diabetic ketoacidosis: Case report and literature review," *Journal of Child Neurology*, vol. 29, no. 11, pp. 1548–1553, 2014.

[6] H. Donnelly, S. Connor, and J. Quirk, "Central pontine myelinolysis secondary to hyperglycaemia," *Practical Neurology*, vol. 16, no. 6, pp. 493–495, 2016.

[7] S. Petzold, T. Kapellen, M. Siekmeyer et al., "Acute cerebral infarction and extra pontine myelinolysis in children with new onset type 1 diabetes mellitus," *Pediatric Diabetes*, vol. 12, no. 5, pp. 513–517, 2011.

[8] J. E. Pitella and H. Gobbi, "Central pontine and extrapontine myelinolysis: report of an autopsied case and review of literature," *Arquivos de Neuro-Psiquiatria*, vol. 45, no. 3, pp. 302–311, 1987.

[9] R. D. Adams, M. Victor, and E. L. Mancall, "Central pontine myelinolysis: a hitherto undescribed disease occurring in alcoholic and malnourished patients," *A.M.A. Archives of Neurology and Psychiatry*, vol. 81, no. 2, pp. 154–172, 1959.

[10] T. Sugimoto, T. Murata, M. Omori, and Y. Wada, "Central pontine myelinolysis associated with hypokalaemia in anorexia nervosa," *Journal of Neurology, Neurosurgery & Psychiatry*, vol. 74, no. 3, pp. 353–355, 2003.

[11] K. Kario, K. Kanatsu, K. Sekita et al., "A case of chronic recurrent portal systemic encephalopathy showing marked diurnal fluctuation of blood ammonia level complicated with central pontine myelinolysis," *The Journal of the Japanese Society of Internal Medicine*, vol. 78, no. 8, pp. 1172–1180, 1989.

[12] L. Sivaswamy and S. Karia, "Extrapontine myelinolysis in a 4 year old with diabetic ketoacidosis," *European Journal of Paediatric Neurology*, vol. 11, no. 6, pp. 389–393, 2007.

[13] J. L. Bonkowsky and F. M. Filloux, "Extrapontine myelinolysis in a pediatric case of diabetic ketoacidosis and cerebral edema," *Journal of Child Neurology*, vol. 18, no. 2, pp. 144–147, 2003.

[14] N. Glaser, P. Barnett, and I. McCaslin, "Risk factors for cerebral edema in children with diabetic ketoacidosis," *The New England Journal of Medicine*, vol. 344, no. 4, pp. 264–269, 2001.

[15] J. A. Edge, R. W. Jakes, Y. Roy et al., "The UK case-control study of cerebral oedema complicating diabetic ketoacidosis in children," *Diabetologia*, vol. 49, no. 9, pp. 2002–2009, 2006.

[16] W. Watts and J. A. Edge, "How can cerebral edema during treatment of diabetic ketoacidosis be avoided?" *Pediatric Diabetes*, vol. 15, no. 4, pp. 271–276, 2014.

[17] P. M. Kochanek, N. Carney, P. D. Adelson et al., "Guidelines for the acute medical management of severe traumatic brain injury in infants, children, and adolescents—second edition," *Pediatric Critical Care Medicine*, vol. 13, supplement 1, pp. S1–82, 2012.

[18] B. Peterson, S. Khanna, B. Fisher, and L. Marshall, "Prolonged hypernatremia controls elevated intracranial pressure in head-injured pediatric patients," *Critical Care Medicine*, vol. 28, no. 4, pp. 1136–1143, 2000.

[19] S. R. Bialo, "Rare complications of pediatric diabetic ketoacidosis," *World Journal of Diabetes*, vol. 6, no. 1, pp. 167–174, 2015.

[20] S. V. Cherian, L. Khara, S. Das, W. A. Hamarneh, A. S. Garcha, and V. Frechette, "Diabetic ketoacidosis complicated by generalized venous thrombosis: a case report and review," *Blood Coagulation & Fibrinolysis*, vol. 23, no. 3, pp. 238–240, 2012.

[21] M. Bilici, B. Tavil, O. Dogru, M. Davutoglu, and M. Bosnak, "Diabetic ketoasidosis is associated with prothrombotic tendency in children," *Pediatric Hematology and Oncology*, vol. 28, no. 5, pp. 418–424, 2011.

[22] K. S. Kamel, M. Schreiber, A. P. C. P. Carlotti, and M. L. Halperin, "Approach to the treatment of diabetic ketoacidosis," *American Journal of Kidney Diseases*, vol. 68, no. 6, pp. 967–972, 2016.

[23] B. Duhon, R. L. Attridge, A. C. Franco-Martinez, P. R. Maxwell, and D. W. Hughes, "Intravenous sodium bicarbonate therapy in severely acidotic diabetic ketoacidosis," *Annals of Pharmacotherapy*, vol. 47, no. 7-8, pp. 970–975, 2013.

[24] S. M. Green, S. G. Rothrock, J. D. Ho et al., "Failure of adjunctive bicarbonate to improve outcome in severe pediatric diabetic ketoacidosis," *Annals of Emergency Medicine*, vol. 31, no. 1, pp. 41–48, 1998.

[25] N. S. Glaser, S. L. Wootton-Gorges, M. H. Buonocore et al., "Subclinical cerebral edema in children with diabetic ketoacidosis randomized to 2 different rehydration protocols," *Pediatrics*, vol. 131, no. 1, pp. e73–e80, 2013.

[26] N. S. Glaser, S. L. Wootton-Gorges, I. Kim et al., "Regional brain water content and distribution during diabetic ketoacidosis," *Journal of Pediatrics*, vol. 180, pp. 170–176, 2017.

[27] C. P. Mahoney, B. W. Vlcek, and M. Delaguila, "Risk factors for developing brain herniation during diabetic ketoacidosis," *Pediatric Neurology*, vol. 21, no. 4, pp. 721–727, 1999.

[28] D. L. Levin, "Cerebral edema in diabetic ketoacidosis," *Pediatric Critical Care Medicine*, vol. 9, no. 3, pp. 320–329, 2008.

[29] D. D. DeCourcey, G. M. Steil, D. Wypij, and M. S. D. Agus, "Increasing use of hypertonic saline over Mannitol in the treatment of symptomatic cerebral edema in pediatric diabetic Ketoacidosis: An 11-year retrospective analysis of mortality," *Pediatric Critical Care Medicine*, vol. 14, no. 7, pp. 694–700, 2013.

[30] A. M. Ranger, N. Chaudhary, M. Avery, and D. Fraser, "Central pontine and extrapontine myelinolysis in children: A review of 76 patients," *Journal of Child Neurology*, vol. 27, no. 8, pp. 1027–1037, 2012.

47

Zinc Chloride Smoke Inhalation Induced Severe Acute Respiratory Distress Syndrome: First Survival in the United States with Extended Duration (Five Weeks) Therapy with High Dose Corticosteroids in Combination with Lung Protective Ventilation

Hafiz Mahboob,[1,2,3] **Robert Richeson III,**[1,2] **and Robert McCain**[3]

[1] *University of Nevada School of Medicine, Reno, NV, USA*
[2] *Renown Regional Medical Center, Reno, NV, USA*
[3] *U.S. Department of Veteran Affairs, Ioannis A. Lougaris Veteran Affairs Medical Center, Reno, NV, USA*

Correspondence should be addressed to Hafiz Mahboob; hmahboob@medicine.nevada.edu

Academic Editor: Kurt Lenz

Zinc chloride smoke bomb exposure is frequently seen in military drills, combat exercises, metal industry works, and disaster simulations. Smoke exposure presents with variety of pulmonary damage based on the intensity of the exposure. Smoke induced severe acute respiratory distress syndrome (ARDS) is often fatal and there are no standard treatment guidelines. We report the first survival of smoke induced severe ARDS in the United States (US) with prolonged use of high dose steroids (five weeks) and lung protective ventilation alone. Previously reported surviving patients in China and Taiwan required extracorporeal membrane oxygenation (ECMO) and other invasive modalities. We suggest that an extended course of high dose corticosteroids should be considered for the treatment of smoke inhalation related ARDS and should be introduced as early as possible to minimize the morbidity and mortality. We further suggest that patients with smoke inhalation should be observed in the hospital for at least 48 to 72 hours before discharge, as ARDS can have a delayed onset. Being vigilant for infectious complications is important due to prolonged steroid treatment regimen. Patients must also be monitored for critical illness polyneuromyopathy. Additionally, upper airway injury should be suspected and early evaluation by otorhinolaryngology may be beneficial.

1. Introduction

Zinc chloride smoke bomb inhalation can induce a severe ARDS which is a lethal condition with an extremely high mortality rate. Two cases of smoke bomb induced severe ARDS survival have been previously reported in China and Taiwan [1, 2]. In the United States (US), a single case series of smoke bomb related ARDS reported two soldiers who succumbed to severe ARDS [3]. No smoke bomb induced severe ARDS survival has been reported in the US, to the best of our literature review. We successfully treated this patient with five weeks of high dose corticosteroids and did not use ECMO or other modalities, required by previously reported surviving patients in China and Taiwan. This case suggests that high doses of corticosteroids for an extended period might be beneficial for treatment of smoke bomb induced ARDS along with protective ventilation.

2. Case Report

A 32-year-old white male was admitted to our facility seventy-two hours after inhalation of emissions from a smoke bomb with very severe hypoxemia with an oxygen index of 58. The exposure was from a smoke bomb 1A, which generates 4000 cubic feet of zinc chloride smoke within thirty seconds. The victim was playing the role of a mock patient during a mining industry drill and was exposed to smoke in an enclosed mine

TABLE 1: Patient characteristics.

Variable	Value
Initial encounter (day 1)	
Pulse	97/minute
Respiratory rate	25/minute
Blood pressure	106/67 mmHg
Oxygen saturation	
Room air	87%
1-2 L oxygen	91%
Second encounter (day 3)	
Pulse	170/minute
Respiratory rate	50/minute
Blood pressure	87/55 mmHg
Temperature	100.5 F
Oxygen saturation	
Room air	48%
100% oxygen	58%
Laboratory data	
WBC	27.8×10^9 /L
Neutrophil	73%
Hemoglobin	16.2 g/dl
Hematocrit	48.8%
Platelets	$76,000 \times 10^9$ /L
Sodium	136 mEq/L
Potassium	5.1 mEq/L
Chloride	98 mEq/L
Bicarbonate	13 mEq/L
BUN	22 mg/dl
Creatinine	2.04 mg/dl
Anion Gap	25 mEq/L
D-dimer	3410 mg/L
Troponin	0.5 ng/mL
BNP	129 pg/mL
ESR	>120 mm/hr
CRP	28.20 mg/L
ABG on 100% oxygen	
pH	7.39
pO2	35 mmHg
pCO2	26 mmHg

ABG: arterial blood gas.

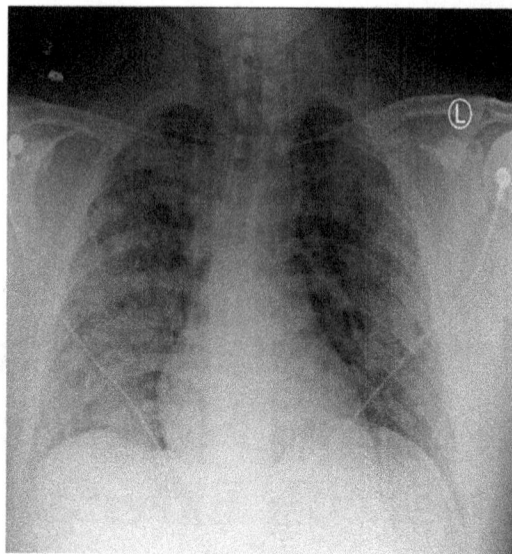

FIGURE 1: Chest X-ray.

analog (container) for approximately ten to fifteen minutes without any protective equipment. He developed shortness of breath and throat and chest discomfort immediately after the exposure and was provided oxygen at site. He then reported to a local emergency room, within one hour of the exposure. On initial presentation, he was tachypneic with a respiratory rate (RR) of 24 per minute and had mild hypoxia with an oxygen saturation of 87% on room air (Table 1). The State Poison Control Center confirmed that the main ingredients of the smoke were zinc chloride and carbon monoxide. He received treatment with bronchodilators (albuterol-ipratropium by nebulization), oxygen, and one dose of intravenous (IV) methylprednisolone 125 mg. His carboxyhemoglobin level

was within normal limits. He was discharged home from the emergency department with a five-day course of oral prednisone 60 mg daily and an albuterol inhaler.

Three days later, he presented to an outside facility for worsening shortness of breath and cough. He had profound hypoxia with an oxygen saturation of 34% on room air, improving only to 58% on 100% oxygen. His pulse was noted to be 170 per minute, and his RR was 50 per minute. At this point, he required intubation due to severe acute hypoxemic respiratory failure. His arterial blood gases (ABG) showed pH of 7.39, pCO2 of 26, and pO2 of 35 on 100% oxygen. His clinical presentation and lab findings are shown in Table 1. Electrocardiogram revealed sinus tachycardia with right axis deviation and nonspecific ST and T-wave changes. Chest X-ray (Figure 1) and chest computed tomography (CT) scan (Figure 2) showed increased opacities in the perihilar region in upper lobes bilaterally with relative sparing of the lower lobes, consistent with ARDS. No lobar consolidation was visible on chest imaging. Patient had normal left ventricular function on echocardiogram. He was placed on mechanical ventilation on volume control mode with PEEP of 20, RR of 20, and tidal volume (TV) of 8 cc/kg and was transferred to our facility.

He was admitted to the intensive care unit (ICU) and treatment was continued with high dose intravenous corticosteroids and lung protective ventilation strategy with low TV 6 cc/kg, PEEP of 18, and peak inspiratory pressure (PIP) of 28 and he was started on inhaled epoprostenol at a rate of 360 mcg/hour. Please refer to the table for complete steroids regimen (Table 2). Piperacillin/tazobactam and vancomycin were administered intravenously for ten days to cover empirically for ventilator associated pneumonia.

After completion of ten days of intravenous antibiotics and initial course of tapering intravenous steroids, he had persistent systemic inflammatory response syndrome (SIRS) criteria, and there was no change in his chest X-ray or

TABLE 2: Details of corticosteroids regimen (day since exposure to smoke, drug and route of administration, frequency and strength, and total number of doses).

Day	Drug and route	Frequency/strength	Total doses
1	Methylprednisolone IV	125 mg	1
2–3	Prednisone oral	60 mg	2
3–6	Methylprednisolone IV	125 mg	1
		62.5 mg every 6 H	10
		50 mg every 8 H	3
7–12	Hydrocortisone IV	100 mg every 12 H	3
		50 mg every 12 H	14
13–21	Methylprednisolone IV	125 mg every 6 H	12
		40 mg every 6 H	12
		40 mg every 8 H	03
		40 mg every 12 H	05
		30 mg	01
28–42	Prednisone oral	40 mg daily	7
		30 mg daily	4
		20 mg daily	3

IV: intravenous, H: hours, day since exposure to smoke.

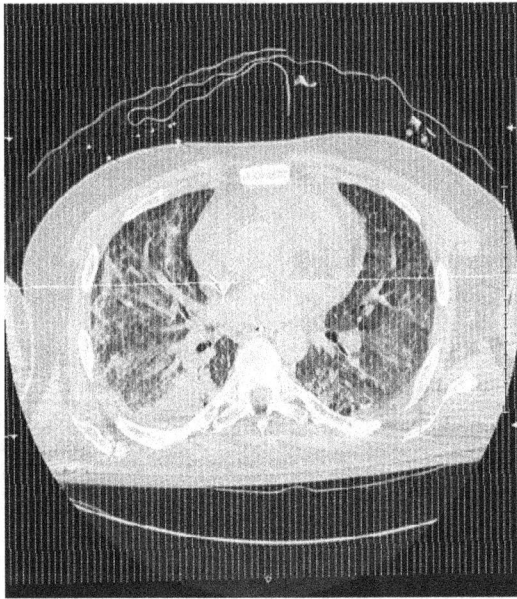

FIGURE 2: Chest CT scan.

ventilator mechanics and his oxygen index was still in the severe range (100–150) but improved from admission oxygen index of 58. All cultures were negative including follow-up bronchoalveolar lavage (BAL) cultures obtained on day eight and day eleven. He was not fluid overloaded clinically and left ventricular function was normal by echocardiogram, although he had mild pulmonary hypertension with an estimated right ventricular systolic pressure (RVSP) of 40. Nonspecific inflammatory markers were extremely elevated with an erythrocyte sedimentation rate (ESR) of greater than 120 and C-reactive protein (CRP) level of 30.97 (Table 1).

Infectious disease consultant agreed that an infectious etiology was unlikely for his ongoing fever and other positive SIRS criteria. The decision was made to resume high dose intravenous steroids on hospital day 13 (Table 2).

On the third week of mechanical ventilation, three to four days after resuming high dose IV steroids, his fraction of inspired oxygen (FiO2) and PEEP along with his inhaled epoprostenol was successfully weaned to levels safe enough to perform elective tracheostomy.

On day sixteen of hospitalization, percutaneous tracheostomy was performed. The proximal trachea revealed minimally inflamed thick whitish eschar/debris and this was partially removed and sent to the laboratory for evaluation and ultimately revealed necrotic debris with fungal elements consistent with aspergillus. CT scan of the head and neck did not reveal invasive disease. Ear nose and throat (ENT) surgeon was consulted and upper airway evaluation and debridement were performed in the operating room on day twenty but only superficial debris was removed from the palate.

While his blood and initial BAL cultures did not show fungal growth, his cultures from tissue biopsy/eschar-debris from the debridement site and later BAL specimens grew aspergillus. He was also found to be positive for serum Beta-D glucan and galactomannan. On day 22, per infectious disease recommendations, he was then empirically initiated on voriconazole for mucosal/mucocutaneous bronchopulmonary aspergillosis. He continued this regimen for a total of 28 days, along with ongoing steroids for chemical pneumonitis/ARDS secondary to smoke. It should be noted that his chest X-ray and oxygenation were already showing some improvement the week before antifungal therapy was started.

Lung protective mechanical ventilation was continued, using PCMV-APV mode, high PEEP (max 20) with inhaled epoprostenol, low TV (6 cc/kg), PIP of 28 initially, and an initial paralysis for first four days using atracurium. Epoprostenol was used as continuous inhalation at dose of 0.05 mcg/kg/min at 12 cc/hour (360 mcg/hour) and was later tapered off over forty-eight hours. He was on epoprostenol inhalation for a total of twelve days. Proning therapy was considered but not employed.

After spending twenty-three days in ICU, he was transferred to a long-term acute care (LTAC) facility for his ongoing need of mechanical ventilation. Steroid therapy was held for one week and then was restarted with oral prednisone for two more weeks. (Last dose of steroids was at end of week 6 of smoke exposure.) He remained in LTAC facility for an additional period of five weeks. Weaning trials with intermittent pressure support and continuous positive airway pressure (CPAP) were initiated from ventilation day thirty and eventually he was liberated from mechanical ventilation. He was on mechanical ventilation for a total period of fifty days.

Of note, his hospital course was further complicated by a left subclavian vein thrombosis, and acute tubular necrosis, later requiring intermittent hemodialysis. The patient recovered completely from his acute tubular necrosis and dialysis was later terminated. He was then discharged to rehabilitation center from LTAC facility without any respiratory complaints and off oxygen. He spent four months in rehabilitation center primarily for critical illness polyneuromyopathy and was then discharged home.

He is now ambulating well without any clinical evidence of dyspnea or oxygen requirements.

3. Discussion

Smoke bombs are commonly used for leak detection in mining, the metal industry, fire simulation exercises, disaster drills, and the military for drills and combat exercises [4–6]. The most commonly used mixture for smoke bombs contains zinc oxide and a chlorine donor, which leads to the formation of fine particles of zinc chloride producing a grey-white smoke [4]. The first case of zinc chloride smoke bomb inhalation injury was reported in 1945 by Evans during World War II, resulting in the demise of ten soldiers [7].

Smoke bomb inhalation is associated with a variety of airway and lung injuries based on the duration and concentration of smoke exposure. Schenker and colleagues described an incident of zinc chloride smoke exposure because of detonation of a smoke bomb in an airport disaster drill. Exposed participants presented with upper respiratory tract symptoms. Frequency of occurrence of the symptoms and severity of the symptoms correlated with proximity to the site and duration of the exposure. In this incident, the exposure was not intense and symptoms resolved over several days without any permanent functional decline [5].

However, sometimes even a modest exposure to zinc chloride smoke can cause significant late and long-term decline in lung functions despite mild initial symptoms. A case series of thirteen soldiers exposed to zinc chloride smoke during a combat exercise showed a statistically significant decline in their lung diffusion capacity and total lung capacity of 16.2% and 4.3%, respectively, four weeks following the

exposure. These findings correlated with elevated plasma zinc levels in all the patients. Lung function and volumes normalized after six to twelve months' postexposure. These patients experienced ongoing dyspnea on exertion despite normalization of lung function and volumes [8].

Intense and prolonged exposure to zinc chloride smoke has been found to cause severe lung injury and severe ARDS with high mortality [3, 6, 7]. The onset and severity of smoke bomb inhalation related lung injury depend on the concentration of the inhaled smoke and duration of exposure. There is one reported case where a patient was exposed to smoke for only 10–15 minutes without wearing a protective breathing apparatus and developed severe ARDS within 48 hours of exposure [1]. In another case series, victims were exposed to hexachloroethane (a chlorine donor for zinc chloride smoke) smoke for only 1-2 minutes without wearing gas masks and developed severe ARDS over the course of two weeks [9].

Our patient was not wearing a mask and was exposed to smoke in a contained space. Symptoms began immediately after the exposure and he was treated with oral prednisone 60 mg as an outpatient, after initial methylprednisolone bolus of 125 mg. Unfortunately, he returned seventy-two hours later with severe ARDS. His second presentation was likely delayed due to outpatient use of steroids.

Zinc chloride smoke bomb exposure is also associated with variety of other pulmonary and airway complications including pneumomediastinum, pneumothorax, and emphysematous bullae [1, 10, 11]. Matarese and Matthews reported another case of zinc chloride inhalation in US, where a patient developed severe emphysematous blebs after smoke inhalation which was complicated by pneumothorax. This patient survived with gradual recovery occurring over several months but chest X-ray remained abnormal with emphysematous blebs [10].

Zinc smoke exposure has also been reported to cause vascular lesions including endothelial cell proliferation and extensive interstitial and intra-alveolar space fibrosis [3, 9, 12]. Milliken with his colleagues reported a case where patient succumbed to acute severe interstitial pulmonary fibrosis after zinc chloride smoke bomb exposure [12].

This patient had a significant upper airway and palatal burn, which required debridement by an ENT surgeon. These burns were complicated by the mucocutaneous aspergillus infection and this complication was likely secondary to steroid and antibiotic treatments. Being on prolonged steroid treatment regimen, it is important to remain vigilant for any infectious complication as well as seeking an ENT evaluation for upper airway injury early on.

Zinc chloride smoke bomb induced severe ARDS has an extremely high mortality rate [3, 6, 7] and only two cases of survival [1, 2] have been reported. However, no smoke bomb induced severe ARDS survival has been reported in the US, to the best of our literature review. There are no standard guidelines available for the treatment of acute respiratory distress syndrome secondary to inhalation of smoke from a smoke bomb.

Traditionally lung protective ventilation strategy and corticosteroids have been the mainstay of treatment for smoke inhalation induced lung injury and both therapies have shown survival benefits [1, 2, 9, 13–15]. Amato and colleagues showed that use of a lung protective ventilatory strategy with low TV, high PEEP, and low plateau pressure of less than 30 cm H_2O increased survival rate up to 62% compared with 29% when conventional ventilation was used [13].

Other pharmacological treatment modalities such as N-acetylcysteine, L-3,4-dihydropyridine, methylene blue, inhaled nitric oxide [2, 9], exogenous surfactants [9], and penicillamine [16] have also been tried in individual cases of smoke exposure induced lung injury. Intravenous and nebulized N-acetylcysteine is thought to increase the urinary excretion of zinc. L-3,4-Dihydropyridine has been proposed to arrest collagen deposition [2] and intravenous methylene blue is used to treat methemoglobinemia and for respiratory support [9]. However, none of these treatment modalities have shown any survival benefits [9]. In addition to pharmacological modalities, other invasive strategies such as videothoracoscopic excision of emphysema bullae and recurrent chemical pleurodesis have been tried for the associated complications of pneumothorax and pleural effusions, respectively [2].

We used epoprostenol as rescue therapy in our patient. Nitric oxide inhalation has shown improved oxygenation for a short period of 48 hours in cases of severe ARDS but it did not show any survival benefits [2, 13, 15, 17]. There are no available strong randomized clinical studies for the effectiveness of inhaled prostaglandins in the treatment of ARDS. One clinical trial, which included 14 critically ill children with ARDS, did not show survival benefits of prostacyclin versus placebo [18]. However, observational studies and case series have shown efficacy of inhaled prostaglandins for improved oxygenation in severe hypoxemia due to ARDS. A recent retrospective chart review, which included 16 patients treated with inhaled epoprostenol, showed that epoprostenol improved oxygenation (defined as an improvement in P_{aO2}/F_{IO2} of >10% from the baseline) in 62.5% of the treated patients [19, 20]. Therefore, inhaled prostaglandins have been increasingly used lately as a rescue therapy for severe refractory hypoxemia in severe ARDS given its cost effectiveness compared to inhaled nitric oxide as well as similar efficacy for improving oxygenation and safety outcomes [21].

There are no prospective trials available on the utility of prone positioning in cases of smoke inhalation induced ARDS. One case report of smoke induced severe ARDS did not show any survival benefit of proning therapy [2]. However, one recent prospective RCT study (PROSEVA trial) has shown mortality benefit for early introduction of prone positioning (implied early within 36 hours, for 18–20 hours daily) as an adjunct therapy with protective lung mechanical ventilation for the treatment of severe ARDS [22]. Early prone positioning leads to effective alveoli recruitment during the acute exudative phase of ARDS, thus improving oxygenation by minimizing the shunt in patients with severe refractory hypoxemia [23]. We started high dose steroids with high PEEP and inhaled epoprostenol as rescue therapy for severe hypoxemia which helped us to wean his FiO2 gradually and improve oxygen index. We would certainly have tried prone positioning if initial rescue modes with epoprostenol, high PEEP, and high dose steroids would have failed. We urge to utilize proning as early adjunct therapy in cases of smoke exposure induced severe ARDS early on and/or in cases of severe refractory hypoxemia despite use of other rescue modalities when there is no contraindication to proning.

ECMO use is not well studied in cases of smoke induced severe ARDS in perspective trials. However, there have been reported cases of severe ARDS due to smoke inhalation who survived with the use of ECMO [1]. Bartlett et al. reported that, among adult patients with ARDS who were treated with ECMO, the survival rate was 61% [24]. ECMO is now being increasingly utilized as a rescue therapy for severe hypoxemia in cases of severe ARDS when there is no absolute or relative contraindication for its use. A recent trial showed a reduction in mortality and severe disability rates at six months following the use of ECMO [25]. Extracorporeal life support organization (ELSO) guidelines suggest considering using ECMO in cases of severe ARDS in adults when there is PaO_2/F_IO_2 ratio of 70–80 mmHg, Murray score > 3, and pH < 7.2 [26–28]. Absolute contraindications to the use of ECMO are irreversible lung disease with no indication for lung transplantation or severe brain damage associated with major cerebral infarction or severe intracranial bleeding. Other situations such as immunosuppression, bleeding, and mechanical ventilation at high settings (F_IO_2 > 0.9, PIP > 30 mmHg) for >7 days are considered as relative contraindication to ECMO therapy [27–30]. For implication of ECMO therapy, a ventilation strategy with a PIP of less than 25 cmH_2O, PEEP of 5–15 cmH_2O, and F_IO_2 of 0.3 is preferred [30–32]. We are well quipped community/university teaching hospital but we are not a recognized ECMO center. We treated our patient with available rescue therapies with epoprostenol and high dose corticosteroid in conjunction with high vent settings (PEEP 20 mx, PIP 28, and FioO2 100% initially) which were weaned down gradually. We considered ECMO as second option and would have transferred him to an outside ECMO center, in case our initial rescue strategy would have failed.

The role of corticosteroids overall in the treatment of acute lung injury and ARDS has been controversial. One study conducted by Bartlett et al. suggests that high dose glucocorticoids do not decrease the frequency of lung injury in patients at risk. It also suggested that high dose glucocorticoids do not modify the disease course [24]. Other studies by Wheeler and Bernard proposed that, in addition to modifying the inflammatory response, high dose corticosteroids reduce mortality. None of these studies included patients with smoke inhalation related ARDS [33]. However, there have been cases reported in English and Asian literature where early introduction of high dose intravenous steroids gave favorable outcomes in zinc chloride smoke inhalation related chemical pneumonitis [1, 2, 9]. Ishimoto and colleagues in Japan reported two cases of inhalational exposure to zinc fumes and zinc powder while working in a boathouse, without using protective equipment. These patients presented early, were admitted to the hospital, and responded well to early administration of intravenous steroids and noninvasive positive pressure ventilation (NIPPV) with favorable clinical outcomes [34]. We did not use NIPPV because of the severity of respiratory distress and profound hypoxemia at presentation. Johnson and Stonehil presented three cases of severe, generalized chemical pneumonitis secondary to zinc chloride smoke exposure [35]. Again, all these patients presented early and responded well. This emphasizes that close, in-hospital observation with early introduction of intravenous steroids can greatly reduce the severity of respiratory failure and thus potentially shorten the duration of hospitalization and decrease the overall morbidity and mortality.

We treated the patient with a 10-day course of intravenous antibiotics to empirically cover for hospital acquired pneumonia (HAP) along with the initial course of steroids [36]. There are no comparative studies available regarding the individual advantages of methylprednisolone versus hydrocortisone for the treatment of ARDS. Both treatment choices have been used in different clinical trials. There is no recommended standard steroid treatment regimen for smoke induced ARDS in the literature. However, there is one recent RCT study which favored the use of intravenous hydrocortisone (for 7 days) over the placebo for improved lung function (duration free from mechanical ventilation, reintubation rate) in patients with ARDS secondary to sepsis. We used intravenous hydrocortisone for one week from day 7 to day 13 [37].

However, he had persistent signs of SIRS with fever and leukocytosis despite optimal empiric coverage for HAP. Microbiology and cultures were negative with extremely elevated ESR and CRP with ongoing signs of inflammation. It was at this point that we went back to a high dose IV methylprednisolone for the continued steroid treatment regimen for smoke induced severe ARDS and he significantly responded and improved over the course of the treatment. Superficial fungal infection was felt to be a minor and secondary complication, mostly in the upper airway eschar/debris secondary to the delayed initial injury, although he did receive treatment for 28 days with voriconazole as per infectious disease recommendations.

In summary, ECMO treatment in addition to steroids and protective lung ventilation has been reported beneficial in individual case reports when treating smoke bomb related ARDS. In our patient, we did not use N-acetylcysteine, L-3,4-dehydroproline, penicillamine proning, or ECMO and the patient did not require any additional invasive procedures. This patient survived with prolonged high dose steroids for five weeks and protective lung ventilation with low tidal volume, high PEEP, and inhaled epoprostenol alone.

The patient also recovered from his acute tubular necrosis. He was discharged to a rehabilitation facility off oxygen without any respiratory complaints, primarily for his critical illness polyneuromyopathy. From the rehabilitation center, he was then discharged home but still has some residual peripheral neuropathy. It should be noted that being vigilant for critical illness polyneuromyopathy is crucial in cases such as these that require prolonged steroid treatments and especially if paralytics are also used [38, 39].

4. Conclusion

High doses of corticosteroids for an extended period might be beneficial for treatment of smoke bomb induced severe ARDS and should be considered as a single agent pharmacologic treatment modality along with protective ventilation. These patients must be observed in the hospital for at least forty-eight to seventy-two hours before discharge, as ARDS can have a delayed onset, especially if treated with steroids early. Being vigilant for any infectious complications and critical illness polyneuromyopathy is prudent due to prolonged steroid treatment regimen. Additionally, upper airway injury should be suspected and early upper airway and proximal trachea evaluation by ENT may be beneficial. Zinc chloride smoke use must be minimized due to the morbidity and mortality associated with the smoke exposure and it should be replaced with another nontoxic or less toxic substance. Future case studies may further enlighten the treatment options for this rare, but frequently lethal condition.

Acknowledgments

The authors want to thank Charles D. Graham, M.D., and Mokshya Sharma, M.D., for reviewing this manuscript. They would also like to acknowledge the permission of patient and family to publish this article.

References

[1] C.-F. Chian, C.-P. Wu, C.-W. Chen, W.-L. Su, C.-B. Yeh, and W.-C. Perng, "Acute respiratory distress syndrome after zinc chloride inhalation: Survival after extracorporeal life support and corticosteroid treatment," American Journal of Critical Care, vol. 19, no. 1, pp. 86–90, 2010.

[2] V. Pettilä, O. Takkunen, and P. Tukiainen, "Zinc chloride smoke inhalation: A rare cause of severe acute respiratory distress syndrome," Intensive Care Medicine, vol. 26, no. 2, pp. 215–217, 2000.

[3] S. Homma, R. Jones, J. Qvist, W. M. Zapol, and L. Reid, "Pulmonary vascular lesions in the adult respiratory distress syndrome caused by inhalation of zinc chloride smoke: A morphometric study," Human Pathology, vol. 23, no. 1, pp. 45–50, 1992.

[4] F. Gil, A. Pla, A. F. Hernández, J. M. Mercado, and F. Méndez, "A fatal case following exposure to zinc chloride and hexachloroethane from a smoke bomb in a fire simulation at a school," Clinical Toxicology, vol. 46, no. 6, pp. 563–565, 2008.

[5] M. B. Schenker, F. E. Speizer, and J. O. Taylor, "Acute upper respiratory symptoms resulting from exposure to zinc chloride aerosol," Environmental Research, vol. 25, no. 2, pp. 317–324, 1981.

[6] M. B. Macaulay and A. K. Mant, "Smoke-bomb poisoning. a fatal case following the inhalation of zinc chloride smoke," Journal of the Royal Army Medical Corps, vol. 110, pp. 27–32, 1964.

[7] E. Evans, "CASUALTIES FOLLOWING EXPOSURE TO ZINC CHLORIDE SMOKE," The Lancet, vol. 246, no. 6369, pp. 368–370, 1945.

[8] B. Zerahn, A. Kofoed-Enevoldsen, B. V. Jensen et al., "Pulmonary damage after modest exposure to zinc chloride smoke," Respiratory Medicine, vol. 93, no. 12, pp. 885–890, 1999.

[9] E. Hjortsø, J. Ovist, M. I. Bud et al., "ARDS after accidental inhalation of zinc chloride smoke," *Intensive Care Medicine*, vol. 14, no. 1, pp. 17–24, 1988.

[10] S. L. Matarese and J. I. Matthews, "Zinc chloride (smoke bomb) inhalation lung injury," *Chest*, vol. 89, no. 2, pp. 308-309, 1986.

[11] P. S. Holmes, "Pneumomediastinum associated with inhalation of white smoke," *Military Medicine*, vol. 164, pp. 751-752, 1999.

[12] J. A. Milliken, D. Waugh, and M. E. Kadish, "Acute interstitial pulmonary fibrosis caused by a smoke bomb," *Canadian Medical Association Journal*, vol. 88, pp. 36–39, 1963.

[13] M. B. P. Amato, C. S. V. Barbas, D. M. Medeiros et al., "Effect of a protective-ventilation strategy on mortality in the acute respiratory distress syndrome," *The New England Journal of Medicine*, vol. 338, no. 6, pp. 347–354, 1998.

[14] R. G. Brower, M. A. Matthay, A. Morris, D. Schoenfeld, B. T. Thompson, and A. Wheeler, "Ventilation with lower tidal volumes as compared with traditional tidal volumes for acute lung injury and the acute respiratory distress syndrome," *The New England Journal of Medicine*, vol. 342, no. 18, pp. 1301–1308, 2000.

[15] J. M. Luce, "Acute lung injury and the acute respiratory distress syndrome," *Critical Care Medicine*, vol. 26, no. 2, pp. 369–376, 1998.

[16] M. B. Allen, A. Crisp, N. Snook, and R. L. Page, "'Smoke-bomb' pneumonitis," *Respiratory Medicine*, vol. 86, no. 2, pp. 165-166, 1992.

[17] R. W. Taylor, J. L. Zimmerman, R. P. Dellinger et al., "Low-Dose Inhaled Nitric Oxide in Patients with Acute Lung Injury: A Randomized Controlled Trial," *Journal of the American Medical Association*, vol. 291, no. 13, pp. 1603–1609, 2004.

[18] A. Afshari, J. Brok, A. M. Moller, and J. Wetterslev, "Aerosolized prostacyclin for acute lung injury (ALI) and acute respiratory distress syndrome (ARDS)," *Cochrane Database of Systematic Reviews*, no. 8, CD007733, 2010.

[19] P. Dahlem, W. M. C. Van Aalderen, M. De Neef, M. G. W. Dijkgraaf, and A. P. Bos, "Randomized controlled trial of aerosolized prostacyclin therapy in children with acute lung injury," *Critical Care Medicine*, vol. 32, no. 4, pp. 1055–1060, 2004.

[20] K. A. Dunkley, P. R. Louzon, J. Lee, and S. Vu, "Efficacy, safety, and medication errors associated with the use of inhaled epoprostenol for adults with acute respiratory distress syndrome: A pilot study," *Annals of Pharmacotherapy*, vol. 47, no. 6, pp. 790–796, 2013.

[21] H. Torbic, P. M. Szumita, K. E. Anger, P. Nuccio, S. LaGambina, and G. Weinhouse, "Inhaled epoprostenol vs inhaled nitric oxide for refractory hypoxemia in critically ill patients," *Journal of Critical Care*, vol. 28, no. 5, pp. 844–848, 2013.

[22] C. Guérin, J. J.-C. Reignier, P. Richard et al., "Prone positioning in severe acute respiratory distress syndrome," *New England Journal of Medicine*, vol. 368, pp. 2159–2168, 2013.

[23] C. M. Romero, R. A. Cornejo, L. R. Gálvez et al., "Extended prone position ventilation in severe acute respiratory distress syndrome: A pilot feasibility study," *Journal of Critical Care*, vol. 24, no. 1, pp. 81–88, 2009.

[24] R. H. Bartlett, D. W. Roloff, J. R. Custer, J. G. Younger, and R. B. Hirschl, "Extracorporeal life support: the University of Michigan Experience," *JAMA: the Journal of the American Medical Association*, vol. 283, no. 7, pp. 904–908, 2000.

[25] M. D. Mitchell, M. E. Mikkelsen, C. A. Umscheid, I. Lee, B. D. Fuchs, and S. D. Halpern, "A systematic review to inform institutional decisions about the use of extracorporeal membrane oxygenation during the H1N1 influenza pandemic," *Critical Care Medicine*, vol. 38, no. 6, pp. 1398–1404, 2010.

[26] Extracorporeal Life Support Organization, https://www.elso.org/.

[27] S. Kolla, S. S. Awad, P. B. Rich, R. J. Schreiner, R. B. Hirschl, and R. H. Bartlett, "Extracorporeal life support for 100 adult patients with severe respiratory failure," *Annals of Surgery*, vol. 226, no. 4, pp. 544–566, 1997.

[28] G. J. Peek, M. Mugford, and R. Tiruvoipati, "Efficacy and economic assessment of conventional ventilatory support versus extracorporeal membrane oxygenation for severe adult respiratory failure (CESAR): a multicentre randomised controlled trial," *The Lancet*, vol. 374, no. 9698, pp. 1351–1363, 2009.

[29] N. Patroniti, A. Zangrillo, F. Pappalardo et al., "The Italian ECMO network experience during the 2009 influenza A(H1N1) pandemic: preparation for severe respiratory emergency outbreaks," *Intensive Care Medicine*, vol. 37, no. 9, pp. 1447–1457, 2011.

[30] D. Brodie and M. Bacchetta, "Extracorporeal membrane oxygenation for ARDS in adults," *New England Journal of Medicine*, vol. 365, no. 20, pp. 1905–1914, 2011.

[31] M. O. Meade, D. J. Cook, G. H. Guyatt et al., "Ventilation strategy using low tidal volumes, recruitment maneuvers, and high positive end-expiratory pressure for acute lung injury and acute respiratory distress syndrome: a randomized controlled trial," *JAMA*, vol. 299, no. 6, pp. 637–645, 2008.

[32] T. Bein, S. Weber-Carstens, A. Goldmann et al., "Lower tidal volume strategy (≈ 3 ml/kg) combined with extracorporeal CO_2 removal versus 'conventional' protective ventilation (6 ml/kg) in severe ARDS: the prospective randomized Xtravent-study," *Intensive Care Medicine*, vol. 39, no. 5, pp. 847–856, 2013.

[33] A. P. Wheeler and G. R. Bernard, "Acute lung injury and the acute respiratory distress syndrome: a clinical review," *The Lancet*, vol. 369, no. 9572, pp. 1553–1564, 2007.

[34] H. Ishimoto, K. Yatera, K. Oda et al., "Two cases of acute respiratory distress syndrome related to zinc fumes and zinc dust inhalation," *Journal of UOEH*, vol. 36, no. 2, pp. 147–152, 2014.

[35] F. A. Johnson and R. B. Stonehil, "Chemical pneumonitis from inhalation of zinc chloride," *Chest*, vol. 40, pp. 619–624, 1961.

[36] A. Ashok Kalanuria and W. Zai, "Email author and Marek Mirski: ventilator-associated pneumonia in the ICU," *Critical Care*, vol. 18, no. 2, 208 pages, 2014.

[37] S. Tongyoo, C. Permpikul, W. Mongkolpun et al., "Hydrocortisone treatment in early sepsis-associated acute respiratory distress syndrome: Results of a randomized controlled trial," *Critical Care*, vol. 20, no. 1, article no. 329, 2016.

[38] R. D. Stevens, D. W. Dowdy, R. K. Michaels, P. A. Mendez-Tellez, P. J. Pronovost, and D. M. Needham, "Neuromuscular dysfunction acquired in critical illness: A systematic review," *Intensive Care Medicine*, vol. 33, no. 11, pp. 1876–1891, 2007.

[39] R. I. Thiele, H. Jakob, E. Hund et al., "Critical illness polyneuropathy: A new iatrogenically induced syndrome after cardiac surgery?" *European Journal of Cardio-thoracic Surgery*, vol. 12, no. 6, pp. 826–835, 1997.

48

Bent Metal in a Bone: A Rare Complication of an Emergent Procedure or a Deficiency in Skill Set?

Mridula Krishnan,[1] **Katherine Lester,**[2] **Amber Johnson,**[2] **Kaye Bardeloza,**[1]
Peter Edemekong,[3] **and Ilya Berim**[4]

[1]*Department of Internal Medicine, CHI Creighton University Medical Center, Omaha, NE, USA*
[2]*Creighton University School of Medicine, Omaha, NE, USA*
[3]*Department of Family Medicine, CHI Creighton University Medical Center, Omaha, NE, USA*
[4]*Department of Pulmonary and Critical Care, CHI Creighton University Medical Center, Omaha, NE, USA*

Correspondence should be addressed to Ilya Berim; ilyaberim@creighton.edu

Academic Editor: Chiara Lazzeri

Intraosseous (IO) access is an important consideration in patients with difficult intravenous (IV) access in emergent situations. IO access in adults has become more popular due to the ease of placement and high success rates. The most common sites of access include the proximal tibia and the humeral head. The complications associated are rare but can be catastrophic: subsequent amputation of a limb has been described in the literature. We report a 25-year-old female presenting with diabetic ketoacidosis (DKA) in whom emergent IO access was complicated by needle bending inside the humerus. Conventional bedside removal was impossible and required surgical intervention in operating room.

1. Introduction

Intraosseous (IO) access can be lifesaving when peripheral vascular access is difficult to obtain and the complications are minimal [1, 2]. Its use is more commonly observed in the pediatric subset of patients due to the ease of access but adult IO placement is becoming a more frequent practice with high success rates [3].

Efficacy of medication administration via intravenous (IV) versus intraosseous (IO) route has been found to be comparable in onset and duration of action of pharmacological agents [1]. We report a case of a 25-year-old female who required placement of an IO needle with the EZ-IO system for treatment of severe dehydration and hemodynamic instability as a complication of diabetic ketoacidosis (DKA).

2. Case Presentation

A 25-year-old female presented to the emergency department with complaints of severe nonradiating epigastric and umbilical pain associated with nausea and vomiting. She was unable to tolerate oral intake. The patient reported this pain to be similar to the abdominal pain that occurred with previous episodes of DKA, although more severe in intensity. Past medical history was significant for type 1 diabetes mellitus with reported noncompliance with insulin and multiple episodes of DKA. Medical history also included asthma, bipolar disorder, ischemic bowel disease status after small bowel resection, methamphetamine abuse, posttraumatic stress disorder, and idiopathic chronic pancreatitis. Her home medications comprised of a long and short acting daily insulin regimen, divalproex, citalopram, and albuterol inhaler. She had no documented allergies.

Vital signs on arrival revealed a heart rate of 115/minute, blood pressure of 132/110 mmHg, respiratory rate of 28/minute, and oxygen saturation of 100% on room air. On physical exam, the patient was noted to be lethargic with dry mucous membranes. Cardiovascular examination revealed sinus tachycardia. Abdominal examination revealed diffuse abdominal tenderness with active bowel sounds with no evidence of guarding or rigidity.

Due to the severity and acuity of her uncontrolled diabetic ketoacidosis with difficulty obtaining IV access, an intraosseous line was obtained in the right humerus for administration of intravenous fluids. A registered nurse, with prior IO access training that included a class and further instruction at hospital orientation when hired, obtained IO access using the EZ-IO system. Initial laboratory studies revealed a blood glucose level of 321 mg/dL, an anion gap of 22, and bicarbonate level of 15 mmol/L. The potassium level was 3.6 without electrocardiographic changes. Urine analysis was positive for ketones and glucose. Arterial blood gas revealed severe metabolic acidosis with the pH being 7.05. Abdominal radiograph was unremarkable. The patient was diagnosed with severe diabetic ketoacidosis and aggressive fluid resuscitation was initiated with normal saline through the intraosseous access, along with insulin infusion as per the hospital's DKA protocol. There were no difficulties with fluid and medication administration through the aforementioned intraosseous needle.

After adequate fluid resuscitation, an attempt at intraosseous line removal in the intensive care unit was unsuccessful due to severe pain in addition to concerns for possible breakage of the needle. A plain radiograph of the right shoulder was significant for an intraosseous needle that appeared bent at the humeral neck, without any evidence of fracture or dislocation on anteroposterior view (Figure 1).

Orthopedics was consulted and the risks and benefits of surgical and nonsurgical options for intraosseous line removal were thoroughly discussed with the patient. The patient opted to undergo surgical removal of the intraosseous line. Intraoperatively, the right arm was abducted and under C-arm guidance, gentle traction on the intraosseous line was placed directly over the bent portion in order to prevent the needle from breaking off inside the bone. The needle was removed in one piece and C-arm images were taken to confirm no pieces of needle were left behind (Figure 2). Intraoperative fluoroscopic images demonstrated removal of the intraosseous needle from the proximal humerus, with no evidence of residual foreign body.

Upon further investigation, the nurse reported two prior successful tibial IO placements. However, the nurse denied having placed a humeral IO line prior to this patient interaction. The nurse noted that the patient refused a stabilizing device to keep her arm stable during the placement. The patient had a history of bent intraosseous needles when removing the needles in the past. The prior incidents did not require surgery to remove the intraosseous needle. After the event, the emergency department nurses received training in obtaining IV access via humeral and tibial IO placement.

3. Discussion

IO infusions are a means of achieving rapid administration of medications into the intravascular compartment in emergency situations [8]. American Heart Association (AHA) and European Resuscitation Council (ERC) both recommend IO access if IV access cannot be obtained especially in emergent

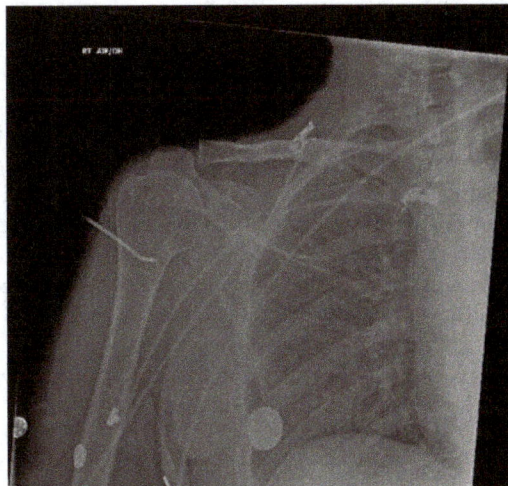

FIGURE 1: Radiograph of the right shoulder with a bent intraosseous needle in the neck of the humerus.

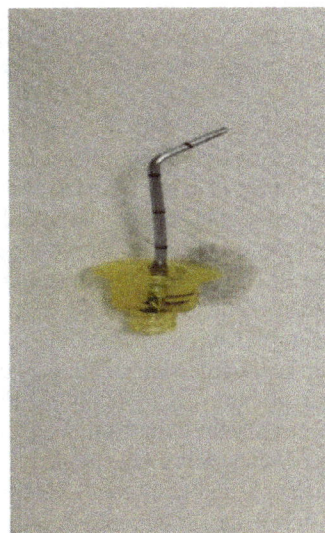

FIGURE 2: Bent EZ-IO after surgical removal from the bone.

situations [9, 10]. IV access failure rates in the emergency department have been reported to be between 10 and 40 percent [11]. The time required to obtain peripheral IV access averages between 2 and 16 minutes in those with difficult peripheral vascular access [6, 11].

There have been multiple large prospective studies based on pediatric literature to assess the safety and efficacy of an intraosseous line placement. The use of semiautomatic IO (EZ-IO) has led to increased use of IOs to obtain peripheral access [12].

In our patient, it was difficult to determine a single event that led to this complication. The various factors that could have contributed to the bend in the needle include patient's inability to maintain appropriate arm position during procedure, level of nurse experience with IO access, incorrect site of placement of the IO, manipulation during removal, improper positioning of the upper limb during and after IO placement, or a defect in manufacturing of the IO needle. There should be major emphasis on correct positioning of the IO needle and also the prevention of dislodgement to prevent such complications. The needle is inserted into the skin perpendicular to the bone and once the needle penetrates the bone marrow cavity, a loss of resistance is detected. When using a power-driven EZ-IO device, the drill has to be stopped within a certain distance so that the needle will remain in the IO space and not penetrate the opposite cortex. In our case, besides the above factors that could have predisposed to the event, it can also be speculated that incorrect size of the needle was used.

Below we will discuss intraosseous access in detail with a focus on the complications of the technique.

3.1. Types of IO.
There are many commercially available intraosseous devices [13]. The ones approved by the Food and Drug Administration (FDA) include the First Access for Shock and Trauma 1 (FAST1), the EZ-IO, and the Bone Injection Gun (BIG). The EZ-IO is a battery operated drill which is most frequently used [2, 13, 14].

The FAST1 is a spring device which was specially designed to obtain IO access through the sternum [14, 15].

3.2. Sites of IO Access.
The sternum was used for IO infusions previously; however, the tibia and humerus have been found to be more advantageous [16]. The tibia and humerus are both long bones and easy to palpate and have easily identifiable landmarks. A nonrandomized, prospective, observational study by Ong et al. compared the infusion rates, rates of successful placement, time to placement, and complications for tibial or humeral IO access using the EZ-IO device. The results indicated no significant difference in flow rates between the two placements. In addition, there were no significant differences in the complication rates between the two different access sites. Advantage of gaining tibial access includes easily palpable and identifiable landmarks [17]. On the other hand, while the aforementioned study found no difference in infusion rates, a cadaveric study by Pasley et al. found advantages to humeral placement to include capability for faster infusion rates and possible decreased time to central circulation. Flow rate in the humerus was found to be greater than in the tibia, with average flow rate of 57.1 mL/min at the humerus and average flow rate of 30.7 mL/min at the proximal tibia [18]. These findings are consistent with previous trials in swine models [19, 20]. Randomized controlled trials comparing time to central circulation have not yet been conducted, but internal report by producers of the EZ-IO suggests that time from injection at humerus insertion site to entry into the superior vena cava is only 2.3 seconds, [21] which may indicate a second advantage of humeral placement.

3.3. Complications Associated with IO Access.
Barlow and Kuhn analyzed the complication rate with the use of IO catheters in a large subset of over 5000 patients and the overall complication rate was as low as 2.1 percent [22].

A bend in the intraosseous line was more commonly observed in manually inserted IOs rather than in cases with the use of a drill-set [5, 23]. Using a live swine model, a study comparing manually placed versus mechanical drill-assisted IO catheters reported 33.3 percent bent needles via manual insertion which made intraosseous infusion impossible. However, no bent needles were reported using mechanical drill-assistance [5]. A study by Brenner et al. reported that 15.4 percent of the time establishing IO access manually resulted in complications such as a bent or broken insertion needle [23]. A Scandinavian study reported bent needles in 4 percent of the patients following insertion of an IO. The most common presenting signs of bent IO needle in these cases were difficulty in penetration of the periosteum and difficult bone marrow aspiration following insertion [2]. The bent needles caused by manual insertion may be explained by increased force when placing the manual IO needle. The complication may also be explained by lack of experience or unfamiliarity with the insertion device [5].

The complication rate with these devices also varies depending on the type of IO used. A bent catheter was the least common complication of the EZ-IO when compared to the other types of IO. Overall minimal complications were reported when using the semiautomatic intraosseous infusion system (EZ-IO) [23].

Uncommonly, life-threatening complications such as limb gangrene and compartment syndrome have been reported with this method of obtaining vascular access. One such event was reported by Greenstein et al. with extravasation of a vasopressor agent from the IO access leading to limb ischemia [8]. Other rare complications are reported such as bending of insertion needle, skin necrosis, retained needle end, and infection manifesting as osteomyelitis (Table 1) [2, 4–8].

3.4. Factors Determining Successful IO Placement in Adults.
Singh et al. demonstrated that the success of IO placement, which was measured by rate of penetration of cortex at the first attempt, was around 66 percent [24]. Another study by Hafner et al. defined successful IO placement by meeting 2 of the 3 following criteria: aspirate bone marrow, infuse 10 mL methylene blue saline solution, and the absence of extravasation. 100 percent of the drill-assisted IO needles were successfully placed [5].

IO access can be difficult to obtain in obese patients. A prospective observational study was done on obese patients in which IO access was preceded by ultrasound guided measurement of soft tissue depth in accessible regions, that is, tibial tuberosity and proximal humerus. A higher BMI was found to be moderately predictive of an increased soft tissue depth at the proximal and distal tibia; however, this was not the case at the distal humerus. The size of the IO needle also determines the success of the procedure in obese patients. The standard IO needle measures 25 mm and is the adequate size for IO access in nonobese patients and for IO access at the proximal tibia and distal tibia if the patient's BMI is less than or equal to 43 and 60, respectively. It is advised that when attempting to gain intraosseous access at the humerus insertion site in an obese patient only a larger 45 mm needle should be used [25]. It has been shown time and again that training imparted to healthcare personnel can significantly

TABLE 1: Complications associated with IO access.

Study	Type of study	Population studied	Number of IO placements	Number/percentage of major or minor complications	Number and type of major or minor complication
Hallas et al. (2013) [2]	Online questionnaire	Newborns to adults	861 (reporting EZ-IO only)	448/52%	25, extravasation 11, bent or broken needle 6, compartment syndrome
Lee et al. (2015) [4]	Prospective observational study	Unspecified, adults	33	3/9.09%	1, extravasation and skin necrosis 1, pain 1, dislodged needle
Hafner et al. (2013) [5]	Randomized prospective crossover experiment	Mixed breed swine	21	4/19%	3, unsuccessful infusion 1, extravasation
Paxton et al. (2009) [6]	Prospective cohort	Unspecified	30	17/57%	11, catheter dislodgement 3, inability to flush 2, failed attempt to place catheter 1, slow flow
Helm et al. (2015) [7]	Retrospective analysis	Newborns to adults	227	4/1.7%	2, needle dislocation 1, needle bending 1, extravasation

improve the efficacy of intraosseous line placement [26]. Levitan et al. demonstrated that minimal training is required for the use of the EZ-IO device. In the study, the participants achieved insertion success after three attempts. The participants received one 5-minute in-service presentation and observed one insertion prior to their attempts [27].

4. Conclusion

Intraosseous access remains safe and easy to use if IV access is difficult and time consuming. There have been rare complications reported such as bending of insertion needle, skin necrosis, retained needle end, and infection manifesting as osteomyelitis [2, 4–8]. Evidence has shown that user training and the device used affect complication rates along with manual and semiautomatic insertion [5, 23]. Our reported case entails a semiautomatic insertion device with evidence of low complications, with limited user experience. Education should be used to facilitate learning experiences for all staff in the hospital for IO insertion. A suggested method of training for healthcare workers includes the initiation of a simulation training protocol for obtaining IO access. Implementation of a hospital wide training program would be relatively low cost and a low time burden. With education and training, EZ-IO may become the preferred method of achieving rapid vascular access for emergent resuscitation with a low risk for complications.

Competing Interests

The authors declare that they have no conflict of interests.

References

[1] J. P. Orlowski, D. T. Porembka, J. M. Gallagher, J. D. Lockrem, and F. VanLente, "Comparison study of intraosseous, central intravenous, and peripheral intravenous infusions of emergency drugs," *American Journal of Diseases of Children*, vol. 144, no. 1, pp. 112–117, 1990.

[2] P. Hallas, M. Brabrand, and L. Folkestad, "Complication with intraosseous access: Scandinavian users' experience," *Western Journal of Emergency Medicine*, vol. 14, no. 5, pp. 440–443, 2013.

[3] P. W. Glaeser, T. R. Hellmich, D. Szewczuga, J. D. Losek, and D. S. Smith, "Five-year experience in prehospital intraosseous infusions in children and adults," *Annals of Emergency Medicine*, vol. 22, no. 7, pp. 1119–1124, 1993.

[4] P. M. J. Lee, C. Lee, P. Rattner, X. Wu, H. Gershengorn, and S. Acquah, "Intraosseous versus central venous catheter utilization and performance during inpatient medical emergencies," *Critical Care Medicine*, vol. 43, no. 6, pp. 1233–1238, 2015.

[5] J. W. Hafner, A. Bryant, F. Huang, and K. Swisher, "Effectiveness of a drill-assisted intraosseous catheter versus manual intraosseous catheter by resident physicians in a swine model," *Western Journal of Emergency Medicine*, vol. 14, no. 6, pp. 629–632, 2013.

[6] J. H. Paxton, T. E. Knuth, and H. A. Klausner, "Proximal humerus intraosseous infusion: a preferred emergency venous access," *The Journal of trauma*, vol. 67, no. 3, pp. 606–611, 2009.

[7] M. Helm, B. Haunstein, T. Schlechtriemen, M. Ruppert, L. Lampl, and M. Gäßler, "EZ-IO® intraosseous device implementation in German helicopter emergency medical service," *Resuscitation*, vol. 88, pp. 43–47, 2015.

[8] Y. Y. Greenstein, S. J. Koenig, P. H. Mayo, and M. Narasimhan, "A serious adult intraosseous catheter complication and review of the literature," *Critical Care Medicine*, vol. 44, no. 9, pp. e904–e909, 2016.

[9] C. D. Deakin, J. P. Nolan, J. Soar et al., "European resuscitation council guidelines for resuscitation 2010 section 4. Adult advanced life support," *Resuscitation*, vol. 81, no. 10, pp. 1305–1352, 2010.

[10] R. W. Neumar, C. W. Otto, M. S. Link et al., "Part 8: adult advanced cardiovascular life support: 2010 American Heart Association guidelines for cardiopulmonary resuscitation and emergency cardiovascular care," *Circulation*, vol. 122, no. 18, supplement 3, pp. S729–S767, 2010.

[11] F. Lapostolle, J. Catineau, B. Garrigue et al., "Prospective evaluation of peripheral venous access difficulty in emergency care," *Intensive Care Medicine*, vol. 33, no. 8, pp. 1452–1457, 2007.

[12] P. Zasko, L. Szarpak, A. Kurowski, Z. Truszewski, and L. Czyzewski, "Success of intraosseous access procedure in simulated adult resuscitation," *Critical Care and Resuscitation*, vol. 18, no. 2, article 134, 2016.

[13] H. J. G. M. Derikx, B. M. Gerritse, R. Gans, and N. J. M. van der Meer, "A randomized trial comparing two intraosseous access devices in intrahospital healthcare providers with a focus on retention of knowledge, skill, and self-efficacy," *European Journal of Trauma and Emergency Surgery*, vol. 40, no. 5, pp. 581–586, 2014.

[14] M. Waisman and D. Waisman, "Bone marrow infusion in adults," *Journal of Trauma-Injury, Infection and Critical Care*, vol. 42, no. 2, pp. 288–293, 1997.

[15] M. D. Calkins, G. Fitzgerald, T. B. Bentley, and D. Burris, "Intraosseous infusion devices: a comparison for potential use in special operations," *Journal of Trauma-Injury, Infection and Critical Care*, vol. 48, no. 6, pp. 1068–1074, 2000.

[16] D. D. Miller, G. Guimond, D. P. Hostler, T. Platt, and H. E. Wang, "Feasibility of sternal intraosseous access by emergency medical technician students," *Prehospital Emergency Care*, vol. 9, no. 1, pp. 73–78, 2005.

[17] M. E. H. Ong, Y. H. Chan, J. J. Oh, and A. S.-Y. Ngo, "An observational, prospective study comparing tibial and humeral intraosseous access using the EZ-IO," *The American Journal of Emergency Medicine*, vol. 27, no. 1, pp. 8–15, 2009.

[18] J. Pasley, C. H. T. Miller, J. J. DuBose et al., "Intraosseous infusion rates under high pressure: a cadaveric comparison of anatomic sites," *Journal of Trauma and Acute Care Surgery*, vol. 78, no. 2, pp. 295–299, 2015.

[19] J. Lairet, V. Bebarta, K. Lairet et al., "A comparison of proximal tibia, distal femur, and proximal humerus infusion rates using the EZ-IO intraosseous device on the adult swine (*Sus scrofa*) model," *Prehospital Emergency Care*, vol. 17, no. 2, pp. 280–284, 2013.

[20] D. W. Warren, N. Kissoon, J. F. Sommerauer, and M. J. Rieder, "Comparison of fluid infusion rates among peripheral intravenous and humerus, femur, malleolus, and tibial intraosseous sites in normovolemic and hypovolemic piglets," *Annals of Emergency Medicine*, vol. 22, no. 2, pp. 183–186, 1993.

[21] Internal study report, Protocol 2013-06: Clinical Studies to Determine the Optimal Technique to Identify the Proximal Humerus Intraosseous Vascular Access Insertion Site, Vidacare Corporation, May 2013.

[22] B. Barlow and K. Kuhn, "Orthopedic management of complications of using intraosseous catheters," *The American Journal of Orthopedics*, vol. 43, no. 4, pp. 186–190, 2014.

[23] T. Brenner, M. Bernhard, M. Helm et al., "Comparison of two intraosseous infusion systems for adult emergency medical use," *Resuscitation*, vol. 78, no. 3, pp. 314–319, 2008.

[24] S. Singh, P. Aggarwal, R. Lodha et al., "Feasibility study of a novel intraosseous device in adult human cadavers," *Indian Journal of Medical Research*, vol. 143, no. 3, pp. 275–280, 2016.

[25] T. Kehrl, B. A. Becker, D. E. Simmons, E. K. Broderick, and R. A. Jones, "Intraosseous access in the obese patient: assessing the need for extended needle length," *The American Journal of Emergency Medicine*, vol. 34, no. 9, pp. 1831–1834, 2016.

[26] J. Cheung, H. Rosenberg, and C. Vaillancourt, "Barriers and facilitators to intraosseous access in adult resuscitations when peripheral intravenous access is not achievable," *Academic Emergency Medicine*, vol. 21, no. 3, pp. 250–256, 2014.

[27] R. M. Levitan, C. D. Bortle, T. A. Snyder, D. A. Nitsch, J. T. Pisaturo, and K. H. Butler, "Use of a battery-operated needle driver for intraosseous access by novice users: skill acquisition with cadavers," *Annals of Emergency Medicine*, vol. 54, no. 5, pp. 692–694, 2009.

49

Use of CytoSorb in Traumatic Amputation of the Forearm and Severe Septic Shock

Heinz Steltzer,[1,2] **Alexander Grieb,**[1] **Karim Mostafa,**[1] **and Reinhard Berger**[1]

[1]*AUVA-Unfallkrankenhaus Meidling, Department of Anesthesiology and Intensive Care Medicine, Vienna, Austria*
[2]*Sigmund Freud Private University, Vienna, Austria*

Correspondence should be addressed to Heinz Steltzer; heinz.steltzer@auva.at

Academic Editor: Kurt Lenz

Severe trauma associated with later disability and mortality still constitutes a major health and socioeconomic problem throughout the world. While primary morbidity and mortality are mostly related to initial injuries and early complications, secondary lethality is strongly linked to the development of systemic inflammatory response syndrome, sepsis, and ultimately multiple organ dysfunction syndrome. We herein report on a 49-year-old male patient who was admitted to the hospital after a traumatic amputation of his right forearm that was cut off while working on a landfill. After initial treatment for shock, he received immediate replantation and was transferred to the ICU. Due to the anticipated risk of a complex infection, continuous renal replacement therapy in combination with CytoSorb was initiated. During the course of the combined treatment, a rapid improvement in hemodynamics was noticed, as well as a significant reduction of IL-6 and lactate levels. Despite a recurring septic episode and the necessity for amputation, the patient clinically stabilized and underwent complete recovery. The early treatment with a combination of CVVHDF and CytoSorb was accompanied by an attenuation of the systemic inflammatory reaction, which subsided without major or permanent organ damage, despite the impressive pathogen spectrum and the pronounced local damage.

1. Introduction

Severe trauma associated with later disability and mortality still constitutes a major health and socioeconomic problem throughout the world [1]. The traumatized patient presents with a series of posttraumatic complications secondary to the traumatic injury itself. While primary morbidity and mortality are mostly related to initial injuries (i.e., severe traumatic brain injury, hemorrhagic shock) and early complications (i.e., acidosis, coagulopathy, hypothermia, oxidative stress, metabolic disorders), secondary lethality is strongly linked to the development of systemic inflammatory response syndrome (SIRS), sepsis, and ultimately multiple organ dysfunction syndrome (MODS) [2]. The poor outcome of these patients is therefore directly related to the association of the aforementioned pathologies.

Several factors may lead to hemodynamic instability and insufficient tissue perfusion, necessitating fluid resuscitation and catecholamine support. Therefore, initial protection of circulation and avoidance of hypoperfusion, initially most often related to blood loss and hypovolemia, is critical in these patients. As blood pressure and heart rate prove partly unreliable to evaluate cardiac output in critically injured patients, increase in lactate levels may help identify a patient whose initially normal vital signs may disguise tissue hypoperfusion [3].

On the other hand, a plethora of cytokines play a role in the inflammatory response subsequent to critical injury. Particularly interleukin-6 (IL-6) appears to play an active role in the postinjury immune response. IL-6 is released in response to an inflammatory stimulus or tissue injury, acting locally and systemically to generate a multitude of physiologic responses. The release of IL-6 in response to traumatic injury mimics that to elective surgery, with IL-6 levels rising early and preceding acute phase protein expression, making it an attractive diagnostic but even more a therapeutic target in attempts to control hyperinflammation-associated organ dysfunction [4].

In this context, extracorporeal blood purification therapy using a recently introduced hemoadsorption device

(CytoSorb) did show promising results in patients with SIRS and sepsis by attenuating the cytokine-driven overwhelming inflammatory response, improving hemodynamic stability as well as other clinically relevant parameters [5–7].

We herein report on a patient who was successfully treated with CytoSorb after a traumatic amputation of his right forearm with subsequent development of severe septic shock due to infection with multiresistant pathogens. Informed consent for data analysis and publication was obtained from the patient.

2. Case Presentation

A 49-year-old male patient was admitted to the hospital via helicopter transport after a traumatic amputation of his right forearm. Earlier, while working on a landfill cleaning surfaces with a high pressure cleaner, the air pressure tube caught his arm and his right forearm was cut off at the elbow joint. The amputate was not damaged macroscopically; however a wide spectrum of various aerobic and anaerobic pathogens was detected in the wound later on, many of which were multiresistant.

On admission, the patient was treated for shock (RR = 69/55 HR 99 and two hours later at RR 71/68, HR 110), followed by X-ray examination and immediate replantation (operation time of approx. 8.5 hours). After successful surgery and a resulting well-perfused transplant, the patient was postoperatively transferred to the intensive care unit intubated, ventilated, and catecholamine-dependent (norepinephrine 0.41 μg/kg/min) with a mean arterial pressure of 65 mmHg. We noticed development of lactic acidosis (3.9 mmol/l) and in the further course a sharp increase in inflammation-relevant parameters (leukocytes 18.700/μl, CRP 13.5 mg/dl, PCT 0.88 ng/ml, IL-6 > 5000 pg/ml). Continuous renal replacement therapy (CRRT) was started due to anuria postshock and the onset of acute renal failure. Detected pathogens included *Aeromonas hydrophila*, an enterotoxin-producing bacterium being endemic in the American tropics; *Stenotrophomonas maltophilia*, a multiresistant nosocomial pathogen detected in dialysis fluid; and *Clostridium subterminale*, which has been described in the medical literature only in nine case reports as being pathogenic. Antibiotic therapy (normal dosages) with sultamicillin 3 × 3 g (first 4 days), piperacillin/tazobactam 4.5 g (for 2 days), clarithromycin (500 mg 2 × 1), and meropenem (3 × 2 g) for 10 days was initiated and hydrocortisone (20 mg/h) plus three red packed blood cells were administered immediately. Due to the anticipated risk of a complex infection because of the location of the accident (landfill), CytoSorb was additionally installed into the CRRT circuit. A total of 6 consecutive treatments with CytoSorb over 3 days with therapy intervals of 12 hours each were carried out. Therapy sessions were partly interrupted by surgical procedures. The CytoSorb treatment was performed in combination with standard continuous hemodiafiltration (CVVHDF, Fresenius Multifiltrate, Fresenius Medical Care AG, Bad Homburg, Germany) using regional citrate anticoagulation and blood flow rates of 100 ml/min. The CytoSorb adsorber was installed in prehemofilter position.

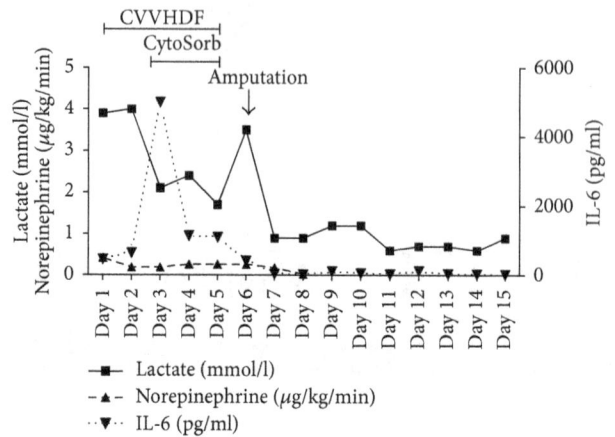

FIGURE 1: Plasma concentrations of IL-6 and lactate and the need of noradrenalin during the course of the eight treatment sessions. Day 1 represents start of treatment directly after postoperative transfer to ICU.

During the course of the combined CVVHDF-CytoSorb treatment we measured demand for catecholamines, inflammatory parameters (IL-6), and lactate levels (Figure 1). We noticed a clear and more importantly rapid improvement in hemodynamics with reduction of norepinephrine dosages from 0.41 down to 0.26 μg/kg/min already within the very first treatment. Norepinephrine infusion rates had to be adjusted at a low scale during the subsequent treatment sessions, which was most likely due to the ongoing infection with multiresistant pathogens and the preceding surgical procedure. Furthermore, we observed a significant reduction of inflammatory parameters, in particular of IL-6, which decreased from >5000 pg/ml to 43 pg/ml one day after the last CytoSorb therapy session.

Initial peak levels of lactate (4 mmol/l) were progressively declining during the next treatments and reached normal values on the third day of CytoSorb treatment. Importantly, after cessation of CytoSorb treatment, we noticed a rebounce of plasma lactate levels in the context of an acute infection and necrosis of the amputate necessitating removal of necrotic tissue and ultimately amputation of the forearm. After amputation, the patient continuously stabilized and improved. Total CRRT time was 5 days, and pressure-controlled ventilation was carried out for 2 days (directly postoperative), was then changed to BiPAP and CPAP ventilation on the following 3 days, and completely stopped on day 5 together with CRRT and CytoSorb. Daily surgical wound care with disinfection and removal of necrotic tissue were performed in the further course. 18 days after initial admission, the patient was transferred to the normal trauma-surgical ward and underwent complete recovery with later adaptation of a robotic prosthesis.

3. Discussion

In the present case report, we treated a critically injured patient after traumatic amputation and subsequent development of severe septic shock with a combination of CVVHDF plus hemoadsorption. Treatment was associated with a rapid hemodynamic stabilization and a decrease in IL-6 as well as blood lactate levels.

One of the most prominent observations in our patient was the promptness in which hemodynamic stabilization occurred. From the data available on CytoSorb in critically ill patients in the context of sepsis and postcardiac surgery SIRS, we found clear conformance as to hemodynamic stabilization with a quick reduction in catecholamine dosages being one of the main effects to be expected from the application of the device [5–7].

In our patient, IL-6 plasma levels could be reduced drastically during the course of the combined treatments. There is evidence that the magnitude of IL-6 elevation after mechanical trauma appears to correlate with the extent of trauma severity, the risk of postinjury complications, and even adverse outcome [4, 8]. Moreover, a study conducted in a cohort of severe trauma patients by Sousa and coworkers showed that several cytokines were associated with outcomes, especially IL-6 and IL-10 at 72 h with MODS and death [9]. Likewise, Guisasola et al. found that patients with MODS had higher plasma levels of IL-6 and TNF-α which therefore suggests a potential role of these mediators as early predictive markers for systemic inflammatory response and clinical complications to stratify patients as to which therapeutic intervention they should receive [10]. Of note, data even suggest IL-6 as a helpful indicator in deciding which primary operation to perform (i.e., external fixator or intramedullary nail) and determining the optimal time for secondary surgery [11].

We monitored a progressive and rapid decline in lactate levels in our patient. With postoperative levels of 3.9–4 mmol/l the patient was still not in full-blown lactic acidosis. However, elevated lactate at this level points towards microcirculatory failure and hypoperfusion of vital organs and requires serious attention. Importantly, studies show that the degree of lactate elevation and the rate of lactate clearance strongly correlate with the risk of MODS and mortality after traumatic injury [12]. As initial lactate levels have been found to be significantly higher in trauma nonsurvivors compared to survivors, lactate levels and its clearance could potentially serve as an endpoint to guide resuscitation [13]. For example, Aslar and colleagues reported a calculated specificity of 86% and sensitivity of 84% for patients with torso trauma and a lactate level > 4 mmol/L to die [14].

After receiving and reviewing the pathogenic spectrum, we did anticipate a high risk of complex infection. Pathogens were rather uncommon and did pose a challenge concerning the right antibiotic therapy to administer.

In conclusion, this case is, to the best of our knowledge, the first published report on the clinical application of CytoSorb hemoadsorption in a patient with severe trauma and septic shock. The early treatment with a combination of CVVHDF and CytoSorb was accompanied by an attenuation of the systemic inflammatory reaction, which subsided without major or permanent organ damage, despite the impressive pathogen spectrum and the pronounced local damage. Treatment was safe and well tolerated. CytoSorb appears to possibly represent a promising adjunctive therapy to treat critically injured patients; however large, controlled studies are urgently required to determine the true benefit of this treatment in this subset of patients.

Disclosure

The work was performed at UKH Meidling, Vienna, Austria, without any financial support.

References

[1] M. M. K. S. G. Peden, *The Injury Chart Book: A Graphical Overview of The Global Burden of Injuries*, World Health Organization, Geneva, Switzerland, 2002.

[2] A. F. Rogobete, D. Sandesc, M. Papurica et al., "The influence of metabolic imbalances and oxidative stress on the outcome of critically ill polytrauma patients: A review," *Burns & Trauma*, vol. 5, no. 8, 2017.

[3] C. C. J. Wo, W. C. Shoemaker, P. L. Appel, M. H. Bishop, H. B. Kram, and E. Hardin, "Unreliability of blood pressure and heart rate to evaluate cardiac output in emergency resuscitation and critical illness," *Critical Care Medicine*, vol. 21, no. 2, pp. 218–223, 1993.

[4] W. L. Biffl, E. E. Moore, F. A. Moore, and V. M. Peterson, "Interleukin-6 in the injured patient: marker of injury or mediator of inflammation?" *Annals of Surgery*, vol. 224, no. 5, pp. 647–664, 1996.

[5] K. Träger, C. Skrabal, G. Fischer et al., "Hemoadsorption treatment of patients with acute infective endocarditis during surgery with cardiopulmonary bypass—A case series," *The International Journal of Artificial Organs*, vol. 40, no. 5, pp. 240–249, 2017.

[6] K. Träger, D. Fritzler, G. Fischer et al., "Treatment of postcardiopulmonary bypass SIRS by hemoadsorption: A case series," *The International Journal of Artificial Organs*, vol. 39, no. 3, pp. 141–146, 2016.

[7] K. Kogelmann, D. Jarczak, M. Scheller, and M. Drüner, "Hemoadsorption by CytoSorb in septic patients: a case series," *Critical Care*, vol. 21, no. 1, 2017.

[8] R. S. Jawa, S. Anillo, K. Huntoon, H. Baumann, and M. Kulaylat, "Interleukin-6 in surgery, trauma, and critical care Part II: Clinical implications," *Journal of Intensive Care Medicine*, vol. 26, no. 2, pp. 73–87, 2011.

[9] A. Sousa, F. Raposo, S. Fonseca et al., "Measurement of cytokines and adhesion molecules in the first 72 hours after severe trauma: association with severity and outcome," *Disease Markers*, vol. 2015, Article ID 747036, 8 pages, 2015.

[10] M. C. Guisasola, A. Ortiz, F. Chana, B. Alonso, and J. Vaquero, "Early inflammatory response in polytraumatized patients: Cytokines and heat shock proteins. A pilot study," *Orthopaedics & Traumatology: Surgery & Research*, vol. 101, no. 5, pp. 607–611, 2015.

[11] M. Van Griensven, "Cytokines as biomarkers in polytraumatized patients," *Der Unfallchirurg*, vol. 117, no. 8, pp. 699–702, 2014.

[12] P. Manikis, S. Jankowski, H. Zhang, R. J. Kahn, and J.-L. Vincent, "Correlation of serial blood lactate levels to organ failure and

mortality after trauma," *The American Journal of Emergency Medicine*, vol. 13, no. 6, pp. 619–622, 1995.

[13] S. R. Odom, M. D. Howell, G. S. Silva et al., "Lactate clearance as a predictor of mortality in trauma patients," *Journal of Trauma and Acute Care Surgery*, vol. 74, no. 4, pp. 999–1004, 2013.

[14] A. K. Aslar, M. A. Kuzu, A. H. Elhan, A. Tanik, and S. Hengirmen, "Admission lactate level and the APACHE II score are the most useful predictors of prognosis following torso trauma," *Injury*, vol. 35, no. 8, pp. 746–752, 2004.

50

Hypoxemic Respiratory Failure from Acute Respiratory Distress Syndrome Secondary to Leptospirosis

Shannon M. Fernando,[1,2] **Pierre Cardinal,**[1] **and Peter G. Brindley**[3]

[1]*Division of Critical Care, Department of Medicine, University of Ottawa, Ottawa, ON, Canada*
[2]*Department of Emergency Medicine, University of Ottawa, Ottawa, ON, Canada*
[3]*Department of Critical Care Medicine, University of Alberta, Edmonton, AB, Canada*

Correspondence should be addressed to Shannon M. Fernando; sfernando@qmed.ca

Academic Editor: Nicolas Nin

Acute respiratory distress syndrome (ARDS), characterized by hypoxemic respiratory failure, is associated with a mortality of 30–50% and is precipitated by both direct and indirect pulmonary insults. Treatment is largely supportive, consisting of lung protective ventilation and thereby necessitating Intensive Care Unit (ICU) admission. The most common precipitant is community-acquired bacterial pneumonia, but other putative pathogens include viruses and fungi. On rare occasions, ARDS can be secondary to tropical disease. Accordingly, a history should include travel to endemic regions. Leptospirosis is a zoonotic disease most common in the tropics and typically associated with mild pulmonary complications. We describe a case of a 25-year-old male with undiagnosed leptospirosis, presenting with fever and severe hypoxemic respiratory failure, returning from a Costa Rican holiday. There was no other organ failure. He was intubated and received lung protective ventilation. His condition improved after ampicillin and penicillin G were added empirically. This case illustrates the rare complication of ARDS from leptospirosis, the importance of taking a travel history, and the need for empiric therapy because of diagnostic delay.

1. Introduction

Acute respiratory distress syndrome (ARDS) is an intense inflammatory lung condition that is triggered by a wide range of pulmonary or systemic insults to the alveolar-capillary membrane [1]. This results in increased vascular permeability, which in turn causes alveolar and interstitial edema and hypoxemia. Prevalence of ARDS in the Intensive Care Unit (ICU) has been estimated as high as 10%, with in-hospital mortality ranging from 30 to 50%, depending on the severity of illness [2]. ARDS is defined by the Berlin Criteria [3], which incorporates four components: (a) acute onset; (b) hypoxemia (defined as a PaO_2/FiO_2 ratio of <300); (c) bilateral infiltrates on chest radiograph; and (d) absence of cardiac failure. While the most common causes include direct lung injury (pneumonia or aspiration), extrapulmonary sepsis, and trauma [2], the etiologic differential for ARDS is large. This means that the clinician should be prepared to undertake a thorough history and remain open to atypical causes.

There are multiple infectious triggers for ARDS. These include the aforementioned pulmonary infections (bacterial, viral, or fungal), and the disseminated inflammatory response associated with sepsis [4]. Various tropical diseases can also cause ARDS, and in such cases, the most commonly implicated etiology is the parasite falciparum malariae [5]. While even more rare, ARDS has also been associated with the tropical disease leptospirosis. This disease is typically associated with nonspecific constitutional symptoms but has the potential to precipitate multisystem organ failure and death [6]. Only a handful of published reports of ARDS secondary to leptospirosis exist [7–9]. We present a case of a patient eventually diagnosed with leptospirosis, but who presented with isolated hypoxemic respiratory failure, and who fulfilled criteria for ARDS. This patient did not get better until he received a full travel history, which in turn led to empiric ampicillin and penicillin G. This case highlights the importance of taking a travel history and considering the rare but potentially deadly diagnosis of leptospirosis.

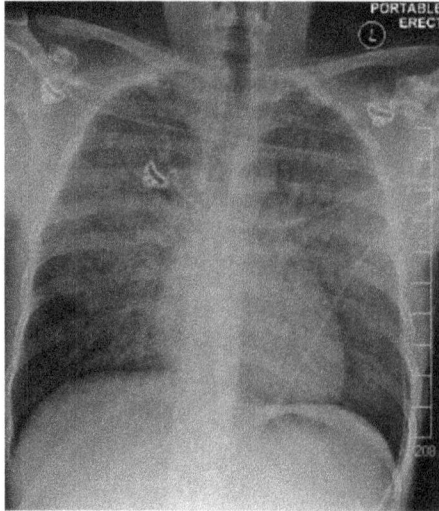

FIGURE 1: Anterior-posterior portable chest radiograph demonstrating bilateral pulmonary opacities, consistent with ARDS.

2. Case Report

A 25-year-old male with no previous medical comorbidities was brought to the Emergency Department (ED) with increasing tachypnea and dyspnea over the previous day. The accompanying partner reported that the patient had been intermittently warm to the touch for the past week, complaining of myalgia and headache. He has never used any medications. The pair had just returned to Canada from two weeks in Costa Rica, where the patient had begun feeling unwell one day before flying home. Immediately upon returning to Canada, the patient saw his primary care physician, who believed he had influenza. In the following days, the patient's condition worsened and he presented to the ED with the following vital signs: blood pressure of 125/75 mmHg, heart rate (HR) of 110 beats/min, respiratory rate (RR) of 35 breaths/minute, temperature of 38.6 degrees Celsius, and oxygen saturation of 82%. Glasgow Coma Scale (GCS) was 15/15. He was in obvious respiratory distress with accessory muscle use. A portable chest radiograph demonstrated bilateral opacities (Figure 1). The patient was placed on a nonrebreather (FiO$_2$ of 1), but his work of breathing did not substantially improve, and he remained hypoxemic. Therefore, the patient was intubated in the ED and an arterial line was inserted. ED bloodwork revealed a pO$_2$ of 65 mmHg on 100% oxygen, but normal electrolytes, renal function, liver enzymes, and coagulation parameters. Following ICU transfer, the patient was diagnosed with ARDS due to his severely depressed PaO$_2$/FiO$_2$ ratio (110 upon ICU admission), bilateral opacities, and no signs that would suggest cardiac dysfunction (i.e., normal blood pressure, no peripheral edema, and normal electrocardiogram). He was ventilated with a standardized ARDSNet protocol that focused on low tidal volume (5 mL/kg of ideal body weight and a target pH > 7.25), plus a positive end-expiratory pressure (PEEP) increased to 10 mmHg [10, 11]. While the etiology for ARDS was unclear, it was presumed infectious in origin, given his

fevers and travel. Blood and urine cultures were performed, along with bronchoalveolar lavage (BAL). Bronchoscopy did not show any pulmonary hemorrhage or purulent secretions. Computed tomography (CT) of the chest confirmed bilateral edema but did not reveal any lobar infiltrate consistent with bacterial pneumonia. Transthoracic echocardiogram revealed normal biventricular function, with no vegetation or valvular regurgitation.

Infectious Diseases consultation led to initiation of broad-spectrum antimicrobials (piperacillin-tazobactam, azithromycin, and vancomycin). Initial blood, urine, and BAL cultures grew no pathogens. Malaria thick and thin smears were performed several times and were negative. Dengue serology was also negative, as was human immunodeficiency virus (HIV) and hepatitis A, B, and C. Despite broad antimicrobial treatment, the patient's respiratory status worsened, which led to prone positioning [12].

Given the recent travel history to Costa Rica, the diagnosis of leptospirosis was considered, but after a delay of 48 hours from presentation. The clue was that, following further questioning, the patient's partner reported that she and the patient had spent several days swimming in freshwater, which they had also drunk. Both are sources of leptospirosis transmission [6, 13]. Leptospirosis serology was sent (specifically, an IgM-detection enzyme-linked immunosorbent assay). Given the prolonged time required to establish leptospirosis diagnosis via serology, the patient was empirically treated with ampicillin and penicillin G [14].

Over the next 48 hours, the patient's condition substantially improved. He became afebrile, his hypoxemia resolved, and his chest radiograph improved. Otherwise, his blood work remained largely unchanged, with normal renal, hepatic, and coagulation function. He was extubated on postadmission day five, was transferred to the medicine ward on day six, and was discharged home on day eight. Diagnosis was confirmed but not until after discharge: due to a positive IgM for *Leptospira* and a *Leptospira canicola* titer of 1 : 200. Diagnosis was further confirmed with microscopic agglutination testing (MAT). He was seen in follow-up by the Infectious Diseases service and never demonstrated any renal dysfunction, hepatic dysfunction, or coagulopathy suggesting Weil's disease.

3. Discussion

Leptospirosis is a zoonotic disease caused by *Leptospira*. These are highly mobile, obligate aerobic spirochetes with features in common with both gram-positive and gram-negative bacteria [6]. This spirochete has been found worldwide, but most commonly in the tropics [13]. It is commonly transmitted from contaminated freshwater in endemic regions, or from animals, such as rodents and bats. The range of disease manifestation is vast and includes those with positive serology but no symptoms or those with minimal symptoms living in endemic regions [15].

Leptospirosis is most often characterized by a nonspecific febrile illness, and therefore it can be difficult to distinguish [16]. The disease can be associated with high mortality, but it is difficult to establish accurate morbidity and mortality rates [13]. Severe leptospirosis can result in Weil's disease: characterized by jaundice, renal dysfunction, and coagulopathy [17]. This can progress to multisystem organ failure, rhabdomyolysis, and death. Definitive diagnosis of leptospirosis requires recovery of leptospires either by culture or by immunohistochemical staining. Serology can also be performed using MAT or IgM-detection. Regardless of the method used, results can take days to weeks, and, therefore, if there is a high degree of suspicion, patients should receive empiric treatment. There is a paucity of evidence regarding optimal antimicrobials for leptospirosis, but sources recommend doxycycline for prophylaxis/mild disease [18, 19] and ampicillin and penicillin G for severe disease [14]. Ceftriaxone is a suitable alternative for treatment of severe disease and in patients with a penicillin allergy [20].

Pulmonary manifestations of leptospirosis have been reported, but are typically mild, and occur in conjunction with other failing organs [8, 21]. Severe ARDS has been described in a few cases reports of leptospirosis [7, 8], though again this is in the context of sepsis and multisystem organ failure. Other cases describe ARDS occurring secondary to pulmonary hemorrhage in leptospirosis [22, 23]. Of note, our patient demonstrated no evidence of hemorrhage on clinical history, CT scan, or bronchoscopy.

The mechanism by which leptospirosis triggered ARDS (in the absence of sepsis) is unclear, though two theories have been proposed to explain the intense inflammatory response [24]. The first is a toxin-mediated capillary vasculitis [25]. This is supported by pathologic evidence that, in patients that die with pulmonary complications, lung tissue has significantly less leptospires than liver and blood counts. In other words, the belief is that pulmonary abnormalities may occur secondary to circulating toxins produced by the pathogen at distant sites [13]. The second proposed mechanism is immune-mediated. Prominent inflammatory mediators, such as cytokines, have been demonstrated to be elevated in leptospirosis [26]. Following this mechanism, postmortem alveolar light microscopy shows a predominance of macrophages, lymphocytes, and plasma cells [27].

Our patient was diagnosed with ARDS but assumed to have a typical bacterial etiology. Leptospirosis was not even contemplated until 48 hours after admission. This is because of its very rare prevalence in North America, coupled with his nonspecific symptoms. Initial diagnostic work-up should include blood cultures, urine cultures, sputum cultures (if available), serological testing (for intracellular bacteria), and microbial sampling of the lung, ideally by BAL [4]. Advanced imaging, such as CT of the chest, may also be considered if the patient is safe for transport.

Community-acquired bacterial pneumonia remains the leading cause of ARDS [1], and therefore antimicrobial coverage of both typical and atypical organisms is prudent. Of note, leptospirosis should be susceptible to piperacillin-tazobactam, though it did not appear to ameliorate our patient. However, it is believed that there is variability in susceptibility to various antimicrobials, based on geographic variation [28]. Special attention should be paid to immuno-compromised individuals, as they have greater propensity for fungal or parasitic organisms. Other history should include

sick contacts, pets, exposures (i.e., farming, occupational), and particularly travel. Our patient's recent travel to an endemic leptospirosis region led to empiric therapy.

There is no evidence that ventilatory management of patients with ARDS from leptospirosis should be any different from other ARDS patients. These patients benefit from a lung protective strategy, marked by low tidal volumes and with the option for increasing PEEP [10, 11]. Fluid therapy should be sufficient to avoid cardiovascular collapse, but should be used with enough caution to avoid worsening pulmonary edema [29]. There is also some evidence for mechanical ventilation in the prone position [12]. Given the patient's age, lack of medical comorbidities, and single-system failure, he may have been considered for extracorporeal membrane oxygenation (ECMO), should his condition have worsened [30].

4. Conclusion

ARDS is a life-threatening condition. In addition to providing mechanical ventilation and fluid therapy that is minimally injurious, clinicians should also identify and target the etiology driving the inflammatory process. A few case reports have identified leptospirosis as the trigger for ARDS. However, given the nonspecific symptoms, diagnosis in North America is only likely to follow a thorough travel history. Furthermore, treatment will need to be empiric, as definitive laboratory diagnosis will be delayed days to weeks. We describe a case of ARDS in a patient with undiagnosed leptospirosis and no other end-organ dysfunction. Making note of the patient's recent travel history, and his exposure to tropical freshwater, heightened suspicion enough that he received timely empiric treatment and made a full recovery.

Authors' Contributions

Shannon M. Fernando, Pierre Cardinal, and Peter G. Brindley all wrote and reviewed the final manuscript.

References

[1] J. Villar and A. S. Slutsky, "GOLDEN anniversary of the acute respiratory distress syndrome: still much work to do!," *Current Opinion in Critical Care*, vol. 23, no. 1, pp. 4–9, 2017.

[2] G. Bellani, J. G. Laffey, T. Pham et al., "Epidemiology, patterns of care, and mortality for patients with acute respiratory distress syndrome in intensive care units in 50 countries," *Journal of the American Medical Association*, vol. 315, no. 8, pp. 788–800, 2016.

[3] V. M. Ranieri, G. D. Rubenfeld, B. T. Thompson et al., "Acute respiratory distress syndrome: the Berlin definition," *The Journal of the American Medical Association*, vol. 307, no. 23, pp. 2526–2533, 2012.

[4] L. Papazian, C. S. Calfee, D. Chiumello et al., "Diagnostic workup for ARDS patients," *Intensive Care Medicine*, vol. 42, no. 5, pp. 674–685, 2016.

[5] W. R. J. Taylor, J. Hanson, G. D. H. Turner, N. J. White, and A. M. Dondorp, "Respiratory manifestations of malaria," *CHEST*, vol. 142, no. 2, pp. 492–505, 2012.

[6] D. A. Haake and P. N. Levett, "Leptospirosis in humans," *Current Topics in Microbiology and Immunology*, vol. 387, pp. 65–97, 2015.

[7] E. S. Panagiotidou, S. V. Akritidou, S. T. Kotoulas et al., "A patient who made an impact on how I practice: severe leptospirosis presenting as ARDS in the ICU," *Journal of Infection and Public Health*, 2017.

[8] M. Clavel, G. Lhéritier, N. Weinbreck et al., "Leptospirosis: an Unusual Cause of ARDS," *Critical Care Research and Practice*, vol. 2010, Article ID 408365, 3 pages, 2010.

[9] V. Chauhan, D. M. Mahesh, P. Panda, J. Mokta, and S. Thakur, "Leptospirosis presenting as acute respiratory distress syndrome (ARDS) in sub-Himalayan region," *Journal of the Association of Physicians of India*, vol. 58, pp. 390-391, 2010.

[10] R. G. Brower, M. A. Matthay, A. Morris, D. Schoenfeld, B. T. Thompson, and A. Wheeler, "Ventilation with lower tidal volumes as compared with traditional tidal volumes for acute lung injury and the acute respiratory distress syndrome," *The New England Journal of Medicine*, vol. 342, no. 18, pp. 1301–1308, 2000.

[11] M. Briel, M. Meade, A. Mercat et al., "Higher vs lower positive end-expiratory pressure in patients with acute lung injury and acute respiratory distress syndrome: systematic review and meta-analysis," *Journal of the American Medical Association*, vol. 303, no. 9, pp. 865–873, 2010.

[12] S. Sud, J. O. Friedrich, N. K. J. Adhikari et al., "Effect of prone positioning during mechanical ventilation on mortality among patients with acute respiratory distress syndrome: a systematic review and meta-analysis," *Canadian Medical Association Journal*, vol. 186, no. 10, pp. E381–E390, 2014.

[13] A. R. Bharti, J. E. Nally, J. N. Ricaldi et al., "Leptospirosis: a zoonotic disease of global importance," *The Lancet Infectious Diseases*, vol. 3, no. 12, pp. 757–771, 2003.

[14] G. Watt, M. Linda Tuazon, E. Santiago et al., "Placebo-controlled trial of intravenous penicillin for severe and late leptospirosis," *The Lancet*, vol. 331, no. 8583, pp. 433–435, 1988.

[15] S. L. Bragg, B. Plikaytis, B. A. Perkins et al., "Asymptomatic infection and risk factors for leptospirosis in Nicaragua.," *The American Journal of Tropical Medicine and Hygiene*, vol. 63, no. 5, pp. 249–254, 2000.

[16] P. R. Torgerson, J. E. Hagan, F. Costa et al., "Global burden of leptospirosis: estimated in terms of disability adjusted life years," *PLOS Neglected Tropical Diseases*, vol. 9, no. 10, Article ID e0004122, 2015.

[17] A. Jansen and T. Schneider, "Weil's disease in a rat owner," *The Lancet Infectious Diseases*, vol. 11, no. 2, p. 152, 2011.

[18] E. T. Takafuji, J. W. Kirkpatrick, R. N. Miller et al., "An efficacy trial of doxycycline chemoprophylaxis against leptospirosis," *The New England Journal of Medicine*, vol. 310, no. 8, pp. 497–500, 1984.

[19] D. M. Brett-Major and R. J. Lipnick, "Antibiotic prophylaxis for leptospirosis," *Cochrane Database of Systematic Reviews*, no. 3, p. CD007342, 2009.

[20] T. Panaphut, S. Domrongkitchaiporn, A. Vibhagool, B. Thinkamrop, and W. Susaengrat, "Ceftriaxone compared with sodium penicillin G for treatment of severe leptospirosis," *Clinical Infectious Diseases*, vol. 36, no. 12, pp. 1507–1513, 2003.

[21] J.-G. Im, K. M. Yeon, M. C. Han et al., "Leptospirosis of the lung: radiographic findings in 58 patients," *American Journal of Roentgenology*, vol. 152, no. 5, pp. 955–959, 1989.

[22] L. Pea, L. Roda, V. Boussaud, and B. Lonjon, "Desmopressin therapy for massive hemoptysis associated with severe leptospirosis," *American Journal of Respiratory and Critical Care Medicine*, vol. 167, no. 5, pp. 726–728, 2003.

[23] T. De Brito, V. De Aiello, L. F. F. da Silva et al., "Human hemorrhagic pulmonary leptospirosis: pathological findings and pathophysiological correlations," *PLoS ONE*, vol. 8, no. 8, Article ID e71743, 2013.

[24] M. Dolhnikoff, T. Mauad, E. P. Bethlem, and C. R. R. Carvalho, "Pathology and pathophysiology of pulmonary manifestations in leptospirosis," *The Brazilian Journal of Infectious Diseases*, vol. 11, no. 1, pp. 142–148, 2007.

[25] A. M. Luks, S. Lakshminarayanan, and J. V. Hirschmann, "Leptospirosis presenting as diffuse alveolar hemorrhage: case report and literature review," *CHEST*, vol. 123, no. 2, pp. 639–643, 2003.

[26] J. M. Estavoyer, E. Racadot, G. Couetdic, J. Leroy, and L. Grosperrin, "Tumor necrosis factor in patients with leptospirosis," *Clinical Infectious Diseases*, vol. 13, no. 6, pp. 1245-1246, 1991.

[27] M. I. Duarte, V. A. Alves, C. F. Takakura, R. T. Santos, E. L. Nicodemo, and A. C. Nicodemo, "Lung lesions in human leptospirosis: microscopic, immunohistochemical, and ultrastructural features related to thrombocytopenia," *The American Journal of Tropical Medicine and Hygiene*, vol. 56, no. 2, pp. 181-187, 1997.

[28] R. A. Ressner, M. E. Griffith, M. L. Beckius et al., "Antimicrobial susceptibilities of geographically diverse clinical human isolates of Leptospira," *Antimicrobial Agents and Chemotherapy*, vol. 52, no. 8, pp. 2750–2754, 2008.

[29] H. P. Wiedemann, A. P. Wheeler, G. R. Bernard et al., "Comparison of two fluid-management strategies in acute lung injury," *The New England Journal of Medicine*, vol. 354, no. 24, pp. 2564–2575, 2006.

[30] B. W. Tillmann, M. L. Klingel, A. E. Iansavichene, I. M. Ball, and A. D. Nagpal, "Extracorporeal membrane oxygenation (ECMO) as a treatment strategy for severe acute respiratory distress syndrome (ARDS) in the low tidal volume era: a systematic review," *Journal of Critical Care*, vol. 41, pp. 64–71, 2017.

51

Fatal Nonhepatic Hyperammonemia in ICU Setting: A Rare but Serious Complication following Bariatric Surgery

Gyanendra Acharya,[1] Sunil Mehra,[2] Ronakkumar Patel,[1]
Simona Frunza-Stefan,[1] and Harmanjot Kaur[3]

[1]Department of Internal Medicine, Wyckoff Heights Medical Center, Brooklyn, NY 11237, USA
[2]Division of Pulmonary and Critical Care Medicine, Department of Internal Medicine, Wyckoff Heights Medical Center, Brooklyn, NY 11237, USA
[3]Department of Medical Education, Wyckoff Heights Medical Center, Brooklyn, NY 11237, USA

Correspondence should be addressed to Gyanendra Acharya; achgyanen@hotmail.com

Academic Editor: Gerhard Pichler

Bariatric surgery is well established in reducing weight and improving the obesity-associated morbidity and mortality. Hyperammonemic encephalopathy following bariatric surgery is rare but highly fatal if not diagnosed in time and managed aggressively. Both macro- and micronutrients deficiencies play a role. A 42-year-old Hispanic female with a history of Roux-en-Y Gastric Bypass Procedure was brought to ED for progressive altered mental status. Physical exam was remarkable for drowsiness with Glasgow Coma Scale 11, ascites, and bilateral pedal edema. Labs showed elevated ammonia, low hemoglobin, low serum prealbumin, albumin, HDL, and positive toxicology. She remained obtunded despite the treatment with Narcan and flumazenil and the serum ammonia level fluctuated despite standard treatment with lactulose and rifaximin. Laboratory investigations helped to elucidate the etiology of the hyperammonemia most likely secondary to unmasking the functional deficiency of the urea cycle enzymes. Hyperammonemia in the context of normal liver function tests becomes diagnostically challenging for physicians. Severe hyperammonemia is highly fatal. Early diagnosis and aggressive treatment can alter the prognosis favorably.

1. Introduction

Bariatric surgery is well established in reducing weight and improving obesity-associated morbidity and mortality. Neurological complication such as hyperammonemic encephalopathy following bariatric surgery is rare but highly fatal if not diagnosed and treated aggressively on time. Both macro- and micronutrients deficiencies seem to play an important role in unmasking the functional deficiency of urea cycle enzymes in an adult woman after bariatric surgery.

2. Case Presentation

A 42-year-old Hispanic female was brought to ED with complaint of progressive altered mental status over the past few days. At ED, the patient was only responsive to painful stimuli but did not appear in acute distress. Her mother, who provided the history, had a conversation with patient three hours prior to the presentation to ED. Patient had decreased oral food intake for the last two weeks. She denied history of fever or illicit drug use except for prescribed medications. Patient had Roux-en-Y Gastric Bypass Surgery (RYGBS) two years ago for morbid obesity and gastrojejunal stent placement procedure two weeks prior to the presentation. Her medications were oral vitamins, dilaudid 4 mg, amitriptyline, and zolpidem.

Physical examinations were remarkable for drowsiness with Glasgow Coma Scale (GCS) 11, ascites, and bilateral pitting pedal edema. Vital signs were within normal range. Initial labs (Table 1) were remarkable for hemoglobin (5.4 gm%), INR (2.15), aPTT (67.5 sec), BUN (11 mg/dL), creatinine (2.1 mg/dL), AST (49 IU/L) and ALT (23 IU/L), CPK (466 IU/L), low HDL cholesterol (<5 mg/dL), and prealbumin (<5 μg/dL) and albumin (1.8 g/dL), and arterial blood

TABLE 1: Basic laboratory investigations.

Lab. test	Results	Ref. range
WBC	8.34	4.5–10.9 k/μL
Hb	**5.4**	12.5–15.0 g/dL
Platelets	116	130–400 k/μL
Sodium	136	135–145 mmol/L
Potassium	4.8	3.6–5.2 mmol/L
BUN	**11**	6–21 mg/dL
Creatinine	**2.1**	0.6–1.1 mg/dL
Glucose	113	70–140 mg/dL
INR	**2.15**	0.8–1.2
aPTT	**67.5**	28–38 sec
CPK	**466**	22–198 IU/L
AST	**49**	13–40 IU/L
ALT	**23**	17–35 IU/L
ALP	116	37–130 U/L
Albumin	**1.8**	3.5–5.0 g/dL
Prealbumin	**<5**	20–40 μg/dL
HDL	**<5**	>50 mg/dL
LDL	95	<100 mg/dL
TG	133	<150 mg/dL
S. NH_3^+	**193**	<30 μmol/L
P. zinc	**23**	60–130 μg/dL
S. copper	57	70–175 μg/dL
24 hr U. Cu	25	15–60 μg/24 hr
Valproate	<1.0	50–100 μg/mL
Lithium	<0.1	0.8–1.2 mmol/L

WBC: white blood cells; Hb: hemoglobin; BUN: blood urea nitrogen; PT: prothrombin time; INR: international normalized ratio; aPTT: activated partial thrombin time; CPK: creatinine phosphokinase; AST/ALT: aspartate/alanine aminotransferase; ALP: alkaline phosphatase; HDL: high-density lipoprotein; LDL: low-density lipoprotein; TG: triglycerides; P.: plasma; S.: serum.

TABLE 2: Special laboratory investigation panel.

Lab test	Results	Ref. range
Plasma amino acid profiles:		
Alanine	350	200–483 μmol/L
Arginine	130	43–407 μmol/L
Asparagine	131	31–64 μmol/L
Aspartic acid	5	1–4 μmol/L
Beta-alanine	3	<5 μmol/L
Citrulline	43	16–51 μmol/L
Glutamine	1363	428–747 μmol/L
Glutamic acid	55	10–97 μmol/L
Glycine	555	122–322 μmol/L
Histidine	129	60–109 μmol/L
Homocysteine	<1	<1 μmol/L
Hydroxyproline	71	4–27 μmol/L
Isoleucine	27	34–98 μmol/L
Leucine	46	73–182 μmol/L
Lysine	359	119–233 μmol/L
Methionine	22	16–34 μmol/L
Ornithine	149	27–83 μmol/L
Phenylalanine	70	40–74 μmol/L
Proline	632	104–383 μmol/L
Serine	156	65–138 μmol/L
Taurine	43	31–102 μmol/L
Tryptophan	5	40–91 μmol/L
Tyrosine	46	38–96 μmol/L
Valine	73	132–313 μmol/L
Serum carnitine levels:		
T. carnitine	88	31–67 nmol/mL
F. carnitine	61	25–55 nmol/mL
Urine orotic acid level:		
Ur. orotic acid	**2.3**	0.4–1.2 mmol/molcr

T.: total; F.: free; Ur.: urine.

gas (ABG) demonstrated PH 7.39. Computed tomography (CT) of the head was unremarkable (Figure 1(a)). EKG shows sinus rhythm. She was empirically treated with Narcan and flumazenil with an impression of prescription drugs overdose as urine toxicology was positive for opiates, benzodiazepines, and Tricyclic Antidepressant (TCA), but she did not improve and remained obtunded. Subsequently, she was intubated to protect her airway. Further investigations revealed elevated ammonia level (193 μmol/L), low zinc level, normal vitamin B12 and folate level, negative immune and viral hepatitis panel, undetectable valproate and lithium level (Table 1), and mild hepatomegaly with fatty infiltration on CT of the abdomen. Blood and urine cultures were negative. Ascitic fluid analysis was negative for spontaneous bacterial peritonitis (SBP).

She received two pints of packed red blood cells, IV pantoprazole, D5% fluid, lactulose/rifaximin via nasogastric tube, and vitamin K subcutaneous. Her mentation and serum ammonia (115 μmol/L) improved over the next day and she was extubated. But, over the next few days, she continued to have fluctuating mental status (in and out of confusion

and delirium) and serum ammonia level (Figure 2). Blood hemoglobin remained stable after the first transfusion. Coagulopathy was corrected after vitamin K supplement. Despite standard treatment for hyperammonemia, her clinical condition deteriorated and she was reintubated.

At this stage, we considered alternative explanation and conducted plasma amino acid profile and urinary orotic acid level (Table 2) to explain the etiology of intractable hyperammonemia. On the 12th day of admission, she developed status epilepticus, which was controlled only with propofol infusion. Repeat CT of the head was consistent with diffuse cerebral edema (Figure 1(b)). Before the results of amino acid profile and urinary orotic acid level came back, she rapidly deteriorated clinically over the short period of time from status epilepticus and coma to multiorgan failure and subsequently died. With elevated urinary orotic acid and serum ornithine levels, normal/low-normal serum arginine and citrulline levels along with other findings, we concluded that her hyperammonemia might have resulted in unmasking of functional deficiency of urea cycle enzyme/s in

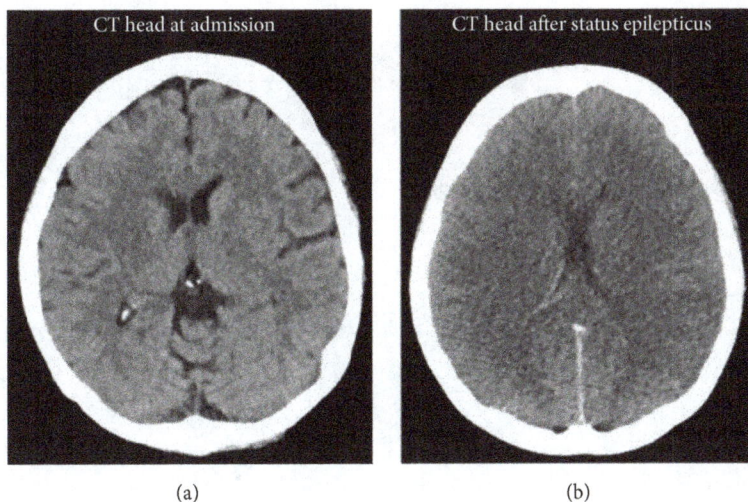

FIGURE 1: Computed tomography of the head at admission and at onset of status epilepticus. Computed tomography (CT) of the head (a) showed no remarkable findings on the day of admission and (b) showed diffused brain swelling consistent with cerebral edema on 12th day.

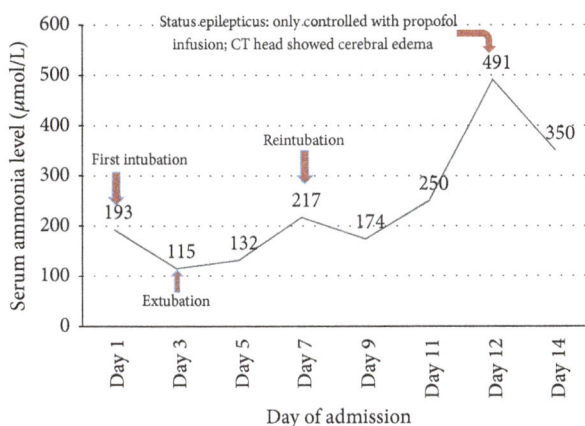

FIGURE 2: Graphical representation of serum ammonia level and associated events. Fluctuation of serum ammonia level during ICU course on this patient. Level of ammonia and mental status did not improve much with conventional treatment of hyperammonemia. The patient showed status epilepticus, which did not improve with midazolam and phenytoin and needed propofol drip to control the seizure. CT of the brain at that stage showed diffused cerebral edema.

this malnourished woman following bariatric surgery. With rapid clinical deterioration followed by death, confirmatory enzymes assay and DNA testing could not be done.

3. Discussion

Hyperammonemia is defined as an increase in the level of ammonia in the blood. Ammonia is a toxic by-product of protein and energy metabolism through biochemical transamination and deamination process in all body tissue. Ammonia is converted to urea (ureagenesis) via urea cycle (Figure 3) primarily in hepatocytes and is excreted through the kidneys and large intestine. Urea can be easily hydrolyzed to ammonia and carbon dioxide by enzyme

urease. So, elevated serum ammonia may result from its increased production, absorption (from intestine or urinary tract), decreased elimination of ammonia, and/or impaired ureagenesis. Hyperammonemia is always a sign of insufficient nitrogen excretion as discussed above, but it does not always necessitate symptomatic presentation. The signs and symptoms of hyperammonemia are usually neurological from mild cognitive and psychomotor changes to altered level of consciousness and coma [1]. Serum ammonia levels above 200 μmol/L are reported to be associated with cerebral edema, herniation, and death [2].

It is imperative not only to diagnose early and manage efficiently but also to find the etiology of symptomatic hyperammonemia. Liver pathology, the most common cause of hyperammonemia, almost always presents with altered liver function tests. Hyperammonemia in the context of unremarkable (or normal) liver function tests becomes diagnostically challenging for physicians. The etiologies of nonhepatic hyperammonemia based on literature are summarized (Table 3). Hyperammonemia has been reported following lung and bone marrow transplantation, portosystemic shunts, ureterosigmoidostomy, chemotherapy of hematological malignancies, and solid organ tumors with 5-fluorouracil [3]. Infections with *urease*-producing bacteria such as *Proteus mirabilis*, *Helicobacter pylori*, *Cornebacterium*, *Klebsiella*, and *Morganella* species cause hyperammonemia presumably due to reabsorption of ammonia (generated from hydrolysis of urea) into the systemic circulation [4]. Hyperalimentation, valproic acid, and carnitine deficiency are reported to cause hyperammonemia [5–8]. In this patient, GI bleeding was initially considered for possible cause of hyperammonemia; however, serum ammonia level remained persistently high even after the treatment of GI bleeding. Elevated INR and aPTT were most likely secondary to vitamin K deficiency. Treatment with vitamin K improved the coagulopathy. All of the other above mentioned causes were essentially excluded with clinical history and relevant laboratory investigations.

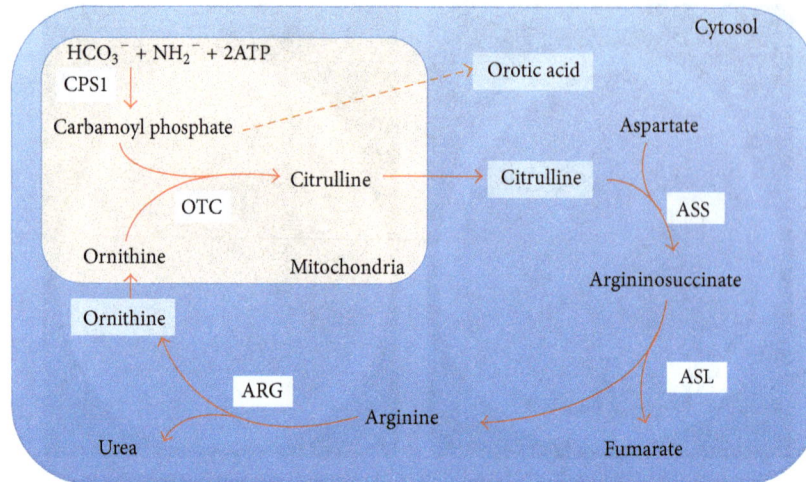

FIGURE 3: Schematic diagram of urea cycle and associated enzymes, CPS1: carbamoyl phosphate synthase 1; OTC: ornithine transcarbamylase; ARG: arginase; ASS: argininosuccinate synthetase; ASL: argininosuccinate lyase; ATP: adenosine triphosphate.

TABLE 3: Differential diagnosis of nonhepatic hyperammonemia based on [3–8].

SN	Ddx	Characteristics
1	Medications	Valproic acid, 5-FU
2	Infections	Urease-producing bacteria: (i) *Proteus mirabilis* (ii) *Helicobacter pylori* (iii) *Cornebacterium*, *Klebsiella*, and *Morganella* species
3	Surgery	(i) Lung transplant (ii) Bone marrow transplant (iii) Ureterosigmoidoscopy (iv) Portosystemic shunts (v) Bariatric surgery
4	Hyperalimentation	Increased nitrogen load in patient receiving parental nutrition
5	Errors in metabolism (a) Fatty acid oxidation defects (b) Urea cycle enzyme defects (c) Amino acid disorders	
6	Gastrointestinal bleeding	
7	Carnitine deficiency	

Inborn errors in metabolism such as fatty acid oxidation defects, amino acid disorders, and urea cycle disorders that cause hyperammonemia are usually present early in childhood [9, 10]. Fatty acid oxidation defects are usually associated with hypoglycemic episodes [11], while amino acid disorders are with metabolic acidosis and ketosis [12, 13]. Both hypoglycemia and metabolic acidosis were not reported in this patient.

Urea cycle disorders (UCDs), as a result of deficiency of or defects in enzymes, usually present with hyperammonemia causing severe morbidity and mortality [14]. Literatures have shown a manifestation of late onset of one or more enzyme functional deficiency/ies unmasking the genetic disorders of the urea cycle in patients after bariatric surgery [15–18]. Markedly increased plasma glutamine, ornithine, and urinary orotic acid levels in the background of severe malnutrition and zinc deficiency may have led to unfolding of the functional deficiency of urea cycle enzyme/s leading to impaired ureagenesis and intractable hyperammonemia. Zinc deficiency can interfere with ornithine transcarbamylase (OTC) function [19, 20], which is possible in this patient. OTC deficiency, an X-linked disorder, is the most common inborn error of the urea cycle [21] and it usually has a fatal outcome soon after birth due to hyperammonemic coma. Heterozygous female may remain asymptomatic until the patient becomes acutely or chronically challenged by enough physiological stress. The recent gastrojejunal stent placement and decreased oral intake in chronically severe Protein-Energy Malnutrition (PEM) state probably led to increased physiological stress and catabolism in our patient. Blind loop syndrome with bacterial overgrowth in the patient with RYGBP (mainly distal type) may lead to illness, decreased oral intake, and increased catabolism. Alternative routes of enteral feeding such as gastrostomy may be needed to keep up with metabolism during an illness in such patients. In this case, no further information on the type of RYGBP was available as the procedure was done in another institution. DNA analysis of urea cycle enzymes would have given more definite etiology, but it was not carried out. Around 20–30% of patients with OTC deficiency are not detected in DNA analysis [22].

The initial goal of treatment should be to reduce ammonia production and absorption and facilitate elimination [23]. Intravenous glucose infusion should be started to provide a source of energy and raise insulin secretion that halts the protein breakdown due to its anabolic property. With the same token, protein intake should be restricted. IV lipid can also be given in increased energy demand. Alternative pathway therapies with sodium benzoate, sodium phenyl butyrate, and arginine have been proposed because these promote the synthesis of nitrogen-containing metabolites with high urinary excretion rates as an alternative to urea to remove waste nitrogen from the body [24]. In cases of uncontrolled hyperammonemia, hemodialysis may be an effective treatment. Due to rapid clinical deterioration and hemodynamic instability, hemodialysis could not be done in our patient. The mainstays of long-term management are dietary protein restriction, arginine or citrulline supplements, and oral alternative pathway medication to facilitate nitrogen excretion. Reversal of bariatric procedure is considered for the failure of weight loss or other complications due to the bariatric surgery itself. The decision of reversal tends to be highly individualized [25]. Consultation with an experienced bariatric surgeon may benefit when a patient presents with the nutritional/metabolic complication of bariatric surgery. This case report contains certain limitations such as being unable to perform DNA tests for urea cycle enzymes, hemodialysis, and use of aggressive scavengers such as sodium benzoate for management of hyperammonemia. Even with optimum therapy, this clinical entity is still associated with high rate of mortality.

In conclusion, hyperammonemia encephalopathy following bariatric surgery in the context of normal liver function tests becomes diagnostically challenging for physicians. The exact mechanism of hyperammonemia in such patient is still not clear but more data are gradually emerging in the support of cause-effect relationship among the triad of hyperammonemia, nutritional complications following bariatric surgery, and functional deficiency of urea cycle enzymes. We emphasize the importance of considering secondary causes of hyperammonemia in an adult woman after bariatric surgery. Early diagnosis and aggressive management are the only keys to improving survival.

Abbreviations

ABG: Arterial blood gas
ALT: Alanine aminotransferase
aPTT: Activated partial thromboplastin time
AST: Aspartate aminotransferase
BUN: Blood urea nitrogen
CT: Computed tomography
D5%: 5% dextrose
DNA: Deoxyribonucleic acid
ED: Emergency Department
EKG: Electrocardiogram
GCS: Glasgow Coma Scale
GI: Gastrointestinal
HDL: High-density lipoprotein
INR: International normalized ratio
IV: Intravenous
OTC: Ornithine transcarbamylase
PEM: Protein-Energy Malnutrition
PRBCs: Pack red blood cells
RYGBP: Roux-en-Y Gastric Bypass Procedure
SBP: Spontaneous bacterial peritonitis
UCD: Urea cycle disorder.

Competing Interests

Authors of this case report declare no competing interests.

References

[1] R. K. Dhiman and Y. K. Chawla, "Minimal hepatic encephalopathy: time to recognise and treat," *Tropical Gastroenterology*, vol. 29, no. 1, pp. 6–12, 2008.

[2] D. Shawcross and R. Jalan, "The pathophysiologic basis of hepatic encephalopathy: central role for ammonia and inflammation," *Cellular and Molecular Life Sciences*, vol. 62, no. 19-20, pp. 2295–2304, 2005.

[3] L. Nott, T. J. Price, K. Pittman, K. Patterson, and J. Fletcher, "Hyperammonemia encephalopathy: an important cause of neurological deterioration following chemotherapy," *Leukemia and Lymphoma*, vol. 48, no. 9, pp. 1702–1711, 2007.

[4] M. Albersen, S. Joniau, H. Van Poppel, P.-J. Cuyle, D. C. Knockaert, and W. Meersseman, "Urea-splitting urinary tract infection contributing to hyperammonemic encephalopathy," *Nature Clinical Practice Urology*, vol. 4, no. 8, pp. 455–458, 2007.

[5] R. E. Grazer, J. M. Sutton, S. Friedstrom, and F. D. McBarron, "Hyperammonemic encephalopathy due to essential amino acid hyperalimentation," *Archives of Internal Medicine*, vol. 144, no. 11, pp. 2278–2279, 1984.

[6] D. M. Felig, S. W. Brusilow, and J. L. Boyer, "Hyperammonemic coma due to parenteral nutrition in a woman with heterozygous ornithine transcarbamylase deficiency," *Gastroenterology*, vol. 109, no. 1, pp. 282–284, 1995.

[7] D. G. Vossler, A. J. Wilensky, D. F. Cawthon et al., "Serum and CSF glutamine levels in valproate-related hyperammonemic encephalopathy," *Epilepsia*, vol. 43, no. 2, pp. 154–159, 2002.

[8] B. N. Limketkai and S. D. Zucker, "Hyperammonemic encephalopathy caused by carnitine deficiency," *Journal of General Internal Medicine*, vol. 23, no. 2, pp. 210–213, 2008.

[9] H. O. de Baulny, A. Slama, G. Touati, D. M. Turnbull, M. Pourfarzam, and M. Brivet, "Neonatal hyperammonemia caused by a defect of carnitine-acylcarnitine translocase," *The Journal of Pediatrics*, vol. 127, no. 5, pp. 723–728, 1995.

[10] N. Longo, C. A. di San Filippo, and M. Pasquali, "Disorders of carnitine transport and the carnitine cycle," *American Journal*

of Medical Genetics—Seminars in Medical Genetics, vol. 142, no. 2, pp. 77–85, 2006.

[11] C. A. Stanley, "New genetic defects in mitochondrial fatty acid oxidation and carnitine deficiency," *Advances in Pediatrics*, vol. 34, pp. 59–88, 1986.

[12] J. M. Kwon and K. E. D'Aco, "Clinical neurogenetics: neurologic presentations of metabolic disorders," *Neurologic Clinics*, vol. 31, no. 4, pp. 1031–1050, 2013.

[13] J. N. Labuzetta, J. Z. Yao, D. L. Bourque, and J. Zivin, "Adult nonhepatic hyperammonemia: a case report and differential diagnosis," *American Journal of Medicine*, vol. 123, no. 10, pp. 885–891, 2010.

[14] O. Braissant, "Current concepts in the pathogenesis of urea cycle disorders," *Molecular Genetics and Metabolism*, vol. 100, supplement 1, pp. S3–S12, 2010.

[15] K. R. Bergmann, J. McCabe, T. R. Smith, D. J. Guillaume, K. Sarafoglou, and S. Gupta, "Late-onset ornithine transcarbamy-lase deficiency: treatment and outcome of hyperammonemic crisis," *Pediatrics*, vol. 133, no. 4, pp. e1072–e1076, 2014.

[16] A. Z. Fenves, O. A. Shchelochkov, and A. Mehta, "Hyperam-monemic syndrome after Roux-en-Y gastric bypass," *Obesity*, vol. 23, no. 4, pp. 746–749, 2015.

[17] W. T. Hu, O. H. Kantarci, J. L. Merritt II et al., "Ornithine tran-scarbamylase deficiency presenting as encephalopathy during adulthood following bariatric surgery," *Archives of Neurology*, vol. 64, no. 1, pp. 126–128, 2007.

[18] J. Estrella, G. Yee, B. Wilcken, M. Tchan, and M. Talbot, "Hyper-ammonemic encephalopathy complicating bariatric surgery: a case study and review of the literature," *Surgery for Obesity and Related Diseases*, vol. 10, no. 3, pp. e35–e38, 2014.

[19] L. C. Kuo, W. N. Lipscomb, and E. R. Kantrowitz, "Zn(II)-induced cooperativity of Escherichia coli ornithine transcar-bamoylase," *Proceedings of the National Academy of Sciences of the United States of America*, vol. 79, no. 7 I, pp. 2250–2254, 1982.

[20] E. Aquilio, R. Spagnoli, D. Riggio, and S. Seri, "Effects of zinc on hepatic ornithine transcarbamylase (OTC) activity," *Journal of Trace Elements and Electrolytes in Health and Disease*, vol. 7, no. 4, pp. 240–241, 1993.

[21] C. L. Pridmore, J. T. R. Clarke, and S. Blaser, "Ornithine transcarbamylase deficiency in females: an often overlooked cause of treatable encephalopathy," *Journal of Child Neurology*, vol. 10, no. 5, pp. 369–374, 1995.

[22] S. Yamaguchi, L. L. Brailey, H. Morizono, A. E. Bale, and M. Tuchman, "Mutations and polymorphisms in the human ornithine transcarbamylase (OTC) gene," *Human Mutation*, vol. 27, no. 7, pp. 626–632, 2006.

[23] A. S. Clay and B. E. Hainline, "Hyperammonemia in the ICU," *Chest*, vol. 132, no. 4, pp. 1368–1378, 2007.

[24] V. Walker, "Severe hyperammonaemia in adults not explained by liver disease," *Annals of Clinical Biochemistry*, vol. 49, no. 3, pp. 214–228, 2012.

[25] E. Chousleb, S. Patel, S. Szomstein, and R. Rosenthal, "Reasons and operative outcomes after reversal of gastric bypass and jejunoileal bypass," *Obesity Surgery*, vol. 22, no. 10, pp. 1611–1616, 2012.

Permissions

List of Contributors

Alexandre Toledo Maciel and Daniel Vitório
Intensimed Research Group, Adult Intensive Care Unit, Hospital São Camilo, Pompéia Avenue, 1178 Pompéia, 05022-001 São Paulo, SP, Brazil

Qi Jin, Erzhen Chen, Jie Jiang and Yiming Lu
Department of Emergency, Shanghai Rui Jin Hospital, Shanghai Jiao Tong University School of Medicine, Shanghai 20025, China

Hafiz Rizwan Talib Hashmi, Gilda Diaz-Fuentes and Misbahuddin Khaja
Division of Pulmonary and Critical Care Medicine, Bronx Lebanon Hospital Center, Bronx, NY 10457, USA

Preeti Jadhav
Department of Internal Medicine, Bronx Lebanon Hospital Center, Albert Einstein College of Medicine, Bronx, NY 10457, USA

Adel Hammodi Ahmed Hanafy and Talal Nakkar
King Fahad Specialist Hospital, Dammam 31444, Saudi Arabia

M. Ali Al-Azem
Critical Care Department, King Fahad Specialist Hospital, Dammam 31444, Saudi Arabia

Saptarshi Biswas and Patrick McNerney
Department of Trauma and Acute Care Surgery, Allegheny Health Network, Pittsburgh, PA, USA

Rachel A. Poley and Daniel W. Howes
Department of Emergency Medicine and Department of Critical Care Medicine, Kingston General Hospital, Queen's University, Kingston, ON, Canada K7L 2V7

Jaime F. Snowdon
Department of Pathology, Queen's University, Kingston, ON, Canada K7L 3N6

Arpit Amin, Saptarshi Biswas and Francis Baccay
Department of Surgery, New York Medical College, Westchester Medical Center, Valhalla, NY 10595, USA

Jérôme Cros and Nathalie Nathan-Denizot
Service d'Anesthésie-Réanimation, Hôpital Mére Enfant, 08 avenue Dominique Larrey, 87000 Limoges, France

Claire Serena and Charles Hodler
Service d'Anesthésie-Réanimation, Hôpital Mére Enfant, 08 avenue Dominique Larrey, 87000 Limoges, France
Service de Réanimation Polyvalente, CIC 0801, CHU Dupuytren, 02 avenue Martin Luther King, 87000 Limoges, France

Emmanuelle Begot Anne Laure Fedou and Marc Clavel
Service de Réanimation Polyvalente, CIC 0801, CHU Dupuytren, 02 avenue Martin Luther King, 87000 Limoges, France

Michael Glas and Thomas Volk
Department of Anesthesiology, Intensive Care and Pain Therapy, Saarland University Hospital, Kirrberger Straße, D-66421 Homburg, Germany

Sigrun Smola and Thorsten Pfuhl
Institute of Virology, Saarland University Hospital, D-66421 Homburg, Germany

Juliane Pokorny and Rainer M. Bohle
Institute of Pathology, Saarland University Hospital, D-66421 Homburg, Germany

Arno Bücker
Department of Diagnostic and Interventional Radiology, Saarland University Hospital, D-66421 Homburg, Germany

Jörn Kamradt
Department of Urology and Pediatric Urology, Saarland University Hospital, D-66421 Homburg, Germany

F. A. Zeiler and J. Silvaggio
Section of Neurosurgery, Department of Surgery, University of Manitoba, Winnipeg, MB, Canada R3A 1R9

Launey Yoann, Nesseler Nicolas, Malledant Yannick and Seguin Philippe
Anesthesiology, Critical Care and Emergencies, Rennes University Hospital, 35000 Rennes, France
Anesthesiology, Critical Care, Emergencies, and SAMU (Service d'Aide Médicale Urgente), Rennes 1 University, Inserm U991, Centre Hospitalier Universitaire (CHU) Pontchaillou, 35000 Rennes, France

Flecher Erwan
Anesthesiology, Critical Care, Emergencies, and SAMU (Service d'Aide Médicale Urgente), Rennes 1 University, Inserm U991, Centre Hospitalier Universitaire (CHU) Pontchaillou, 35000 Rennes, France
Department of Cardiovascular and Thoracic Surgery, Rennes University Hospital, 35000 Rennes, France

J. I. Alonso-Fernández J. R. Prieto-Recio C. García-Bernardo I. García-Saiz J. Rico-Feijoo and C. Aldecoa
Anesthesiology and Postoperative Critical Care Department, Río Hortega Universitary Hospital, 47009 Valladolid, Spain

Syed Amer, Ali Shafiq, Waqas Qureshi and Syed Hassan
Department of Medicine, Henry Ford Hospital, Detroit, MI 48202, USA

Mohammed Muqeetadnan
Department of Medicine, University of Oklahoma Health Sciences Center, Oklahoma City, OK 73104, USA

Nadine Monteiro, Camila Tapadinhas and VitorMendes
Polyvalent Intensive Care Unit, São Francisco Xavier Hospital,West Lisbon Hospital Centre, 1449-005 Lisbon, Portugal

Joana Silvestre, João Gonçalves-Pereira and Pedro Póvoa
Polyvalent Intensive Care Unit, São Francisco Xavier Hospital, West Lisbon Hospital Centre, 1449-005 Lisbon, Portugal
Faculty of Medical Sciences, New University of Lisbon, 1169-056 Lisbon, Portugal

Faisal A. Khasawneh
Division of Critical Care Medicine, Department of Internal Medicine, Texas Tech University Health Sciences Center, 1400 S. Coulter, Amarillo, TX 79106, USA

Roger D. Smalligan
Department of Internal Medicine, Texas Tech University Health Sciences Center, 1400 S. Coulter, Amarillo, TX 79106, USA

F. A. Zeiler and M. West
Section of Neurosurgery, Department of Surgery, University of Manitoba,Winnipeg, MB, Canada R3A 1R9

L. M. Gillman
Section of Critical Care Medicine, Department of Medicine, University of Manitoba,Winnipeg, MB, Canada R3A 1R9

Section of General Surgery, Department of Surgery, University of Manitoba,Winnipeg, MB, Canada R3A 1R9

J. Teitelbaum
Section of Neurocritical Care, Montreal Neurological Institute, McGill University, Montreal, QC, Canada H3A 2B4
Section of Neurology, Montreal Neurological Institute, McGill University,Montreal, QC, CanadaH3A 2B4

Alawi Luetz, Bjoern Weiss and Claudia D. Spies
Department of Anesthesiology and Intensive Care Medicine, Charité-Universitätsmedizin Berlin, Campus Charité Mitte and Campus Virchow-Klinikum, Augustenburger Platz 1, 13353 Berlin, Germany

P. Henin, A. Molderez, V. Huberlant and H. Trine
Groupe Jolimont, Centre Hospitalier de Jolimont, 159 rue Ferrer, 7100 Haine Saint Paul, Belgium

Shiwan K. Shah
Department of Internal Medicine and Pediatrics, University of Texas Medical Branch, 301 University Boulevard, Route 0354, Gaveston, TX 77555, USA

Sanjeev Kumar Goswami, Rajesh V. Babu, Gulshan Sharma and Alexander G. Duarte
Department of Pulmonary, Allergy, and Critical Care, University of Texas Medical Branch, Gaveston, TX 77555, USA

Pedro Gaspar-da-Costa
Department of Internal Medicine, Hospital de Santa Maria and Faculty of Medicine of Lisbon, Lisbon, Portugal

Sandra Braz, João Meneses Santos and Rui M. M. Victorino
Department of Internal Medicine, Hospital de Santa Maria and Faculty of Medicine of Lisbon, Lisbon, Portugal
Faculty of Medicine of Lisbon, Lisbon, Portugal

Sofia Reimão
Department of Neurologic Imaging, Hospital de Santa Maria and Faculty of Medicine of Lisbon, Lisbon, Portugal
Faculty of Medicine of Lisbon, Lisbon, Portugal

Muhammad Kashif, Hafiz Rizwan Talib Hashmi and Misbahuddin Khaja
Division of Pulmonary and Critical Care Medicine, Department of Medicine, Bronx Lebanon Hospital Center, Bronx, NY 10457, USA

Narjis AL Saif, Adel Hammodi, M. Ali Al-Azem, and Rasheed Al-Hubail
Critical Care Department, King Fahad Specialist Hospital, Dammam 31444, Saudi Arabia

Julia Park, Josh Tan, Sylvia Krzeminski and Meghana Bandlamuri
Department of Medicine, Maricopa Medical Center, Phoenix, AZ, USA

Richard W. Carlson
Department of Medicine, Maricopa Medical Center, Phoenix, AZ, USA
College of Medicine, University of Arizona, Phoenix, AZ, USA
College of Medicine, Mayo Clinic, Scottsdale, AZ, USA

Maryam Hazeghazam
Department of Psychiatry, Maricopa Medical Center, Phoenix, AZ, USA

Aristide Ntahe
Département d'Anesthésie-Réanimation, Hôpital Saint-Louis, Assistance Publique-Hôpitaux de Paris, 1 Avenue Claude Vellefaux, 75010 Paris, France

Lam-Phuong Nguyen, Narin Sriratanaviriyakul and Christian Sandrock
Division of Pulmonary, Critical Care, and Sleep Medicine, University of California, Davis, Suite #3400, 4150 V Street, Sacramento, CA 95817, USA
Department of Internal Medicine, University of California, Davis, Sacramento, USA
VA Northern California Health Care System, Mather, USA

Erin N. Frazee and Heather A. Personett
Hospital Pharmacy Services, Mayo Clinic, 200 1st SW, Rochester, MN 55905, USA

Sarah J. Lee and Darlene R. Nelson
Division of Pulmonary and Critical Care Medicine, Mayo Clinic, 200 1st SW, Rochester, MN 55905, USA

Ejaaz A. Kalimullah
Department of Emergency Medicine and Division of Pulmonary and Critical Care Medicine, Loyola University Medical Center, 2160 S 1st Avenue, Maywood, IL 60153, USA

Evgeni Brotfain, Leonid Koyfman, Ruslan Kutz, Amit Frenkel, Alexander Zlotnik and Moti Klein
Department of Anesthesiology and Critical Care, General Intensive Care Unit, Soroka Medical Center, Ben-Gurion University of the Negev, 85102 Beer-Sheva, Israel

Shaun E. Gruenbaum
Department of Anesthesiology, Yale University School of Medicine, New Haven, CT 06511, USA

Caroline Phillips and Nathaniel Broughton
Department of Anaesthesia and Critical Care, West Suffolk NHS Foundation Trust, Bury St Edmunds, UK

Clare Harris and Thomas Pulimood
Department of Respiratory Medicine, West Suffolk NHS Foundation Trust, Bury St Edmunds, UK

Liam Ring
Department of Cardiology, West Suffolk NHS Foundation Trust, Bury St Edmunds, UK

Alison Markland
University of Saskatchewan, Saskatoon, SK, Canada

Gregory Hansen
Division of Pediatric Intensive Care, University of Saskatchewan, Saskatoon, SK, Canada

Anke Banks
Department of Pediatrics, Cumming School of Medicine, University of Calgary, Calgary, AB, Canada

Rajni Chibbar
Department of Laboratory Medicine, University of Saskatchewan, Saskatoon, SK, Canada

Darryl Adamko
Division of Pediatric Respirology, University of Saskatchewan, Saskatoon, SK, Canada

Mohsin Ijaz and Dmitry Lvovsky
Division of Pulmonary and Critical Care Medicine, Department of Medicine, Bronx Lebanon Hospital Center, 1650 Selwyn Avenue, Suite 12F, Bronx, NY 10457, USA

Naeem Abbas
Department of Medicine, Bronx Lebanon Hospital Center, 1650 Selwyn Avenue, Suite 10C, Bronx, NY 10457, USA

Jan-Thorben Sieweke, Jörn Tongers, Andreas Schäfer, Johann Bauersachs and L. Christian Napp
Cardiac Arrest Center, Department of Cardiology and Angiology, Hannover Medical School, Hannover, Germany

Jens Vogel-Claussen
Institute for Diagnostic and Interventional Radiology, Hannover Medical School, Hannover, Germany

Andreas Martens
Department of Cardiothoracic, Transplantation and Vascular Surgery, Hannover Medical School, Hannover, Germany

Kenichiro Ishida, Mitsuhiro Noborio, Nobutaka Iwasa, Taku Sogabe, Yohei Ieki, Yuki Saoyama, Kyosuke Takahashi, Yumiko Shimahara and Daikai Sadamitsu
Traumatology and Critical Care Medical Center, National Hospital Organization, Osaka National Hospital, 2-1-14 Hoenzaka, Chuo-ku, Osaka 540-0006, Japan

Pratik Patel and Cristina Varallo-Rodriguez
Department of Medicine, St. John's Riverside Hospital, 967 N. Broadway, Yonkers, NY 10701, USA

Mikhael Bekkerman
Department of Medicine, St. John's Riverside Hospital, 967 N. Broadway, Yonkers, NY 10701, USA
Lake Erie College of Osteopathic Medicine, 1858WGrandview Blvd, Erie, PA 16509, USA

Rajendra Rampersaud
Pulmonary and Critical Care, St. John's Riverside Hospital, 967 N. Broadway, Yonkers, NY 10701, USA

Hafiz B. Mahboob and Bruce W. Denney
University of Nevada School of Medicine, Reno, NV, USA
Renown Regional Medical Center, Reno, NV, USA

Tomohiro Shoji, Takeshi Umegaki, Kota Nishimoto, Natsuki Anada, Akiko Ando, Takeo Uba, Munenori Kusunoki, Kanako Oku and Takahiko Kamibayashi
Department of Anesthesiology, Kansai Medical University Hospital, Osaka, Japan

Kirsten S. Deemer
Department of Critical Care Medicine, South Health Campus ICU, 4448 Front Street SE, Calgary, AB, Canada T3M 1M4

George F. Alvarez
Department of Critical Care Medicine, University of Calgary, AB, Canada

Rashmi Mishra and Richard Duncalf
Division of Pulmonary and Critical Care Medicine, Bronx Lebanon Hospital Center, 1650 Grand Concourse, Bronx, NY 10457, USA

Nupur Sinha
Division of Pulmonary and Critical Care, Community Hospital of the Monterey Peninsula, 23625 Pacific Grove-Carmel Highway, Monterey, CA 93942, USA

Kwadwo Kyeremanteng and Gianni D'Egidio
The Ottawa Hospital, Ottawa, ON, Canada
Division of Critical Care, Department of Medicine, The University of Ottawa, Ottawa, ON, Canada

Alan Baxter
The Ottawa Hospital, Ottawa, ON, Canada
Department of Anesthesiology, The University of Ottawa, Ottawa, ON, Canada

Hans Rosenberg
The Ottawa Hospital, Ottawa, ON, Canada
Department of Emergency Medicine, The University of Ottawa, Ottawa, ON, Canada

Cynthia Wan
School of Psychology, The University of Ottawa, Ottawa, ON, Canada

Dominick Roto
Department of Medicine, University of Rochester Medical Center, 601 Elmwood Avenue, Rochester, NY 14642, USA

Michelle L. Malnoske and Steve N. Georas
Division of Pulmonary and Critical Care, Department of Medicine, University of Rochester Medical Center, 601 Elmwood Avenue, Rochester, NY 14642, USA

Shira Winters
Department of Pathology, University of Rochester Medical Center, 601 Elmwood Avenue, Rochester, NY 14642, USA

A. Thakkar
Department of Internal Medicine, Mount Sinai St. Luke's-West Hospital, New York, NY, USA

K. Parekh and E. M. Mohanraj
Division of Pulmonary, Critical Care and Sleep Medicine, Mount Sinai St. Luke's-West Hospital, New York, NY, USA

K. El Hachem
Division of Nephrology, Mount Sinai St. Luke's-West Hospital, New York, NY, USA

Grant A. Miller, Yousef M. Ahmed and Nicki S. Tarant
Department of Critical Care Medicine, Naval Medical Center Portsmouth, Portsmouth, VA, USA

Hafiz B. Mahboob, Kazi H. Kaokaf and Jeremy M. Gonda
University of Nevada School of Medicine, Reno, NV, USA
Renown Regional Medical Center, Reno, NV, USA

Iouri Banakh
Department of Pharmacy, Frankston Hospital, Peninsula Health, Frankston, VIC 3199, Australia

Ross Kung
Department of Intensive Care Medicine, Frankston Hospital, Peninsula Health, Frankston, VIC 3199, Australia

Kavi Haji, Sachin Gupta and Ravindranath Tiruvoipati
Department of Intensive Care Medicine, Frankston Hospital, Peninsula Health, Frankston, VIC 3199, Australia
School of Public Health, Faculty of Medicine, Nursing and Health Sciences, Monash University, Clayton, VIC 3800, Australia

Erin K. Yeung and Mark Wong
Department of Pharmacy Services, South Texas Veterans Health Care System, 7400 Merton Minter, San Antonio, TX 78229, USA
Pharmacotherapy Education and Research Center, The University of Texas Health San Antonio, 7703 Floyd Curl Dr., MSC 6220, San Antonio, TX 78229-3900,USA

Haritha Saikumar and Jose Castaneda-Nerio
3Medicine Service, Pulmonary/Critical Care Division, South Texas Veterans Health Care System, 7400 Merton Minter (111E), San Antonio, TX 78229, USA

Sandra G. Adams
Medicine Service, Pulmonary/Critical Care Division, South Texas Veterans Health Care System, 7400 Merton Minter (111E), San Antonio, TX 78229, USA
Department of Medicine, Pulmonary/Critical Care Division, The University of Texas Health San Antonio, 7703 Floyd Curl Dr., MSC 7885, San Antonio, TX 78229-3900, USA

Juan G. Ripoll
Department of Critical Care Medicine, Mayo Clinic, 4500 San Pablo Road, Jacksonville, FL, USA

Robert A. Ratzlaff
Department of Critical Care Medicine, Mayo Clinic, 4500 San Pablo Road, Jacksonville, FL, USA
Department of Anesthesiology, Mayo Clinic, 4500 San Pablo Road, Jacksonville, FL, USA

José L. Díaz-Gómez
Department of Critical Care Medicine, Mayo Clinic, 4500 San Pablo Road, Jacksonville, FL, USA
Department of Anesthesiology, Mayo Clinic, 4500 San Pablo Road, Jacksonville, FL, USA
Department of Neurosurgery, Mayo Clinic, 4500 San Pablo Road, Jacksonville, FL, USA

David M. Menke and Maria C. Olave
3Department of Pathology, Mayo Clinic, 4500 San Pablo Road, Jacksonville, FL,USA

Joseph J. Maleszewski
Division of Anatomic Pathology, Mayo Clinic, 200 First St SW, Rochester, MN, USA

Hannah Kinoshita
University of Hawaii Pediatric Residency Program, USA

Leon Grant
Department of Pediatric Neurology, Kapiolani Medical Center for Women and Children, USA

Konstantine Xoinis and Prashant J. Purohit
Department of Pediatric Critical Care, Kapiolani Medical Center for Women and Children, USA

Hafiz Mahboob
University of Nevada School of Medicine, Reno, NV, USA
Renown Regional Medical Center, Reno, NV, USA
U.S. Department of Veteran Affairs, Ioannis A. Lougaris Veteran Affairs Medical Center, Reno, NV, USA

Robert Richeson III
1University of Nevada School of Medicine, Reno, NV, USA
Renown Regional Medical Center, Reno, NV, USA

Robert McCain
U.S. Department of Veteran Affairs, Ioannis A. Lougaris Veteran Affairs Medical Center, Reno, NV, USA

Mridula Krishnan and Kaye Bardeloza
Department of Internal Medicine, CHI Creighton University Medical Center, Omaha, NE, USA

Katherine Lester and Amber Johnson
Creighton University School of Medicine, Omaha, NE, USA

Peter Edemekong
Department of Family Medicine, CHI Creighton University Medical Center, Omaha, NE, USA

Ilya Berim
Department of Pulmonary and Critical Care, CHI Creighton University Medical Center, Omaha, NE, USA

Alexander Grieb, Karim Mostafa and Reinhard Berger
AUVA-Unfallkrankenhaus Meidling, Department of Anesthesiology and Intensive Care Medicine, Vienna, Austria

Heinz Steltzer
AUVA-Unfallkrankenhaus Meidling, Department of Anesthesiology and Intensive Care Medicine, Vienna, Austria
Sigmund Freud Private University, Vienna, Austria

Pierre Cardinal
Division of Critical Care, Department of Medicine, University of Ottawa, Ottawa, ON, Canada

Shannon M. Fernando
Division of Critical Care, Department of Medicine, University of Ottawa, Ottawa, ON, Canada

Department of Emergency Medicine, University of Ottawa, Ottawa, ON, Canada

Peter G. Brindley
Department of Critical Care Medicine, University of Alberta, Edmonton, AB, Canada

Gyanendra Acharya, Ronakkumar Patel and Simona Frunza-Stefan
Department of Internal Medicine, Wyckoff Heights Medical Center, Brooklyn, NY 11237, USA

Sunil Mehra
Division of Pulmonary and Critical Care Medicine, Department of Internal Medicine, Wyckoff Heights Medical Center, Brooklyn, NY 11237, USA

Harmanjot Kaur
Department of Medical Education, Wyckoff Heights Medical Center, Brooklyn, NY 11237, USA

Index